Latest in Healthcare Management

Pradeep Bhardwaj
(IIM-A and ISB Alumnus/5 National Awards/Listed under India's top 10 doctors)
DP (IIM Ahmedabad) FNF (ISB Hyderabad) PhD (Healthcare Strategy Management)
M Phil (Management) MBA (Hospital Management) MHA MPH LLB (Hons)
PG (Hospital Administration) PG (Medicolegal) PG (Materials Management—Amity)
NABH NABL JCI NABET Cyber Law–ILI

Executive Director and CEO
Six Sigma Star Healthcare Limited and
Global Institute of Healthcare Management
New Delhi, India

Chairman
Six Sigma Accreditation Board (SSAB)

Chief Editor
Six Sigma Health Express Magazine
Medgate Today Magazine

Visiting Professor and Faculty/Panel Expert/Assessor
IIM (Ahmedabad), IIM (Lucknow), ISB (Hyderabad), Amity University
Symbiosis, GIHM, YMCA, AIIMS, National Board of Examination, NABH, CGHS
NABET, JCI, IMA, Bhartiya Vidya Bhavan, New Delhi, India

Formerly at
Sir Ganga Ram Hospital
Apollo Hospitals Group
Fortis Healthcare Limited
Indian Spinal Injuries Hospital
New Delhi, India

Forewords

DS Rana
Maj. Gen. SB Akali (Retd)

JAYPEE *The Health Sciences Publisher*
New Delhi | London | Philadelphia | Panama

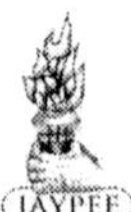 **Jaypee Brothers Medical Publishers (P) Ltd**

Headquarters
Jaypee Brothers Medical Publishers (P) Ltd.
4838/24, Ansari Road, Daryaganj
New Delhi 110 002, India
Phone: +91-11-43574357
Fax: +91-11-43574314
Email: jaypee@jaypeebrothers.com

Overseas Offices

J.P. Medical Ltd.
83, Victoria Street, London
SW1H 0HW (UK)
Phone: +44 20 3170 8910
Fax: +44 (0)20 3008 6180
Email: info@jpmedpub.com

Jaypee-Highlights Medical Publishers Inc.
City of Knowledge, Bld. 237, Clayton
Panama City, Panama
Phone: +1 507-301-0496
Fax: +1 507-301-0499
Email: cservice@jphmedical.com

Jaypee Medical Inc.
The Bourse
111, South Independence Mall East
Suite 835, Philadelphia, PA 19106, USA
Phone: +1 267-519-9789
Email: jpmed.us@gmail.com

Jaypee Brothers Medical Publishers (P) Ltd.
17/1-B, Babar Road, Block-B, Shaymali
Mohammadpur, Dhaka-1207, Bangladesh
Mobile: +08801912003485
Email: jaypeedhaka@gmail.com

Jaypee Brothers Medical Publishers (P) Ltd.
Bhotahity, Kathmandu, Nepal
Phone: +977-9741283608
Email: kathmandu@jaypeebrothers.com

Website: www.jaypeebrothers.com
Website: www.jaypeedigital.com

Inquiries for bulk sales may be solicited at: jaypee@jaypeebrothers.com

Latest in Healthcare Management

First Edition: **2015,** Reprint: 2025

ISBN: 978-93-5152-859-3

Printed in India

Latest in
Healthcare Management

Dedicated to

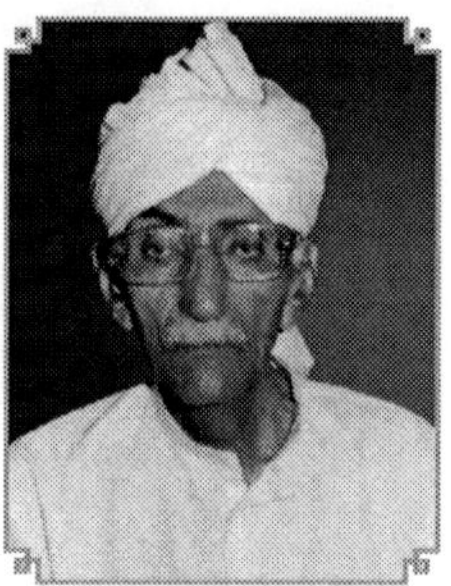

My Grandfather Shri Ramgopal Bhardwaj for being my North Star and my father and mother—the sources of my inspirations.

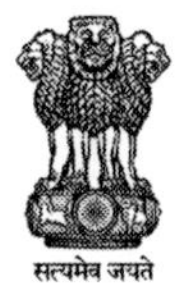

प्रधान मंत्री

Prime Minister

Message

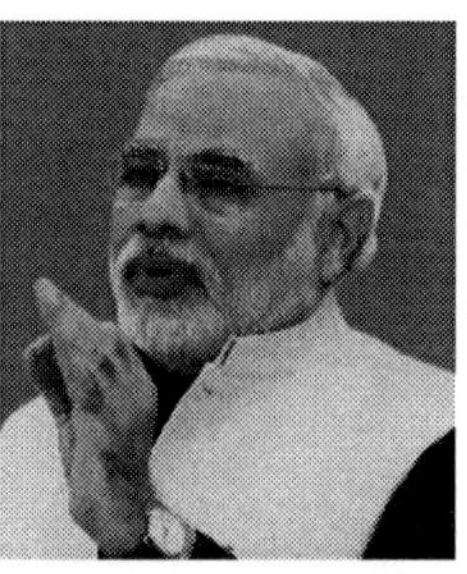

I am very glad to know that Dr Pradeep Bhardwaj, CEO, Six Sigma Star Healthcare Ltd., New Delhi, India, has written the book *Latest in Healthcare Management*. The Indian hospital and healthcare industry has the potential to become a global hub for healthcare services. An increasing number of global players in healthcare industry is focusing on the Indian market. The need for efficiency, latest technology in healthcare delivery has led to the emergence of organized and professionally managed primary care set-ups. A large number of providers is setting up chains of multispecialty outpatient clinics across India.

I hope, this book will be useful to all healthcare professionals associated with the medical management of hospitals.

I convey my good wishes and great success in this venture.

Narendra Modi
Hon'ble Prime Minister of India

P.D. Rai
Member of Parliament
(Lok Sabha)
SIKKIM

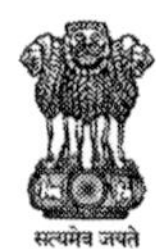

13-E, Ferozeshah Road, New Delhi - 110 001
Tel. : 011-23782461 * Fax : 011-23782214
E-mail : mpsikkim@gmail.com

J-155, Tadong, Gangtok -737 102, Sikkim
Tel. :03592-231181

Message

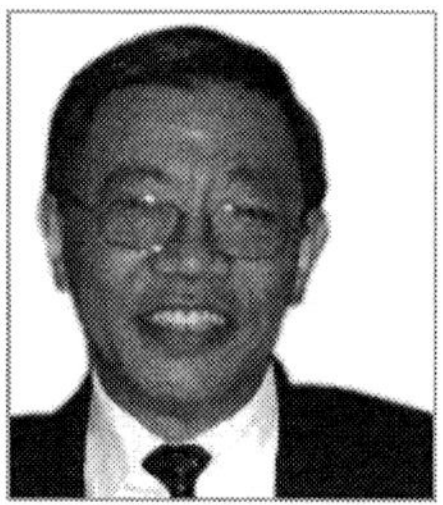

The book *Latest in Healthcare Management* authored by Dr Pradeep Bhardwaj deserves appreciation and recognition in the field of healthcare management. The book is designed to provide comprehensive and latest knowledge of quality in healthcare including Six Sigma, laws applicable in health, latest management techniques and tools in the changing scenario of hospital management.

Whether you are a new CEO, Medical Director, a Manager seeking to expand your skills or a seasoned professional looking to broaden your knowledge base, this solution-oriented book puts reliable answers in your fingertips.

Do you need smart, latest, actionable management knowledge in the Healthcare sector? Then you must read this book.

I wish Dr Bhardwaj a great success in this leadership venture.

PD Rai
Member of Parliament (Lok Sabha)

प्रवेश साहिब सिंह

संसद सदस्य
(लोक सभा)

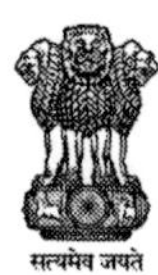

1/14B,शान्ति निकेतन
नई दिल्ली
011-24111541

Message

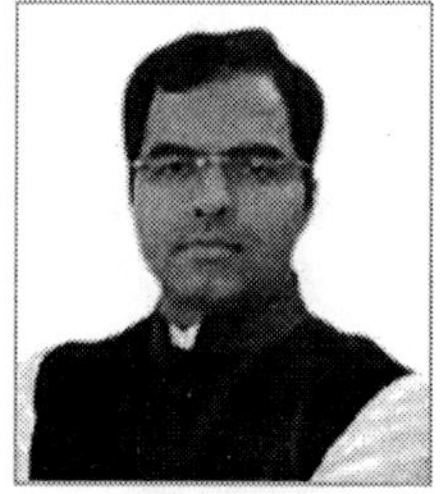

Latest in Healthcare Management written by Dr Pradeep Bhardwaj, CEO, Six Sigma Star Healthcare Ltd., New Delhi, India, is an excellent book of its kind covering the latest aspect of Healthcare Management.

Today's hospital administrator plays a vital role in saving lives, without scalpel in hand. Medical directors and hospital administrators manage hospitals, outpatient clinics and drug-abuse treatment centers by possessing the latest knowledge of tools and techniques. Hospitals are open round the clock—24/7—and administrators may be called in at any hour to make decisions and resolve disputes. Hospital administration is all about the knowledge management and I am sure that this book will provide the latest knowledge in the changing arena of health sector.

Well done Dr Bhardwaj!

I wish you the best wishes from the core of my heart!

Pravesh Sahib Singh
Member of Parliament (Lok Sabha)

Dr DS RANA
CHAIRMAN, BOARD OF MANAGEMENT
PADMASHRI AWARDEE

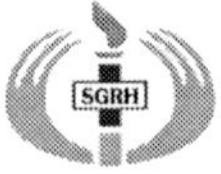

Sir Ganga Ram Hospital
Accumulating trust for over fifty years

Message

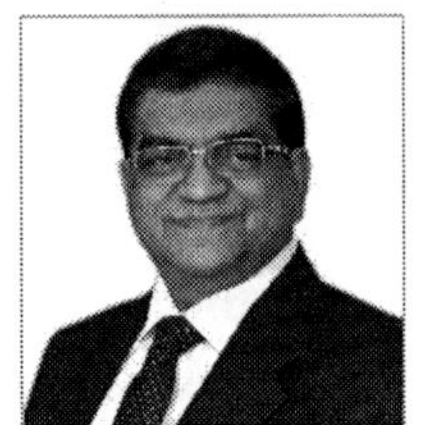

I congratulate and appreciate Dr Pradeep Bhardwaj, for authoring an excellent text-cum-reference book titled *Latest in Hospital Management* under Jaypee Brothers Medical Publishers (P) Ltd., New Delhi.

Hospital administration is one of the most competitive and challenging careers you can embark on and one of the most rewarding professions. Healthcare is a more complex business now than ever before—and it is changing rapidly. Skilled hospital administrators are vital to ensure that medical facilities run efficiently and deliver quality patient care. The hospital administrator liaisons between management, doctors, patients, staff and health insurance companies. I am sure that this book will add values in the profession of hospital management.

I convey my best wishes to the author and readers of this book.

DS Rana
Chairman, Board of Management
Sir Ganga Ram Hospital
New Delhi, India

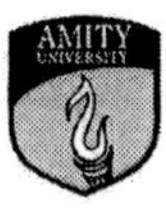

AMITY UNIVERSITY

Maj. Gen. K Jai Singh (Retd)
MSc (UK), sdmc, FIE, FIETE, FNTF, SMCSI, FIMA
Group Vice Chancellor and
Executive Senior Vice President, RBEF

Message

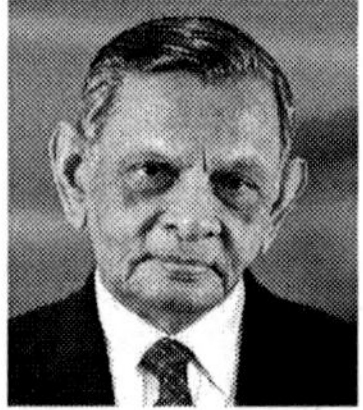

You are the source of inspiration in healthcare and I feel proud on you for authoring reference book on *Latest in Healthcare Management* under a leading publisher M/s Jaypee Brothers Medical Publishers (P) Ltd., New Delhi, India. I am sure that, this book will guide all our future and current medical professionals in the arena of healthcare administration.

Hospital management is all about knowledge management. A healthcare leader is a person with clear, long-term vision full of latest knowledge. He is articulate and acts as a motivational force for sustainable growth for the healthcare organization. The most important trait of a health leader is skill to manage all stakeholders, medicos, command respect and be receptive to change. In addition to these, the leader must be a person of very high integrity to be able to inculcate the right value system in the hospital. He or she should be industrious and set benchmarks for his medical and non-medical team. A leader should be able to sell his dreams for the team to others—peers, superiors, doctors, managers and stakeholders. This book covers all the above aspects and will be handy tool for any Medical Director, CEO, Administrator and Doctor, etc.

Please accept my good wishes and great success.

Maj. Gen. K Jai Singh
Group Vice Chancellor
Amity University and
Executive Senior Vice President, RBEF

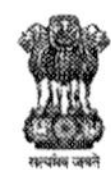

भारत के राष्ट्रपति का चिकित्सक
Physician to the President of India

Message

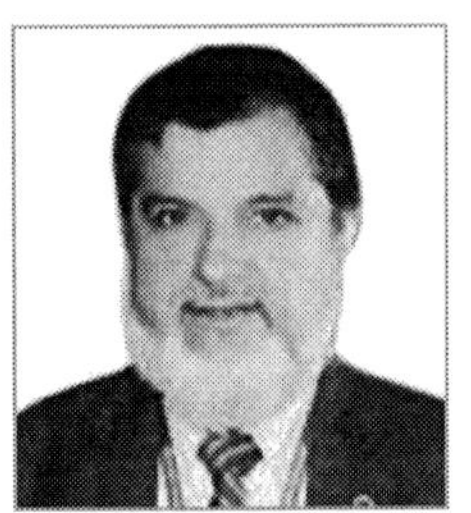

I am very happy to know that Dr Pradeep Bhardwaj, CEO, Six Sigma Star Healthcare Ltd., New Delhi, India has composed the book *Latest in Healthcare Management* being published by Jaypee Brothers Medical Publishers (P) Ltd., New Delhi, India.

The book covers all the latest aspects of medical science. I hope, this book will be useful to healthcare professionals associated with the medical and healthcare management. *Latest in Healthcare Management* covers topics of healthcare including Entrepreneurship, Quality Management, NABH, NABL, JCI, Six Sigma Accreditation, Latest Medical Laws, Latest Healthcare Architect and Hospital Planning, Green Buildings, Public Health, Outsourcing, IVF, Paramedical, TPA, High Altitude Medical Services, Latest of Medical Education and Opportunities in Healthcare, etc. The Indian healthcare industry has the potential to become a global hub for medical services.

I convey my good wishes and great success in this venture.

M Wali
Physician to the President of India

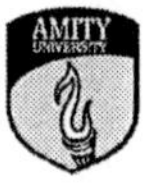

AMITY UNIVERSITY

UTTAR PRADESH

Prof (Dr) Ramesh C Deka
MS FIAO, FIMSA, FAAO (USA)
Advisor to the Founder President
Distinguished Professor
Chair, Medical Education & Research
(Past Dean, Director, AIIMS, New Delhi)

Message

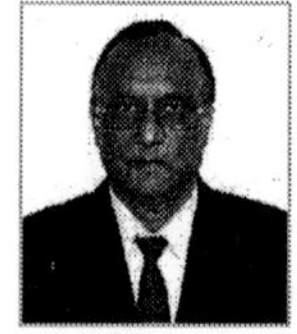

I am happy to know that Dr Pradeep Bhardwaj, a distinguished healthcare practitioner as well as a renowned healthcare leader in the country and also CEO of Six Sigma Star Healthcare, New Delhi, India, along with his team consisting of colleagues and experts from different domains of healthcare sector has served humanities, especially to those who had suffered significantly during the Uttarakhand flood and many other natural calamity situations in the country during past few years.

On the basis of his practical experiences, he has been able to write a book on *Latest in Healthcare Management*. I feel, the book will be motivating many people including nurses and other health workers and also ordinary people who will work under such difficult situations for the welfare of public at large. I congratulate Dr Bhardwaj and his colleagues on their excellent work in this field of public health.

I wish the 'Book Release Function' a great success.

Ramesh C Deka
Advisor to the Founder President
Distinguished Professor
Chair, Medical Education and Research
(Past Dean, Director, AIIMS, New Delhi)

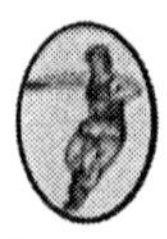

PRAVEEN KUMAR (BHEEM)

Former Olympian and Asian Champion

Winner of Arjuna Award (Athletics)

'Bheem' of BR Chopra's legendary television series **'Mahabharata'**

Star of Indian athletics in the 1960s & 1970s Asian Games

(Indian Athlete, Actor in 50 Films, Arjuna Awardee)

Message

"Winner does not follow other's footsteps, they create their own and you did it in healthcare".

Nice to see the fantastic book of *Latest in Healthcare Management* authored by you. I am proud of your success in hospital and healthcare management. The book on hospital management authored by you is like the 'Bible of Healthcare Management'. Good to see a different and new book on the management of health.

Leadership is the capacity to translate vision into reality. You are the source of encouragement and inspiration in healthcare industry. I wish to express my most sincere gratitude and heartfelt thanks to you and your family. My blessings are always with you. Please accept my good wishes and great success ahead.

Praveen Kumar
Former Olympian and Asian Champion
Winner of Arjuna Award (Athletics)

Reviewers

This book covers all the latest of healthcare and will be handy tool for Medical Directors, CEOs, Administrators, Managers and Doctors. I am sure that book will guide all our future and current medical professionals.

Maj. Gen. K Jai Singh
Group Vice Chancellor—Amity University, India

The book deserves appreciation and recognition in the field of healthcare management. The book is designed to provide comprehensive and latest knowledge in the changing scenario of hospital management. This solution-oriented book puts reliable answers in your fingertips.

Do you need smart, latest, actionable management knowledge in the healthcare sector? Then you must read this book.

PD Rai, MP—Lok Sabha
Sikkim (First IIM-A Alumni as MP)

Hospital administration is the most competitive and challenging career. I am sure that, this book will add values in the profession of hospital management. I am proud of you. God bless you.

DS Rana, Chairman
Sir Ganga Ram Hospital, New Delhi (Padmashri Awardee)

Congratulations! This book is an excellent initiative of Dr Bhardwaj.

Harsh Vardhan, Minister of Science and Technology, Govt of India

I am sure that this book will inspire everyone in general and entire healthcare professionals across the nation.

SK Srivastava, IAS, Former Chief Secretary, Govt of NCT of Delhi

The country can feel proud of you. The book written by you not only motivates persons from medical field but also from other areas for doing human services.

Ashok K Chauhan, Founder President—RBEF, Chairman—Amity University and AKC Group

This book is the 'Bible of Healthcare Management'. Good to see a different and new book on hospital management as career.

Praveen Kumar (Bheem), Arjuna Awardee

Foreword

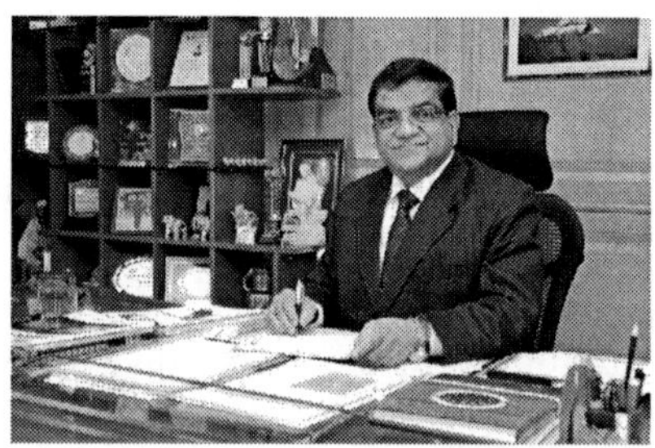

I take great pride to introduce a wonderful and high-knowledge power-dose book on healthcare management authored by Dr Pradeep Bhardwaj, Ambassador of Sir Ganga Ram Hospital and renowned leader of today's healthcare industry. This book is one of the unique reference book-cum-handbook, which includes all important issues like NABH, NABL, JCI, Six Sigma, Medicolegal, Laws, new techniques, such as NLP, Green Buildings, IVF Management, Paramedical, TPA, EMR, KPO, Medical Education, Entrepreneurship, High Altitude Medical Services, Clinical Research, Hospital Administration, Consultancy Services, etc.

The Indian hospital and healthcare industry has the potential to become a global hub for healthcare services. An increasing number of global players in healthcare is focusing on the Indian market. The healthcare industry is expected to grow rapidly over the next decade to reach ₹ 7.9 trillion by 2024. The size of the Indian hospital industry is presently estimated at ₹ 3.7 trillion. This industry is growing at an annual rate of 13%. According to a WHO report, India needs to add 80,000 hospital beds each year for the next 5 years to meet the demands of its growing population. The private sector accounts for nearly 86% of the healthcare market, while the public sector accounts for the rest. With over a 350 million strong middle class demanding quality healthcare, the Indian hospital industry is poised to grow at an even faster pace. The number of medical tourists visiting India is also increasing every year.

The last couple of years have seen a rapid increase of private equity and venture capital funds available for entrepreneurs in healthcare, which has enabled scale-up of some new interesting models for providing healthcare.

There are countless new developments cropping up regularly, but certain strategies, systems and trends are set to reach a tipping point of adoption and popularity in the coming years. Some of the emerging trends in this sector will have widespread effects and the potential to change the landscape significantly.

Technology is rapidly changing the way healthcare is delivered across the country. It is making healthcare more pervasive and has integrated it more seamlessly into our everyday life. Technology, for instance, in diagnostics, genomics and invasive procedures, has revolutionized clinical practice. While product innovations have been exponential in the last decade, and are only going to grow, process innovations through technologies in healthcare are a recent emerging trend—making management of healthcare more efficient, cost effective and accessible. Innovations in delivering what services are available, and delivering them better is going to be the defining shift in the coming years.

Increasing access to reach the unreached, while controlling costs, is made possible through the induction of technology in healthcare. Telemedicine is being used to connect remote rural populations to medical advice from specialists, which were until now, unavailable to them. Besides this, telemedicine technology also allows physicians easier access to their colleagues in multiple locations across health facilities, thus, offering the possibility of creating a network of health service providers.

Another area where technology will be used increasingly is in healthcare and hospital management to improve efficiency. Technology is offering comprehensive clinical and financial solutions that enable better decisions and outcomes for both businesses and patients, improve revenue cycle, drive quality outcomes and accelerate image management and workflow.

Now this book is in your hand to take maximum benefit from it. I once again appreciate and congratulate Dr Pradeep Bhardwaj for authoring this great book on Healthcare Management.

Best wishes!

DS Rana
Chairman, Board of Management
Sir Ganga Ram Hospital
New Delhi, India

Foreword

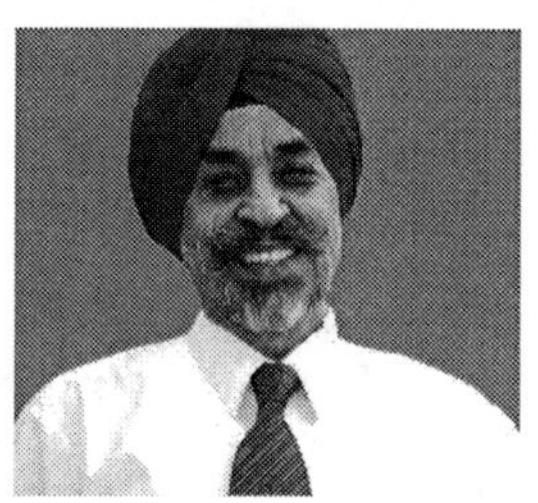

Healthcare and Hospital Management is a vast, challenging, progressive, complex and an ever-changing field and a very interesting one too.

Advances in technology in almost all healthcare-related fields are making changes at an exponentially fast pace. Technological advances in diagnostic equipment, instrumentation, life-sustaining devices, explosion in communication media, electronics, metallurgy, medicines and awareness among the population directly impinges on quality of healthcare, demands on expertise of doctors and provision and upgradation of excellent infrastructure. This makes the role of healthcare professionals more challenging. They are expected to keep themselves abreast of these changes.

While medical personnel are the frontline of any healthcare organization, there are other healthcare professionals (generally in the background) in whom patients invest their trust and hope—even though they are not always aware who these people are or the roles they play. These professionals are healthcare executives/administrators/managers. They are the men/women who while staying in the background, manage today's highly complex hospitals and healthcare organizations. They help to create and maintain the facilities and environment for medical professionals to deliver the required patient care. They ensure their organizations have strong medical, operational, and financial footing to serve the needs of all stakeholders—patients, their families, community, owners, government agencies, employees, insurance companies, pharmaceutical agencies, etc.

Hospital and healthcare managers are qualified and highly trained professionals, who care deeply about the quality of care, their patients receive. They partner with physicians, nurses, and other professionals to provide desired medical care. They help in educating community members about important health issues and ensure that hospitals and other healthcare organizations serve as 'safety nets' in their communities by providing emergency and ongoing care, as well as accurate, timely information about public threats in times of crisis.

In today's scenario, a career as a Healthcare/Hospital Management professional may be right for one who enjoys facing challenges and solving problems. It makes one's work meaningful. While it entails good financial compensation, it also involves the concept of "SEVA"—to help people in distress, pain and agony, care about health of individuals and community. It has excellent compensation and growth opportunities.

The government today has come forward with directives/drives to bring about changes highlighting the importance of good quality/ accredited, efficient and effective healthcare services to transform the old deeply entrenched *Chalta-hai* systems to a modern state-of-the-art system through Quality Accreditations. This would necessitate changes in existing perceptions, policies and practices. Further, it would entail commitment of additional resources without immediate returns in a tangible form. It is a known fact that after government schemes like CGHS, ECHS, ESI, etc. (many more may follow) have declared much higher rates for treatment of their beneficiaries from Quality Accredited Hospitals, there has been a distinct urgency for accreditations through the NABH.

It is assumed that the managements of government hospitals would also jump into the quality accreditation plan and many more from the private sector in the tier-II cities would follow soon. The problem is much more acute with the healthcare set-ups in tier-II cities and in the rural sector. The government hospitals, therefore, need to be not only educated about the need for quality accreditation but also to be guided continuously. Those in the smaller cities and rural areas would need some extra consideration—like the different yardsticks/policies for the differently endowed population of our country (like reservations based on the economic or social background of the population)—providing 'incentives' could be one, lowering application fees could be another (e.g. application amount made 'zero', i.e. made free).

In today's competitive and fast moving environment, one cannot be dogmatic in its approach. Being pragmatic in implementation of the directives/policies of the government, all across, one has to be appreciative and understanding of the fact that different approaches need to be followed, based on the environment of the entity concerned.

For example, there is an acute shortage of allopathic qualified RMO/ CMO/Residents, etc. even in metropolitan cities. There could be some relaxation not only in this category but in other manpower categories. Further, the quality expectations from other areas too may need to be suitably relaxed. There is a dire need to have a "mix and match approach" to healthcare by different schools of medicine available in our country. While some practitioners of medicine in streams other than allopathic have started depending on diagnostics prevalent in allopathic system to base their treatment on, the same is not readily accepted by those practicing allopathy.

Requirements for ancillary facilities like diagnostics, pharmacy and blood bank, etc. may also have to be relaxed to allow them to proliferate to larger areas. We may consider having a blood storage center instead of blood bank. Services like nutrition and dietary services and dedicated ambulance(s) also may require a re-think for upgrading the government hospitals to the 'benchmark' levels. All these changes add to the 'woes' of a healthcare manager.

For diverse requirements of a manager in hospital or in healthcare sector, no comprehensive reference book was available in the Indian market for one to refer to. Dr Pradeep Bhardwaj's book, *Latest in Healthcare Management* is likely to fill that gap. It is a wide-ranging anthology of almost all the subjects on hospital and healthcare management. Having been professionally associated with Dr Bhardwaj for a long time, I can vouch for the fact that he would not have spared any effort to ensure that a healthcare-management practitioner gets not only a comprehensive and reliable book for healthcare-related subjects but also the latest data on such subjects.

The book is bound to be accepted by one and all in the healthcare management arena.

Maj. Gen. SB Akali (Retd)
Director General
Six Sigma Star Healthcare and
Global Institute of Healthcare Management
New Delhi, India

From the Editor's Desk

Dear Friends,

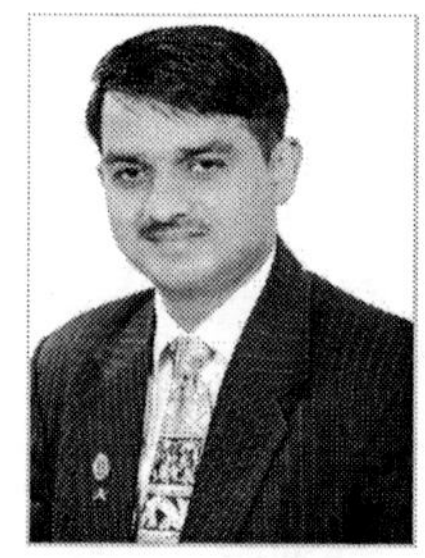

The Indian healthcare sector currently represents a US$ 40 billion industry. The industry is expected to grow to US$ 280 billion by 2020. India has an average 0.6 doctors per 1000 population against the global average of 1.23. Nowadays, almost all corporate hospitals are realizing the importance of leadership in the management. A leader should be able to influence people to act with zeal and enthusiasm to achieve the target goal. He should be able to lead people and not seek directions from them in difficulty. He should inspire confidence—encourage them to give suggestions. He should take responsibility for the mistakes of his subordinates, if committed without motive, i.e. he should be able to know his men. While facing problems or difficulties, he should be able to keep cool even in scary situations. When chips are down, he should be able to stand, i.e. hold his ground and be counted. It should be able to cope with change effortlessly in today's ever-changing environment and should not feel rattled by change.

Latest in Healthcare Management covers the latest topics of healthcare including Entrepreneurship, Quality Management, National Accreditation Board for Hospitals and Healthcare Providers (NABH), National Accreditation Board for Testing and Calibration Laboratories (NABL), Joint Commission International (JCI), Six Sigma Accreditation, Latest Medical Law, Latest Healthcare Architect, Hospital Planning, Green Buildings, Public Health, Outsourcing, IVF, Paramedical, TPA, High Altitude Medical Services, Latest of Medical Education, Opportunities in Healthcare Consultancy, etc. This book is full of latest information in healthcare and also contains the list of important magazines and journals that are useful in health management.

Nowadays, in the world of advancing technology, healthcare delivery represents an extremely complex collection of diagnostic, operational and administrative processes. Management skills in Six Sigma, NABH, NABL, JCI, Planning, Operation, Marketing, Materials, Telemedicine, HIS and Human Resource Management are the need of the hour. Today, we have about 3.5 lakh health institutions in India (large, medium, small). Our health system is unique as compared to other countries—there are Government,

Private, Religious, Industrial, MNCs, Allopathic, *Ayurveda*, Homeopathy, Paramedicals and Nature Cure Hospitals and Institutions. There are newer diseases, newer diagnostic technology, etc.

The book is foreworded along with messages by the Hon'ble Prime Minister Shri Narendra Modi Ji; PD Rai Ji, First MP from IIMA; Dr DS Rana, Chairman, Sir Ganga Ram Hospital; Maj. Gen. K Jai Singh, Group Vice Chancellor, Amity Universities; Maj. Gen. SB Akali, Director General, Six Sigma Healthcare.

Ability to deal with people from diverse background is an essential quality of hospital administrators. They should hence be sympathetic, tactful and patient listeners. Problem solving is required at all times hence the ability to be a team leader with a positive approach is essential. Hospital administrators must understand organizational development, financial budgeting, material management, medical purchasing and maintenances, building regulations and above all must have good public relations skills. Interest in service, in healthcare and in welfare are at the core of this profession. Hospital administrators convene meetings at various levels and hence need good communication skills.

Think, Feel and Do.

Enjoy *Latest in Healthcare Management*.

With Best Wishes!

Pradeep Bhardwaj
pradeepkb28@gmail.com
www.drpradeepbhardwaj.com

Preface

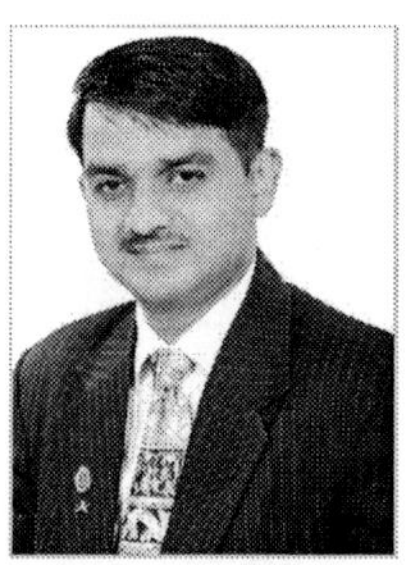

A warm welcome to the 1st edition of the book *Latest in Healthcare Management.*

Hospitals are becoming a highly scientific and complex medical center and are becoming hub of whole system of healthcare. The Hospital Administrator and population ratio in India is 1:1,65,000. This is the right and exciting time to ensure an international future in the recession-proof world's largest and fastest growing industry. Leaders within hospital and health systems must be equipped to face today's daunting challenges and other tests that will emerge in the next decade. At present, 42% doctors in America are Indians and 2% hospital administrators are Indians in America.

Hospital and healthcare is one of the toughest managements on earth. Hospital administration is a serious business, since it covers a large number of activities. The profession of hospital and healthcare administration is unique because hospitals involve highly qualified professionals dealing with the question of life and death. Hospital administration is more complex than administration of any other business institute or organization. The health sector is in dire need for managers who have an in-depth understanding of general management principles combined with the ability to apply them appropriately to healthcare delivery system. Healthcare leaders need knowledge, operational efficiency while meeting day-to-day challenges. Vibrant and successful organizations require innovative and strong leadership at all levels and hospital administration is a convenient passport to a disciplined approach towards hospital and healthcare management and decision-making leadership.

"Leading-edge technologies, innovative treatment and state-of-the-art facilities may be the hallmark of modern healthcare; but, ultimately, a healthcare organization is defined by the strength of a single resource—its people".

In today's world of advancing technology healthcare delivery represents an extremely complex collection of diagnostic, operational and administrative processes. Management skills in Six Sigma, NABH, NABL, JCI, Planning, Operation, Marketing, Materials, Telemedicine, HIS and Human Resource Management are the need of the hour. Today, we have about 3.5 lakh health institutions in India (large, medium, small). Our health system is unique as compared to other countries—there are Government, Private, Religious, Industrial, MNCs, Allopathic, *Ayurveda*, Homeopathy, Paramedicals and Nature Cure Hospitals and institutions. There are newer diseases, newer diagnostic technology, etc.

The purpose of life is to grow and to share. When you come to look back on all that you have done in life, you will get more satisfaction from the pleasure you have brought to other people's lives than you will from the times that you outdid and defeated them.

Rising costs, expanding demand, and increasing customer expectations characterize healthcare today and are redefining the roles of patients, providers and payers. This is especially true as health facilities across the chain (primary, secondary, tertiary) are increasingly being run by corporates and funded through private equity that demands better management practices and accountability mechanisms. The need for efficiently managed health systems, while containing costs and increasing access and profitability, has brought about a shift in focus from just medical expertise to principles of business and management. Apart from clinical specialization, corporate hospitals are focusing on internal business functions, such as inventory, asset, financial and human resource management, as well sales and marketing, and customer relationship management (CRM). This trend will continue and create a demand for a specialized resource base.

The striking feature of the healthcare sector is its potential to grow at an exponential rate in the foreseeable future and present new opportunities within related industries, which will emerge as growth drivers. There is immense potential for each stakeholder (e.g. government, entrepreneurs, healthcare service providers, pharmaceutical companies, medical equipment manufacturers) to invest in and grow with the sector. However, given the complex and interdependent nature of the sector there is a need for a cohesive and collaborative approach, where all stakeholders effectively work synergistically and leverage the opportunities to create a lasting impact.

The book in your hand covers the latest issues of healthcare management.

Pradeep Bhardwaj

Acknowledgments

"No one walks alone when one is walking on the journey of life just where you start to thank those who joined you, walked besides you, and helped you along the way".

The book *Latest in Healthcare Management* in your hand has become a reality as a result of contribution from many people, professionals, and hospitals. Foremost are my wife Dr Anita Bhardwaj, daughter Parikul Bhardwaj and son Angad, who were instrumental in inspiring me to write on the subject which they felt is of great importance in today's changing scenario of hospital and healthcare administration.

My all efforts fail to pen the words that could precisely articulate my deep sense of gratitude towards my parents, sisters and especially my brother "Er Darshan Deep Bhardwaj" for their prolific support, spirited inspiration and tremendous concern that worked as a beacon of light to me.

I feel privileged to express my gratitude to Dr DS Rana, Chairman, Sir Ganga Ram Hospital; Dr K Raj Kapoor, Dr Rajat Mohan, Senior Cardiologist, Sir Ganga Ram Hospital.

My special thanks to Maj. Gen. SB Akali, Director General, Six Sigma Star Healthcare; Sh. Bhim Bhadur Pun, Dr Braj Kishore Rajoriya, Sh. Maninder Singh, Sh. Ashish Sharma, Sh. Bharat Sharma, Dr SP Bayotra and all friends whose diligent effort, valuable contribution made this book successful.

Many thanks to all my students of PhD, DNB, MPhil, MBA, MHA, BHM, MPH courses, my clients, hospitals, institutes and readers, without you this book would not exist.

I express my appreciation and gratitude to Shri Jitendar P Vij (Group Chairman) and Mr Ankit Vij (Group President) of M/s Jaypee Brothers Medical Publishers (P) Ltd., New Delhi, India, which is one of the largest medical publishers in the world, for their assistance and help. Mr Tarun Duneja (Director-Publishing) and Ms Samina Khan (Executive Assistant to Director-Publishing) have been instrumental in getting the final shape of the book. Also, my acknowledgments to Mr KK Raman (Production Manager), Mr Sunil Kumar Dogra (Production Executive), Mr Neelambar Pant (Production Coordinator), Mr Anil Sharma (Graphic Designer), Mr Varun Rana and Mr Pramod Kumar Rout (Typesetters), Mr Akhilesh Kumar Dubey (Proofreader) and other members for their immense patience to bring out the book.

Contents

PLATE 1

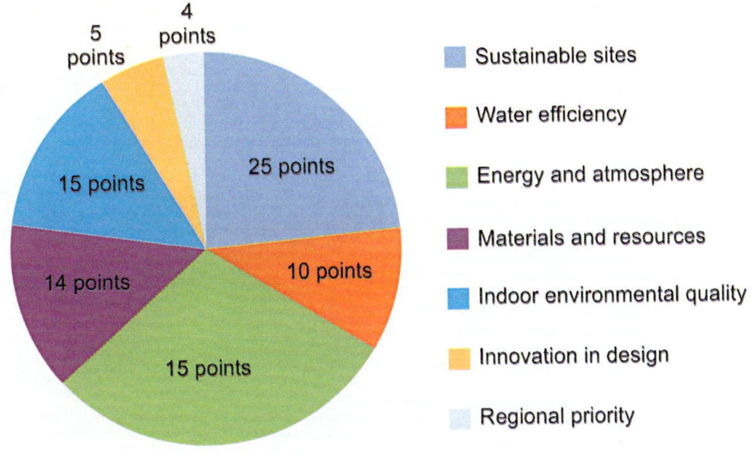

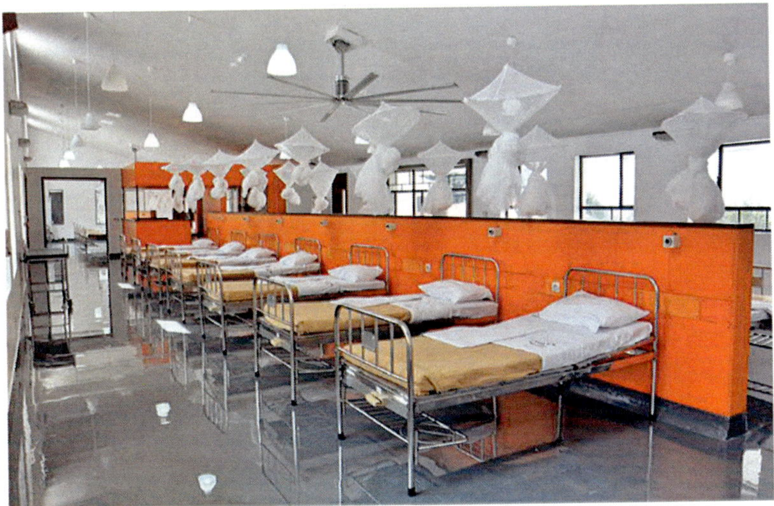

Fig. 19.2: Natural light-friendly wards

PLATE 2

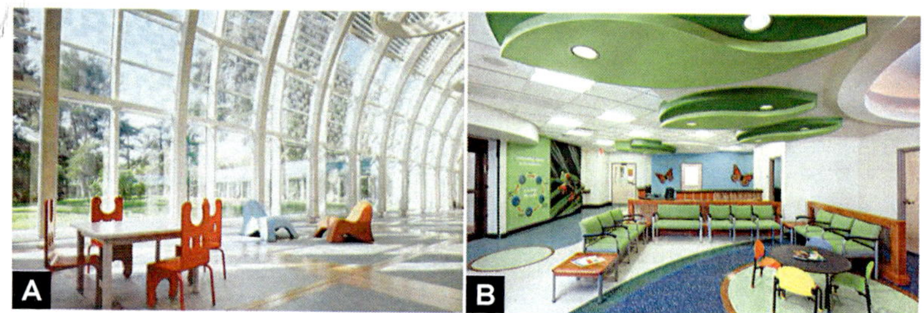

Figs 19.4A and B: Environment-friendly patient area

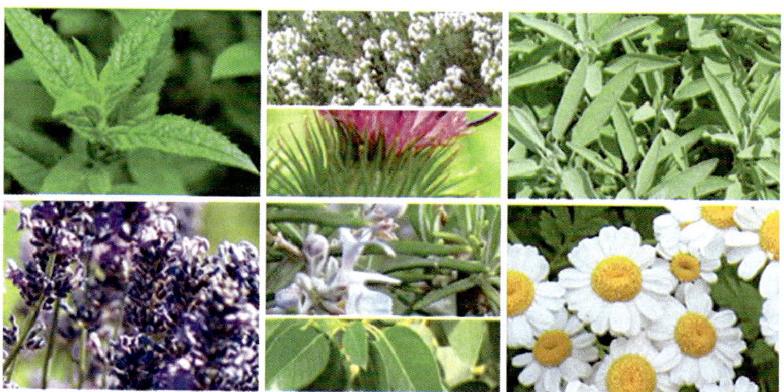

Fig. 19.6: Eco-friendly environment

■■■ Chapter 1

Public Health and its Scope

INTRODUCTION

Now is a great time to pursue a career in Public Health. A diverse and rewarding field, public health offers meaningful career opportunities for people at all educational levels. No matter what your interests, odds are you will be able to find a position you enjoy in public health. The Master of Public Health (MPH) degree is the most demanding widely recognized professional credential for leadership in the Public Health. The MPH program is designed for public health leaders who aspire to high-level roles in State, Federal, and International Health Organizations, Research and Academic Institutions, or the Private Sector.

Master of Public Health (MPH) is a multidisciplinary professional degree awarded for studies in areas related to public health. The MPH degree is the most widely recognized professional credential for leadership in public health.

The program emphasizes active, student-directed learning, problem solving, and the acquisition of skills essential to the practice of public health.

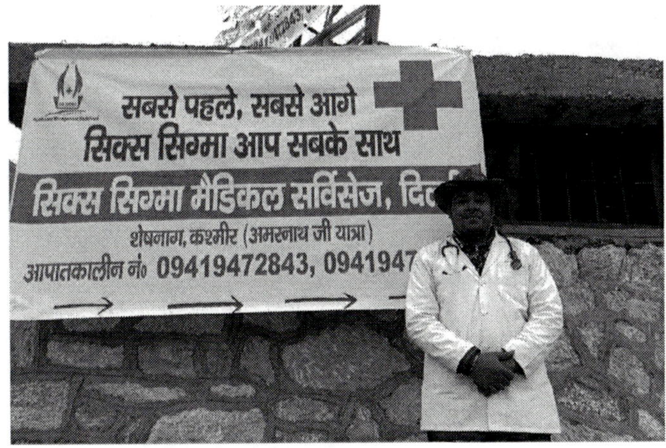

Public Health Services at Shri Amarnath ji Yatra, JK

Master of public health degrees may also intersect with fields such as urban planning, policy, advocacy, community organizing, communications, integrated health, social work and social sustainability.

WHAT IS THE SCOPE OF MPH COURSE?

- Job availability in international organizations like WHO, UNICEF, Red Cross, All Government Agencies, NGOs, Societies, Hospitals, International and National Healthcare Organizations, etc.
- Work for improvement of the various aspects of environment which may include prevention of all types of pollution-water, air, noise, etc.
- Prevention of communicable diseases which can be easily done by screening the surroundings and also screening the chronic ailments before it becomes too late.
- Work for improvement of conditions of employment for prevention of occupational hazards.
- Work for the prevention of conditions which may lead to disturbances of growth and development in maternity, infancy and childhood. Disturbances and defects of mentality, personality, emotions, behavior or interpersonal relationships now begin to receive the attention they warrant as we shift emphasis from concern chiefly with institutional care of the already mentally sick or socially inadequate to guidance by sympathetic education in the natural history of mental health.
- Some Designations/Career Options—Public Health Writer, Public Health Inspectors, Faculty, Public Health Journalist, Medical Investigator, Biostatical, Public Health Consultant, NGO Director, Health Researchers, Community Health Worker, *Anganwadi* Manager, Disease Ecologist, Public Health Information Officer, Disaster Management, etc.

Why Pursue a Career in Public Health?

- *Public health is an exciting and growing field of study*: The field challenges its professionals to confront complex health issues, such as improving access to healthcare, controlling infectious disease, and reducing environmental hazards, violence, substance abuse, and injury.
- *Public health is a diverse and dynamic field*: Public health professionals come from varying educational backgrounds and can specialize in an array of fields. A host of specialists, including teachers, journalists, researchers, administrators, environmentalists, demographers, social workers, laboratory scientists, and attorneys, work to protect the health of the public.

- *Public health is a field geared toward serving others*: Public health professionals serve local, national, and international communities. They are leaders who meet the many exciting challenges in protecting the public's health today and in the future.
- *Public health is a rewarding field*: The field of public health offers great personal fulfillment-working towards improving people's health and well-being is a rewarding day's work.

Who should Consider a Degree in Public Health?

Public health is a field that offers an abundance of job opportunities to suit a variety of interests and skills. Whether you are more interested in crunching numbers, conducting research, or working with people, there is a place for you in the field of public health. Recent college graduates and those that have been in the field for years have something to offer and to gain in this field. Public health is ideal for those that gain satisfaction knowing that they are working to improve the lives of others.

How can a Graduate Degree in Public Health Enhance my Career Opportunities?

Many public health jobs require a graduate degree in public health. A graduate degree gives public health professionals a competitive edge over other professionals and enables professionals to:

- Gain knowledge of the factors which influence local, national and global legislative and social polices.
- Apply broad-based, state-of-the-art quantitative and qualitative skills needed for problem solving.
- Develop multidisciplinary and collaborative strategies for solving health-related problems.
- Enhance communication skills by working with diverse populations; and, be positioned for a leadership role in health promotion and disease prevention.

Where do Public Health Professionals Work?

Public health professionals work in both the public and private sectors. Many public health graduates will find work in the public sector in WHO, International Health Agencies, Local, State, or Federal Health Departments. The jobs available at health departments range from Food Safety Inspectors to Health Educators; from Policy Analysts to Epidemiologists. Other public health professionals will find work in university systems as researchers.

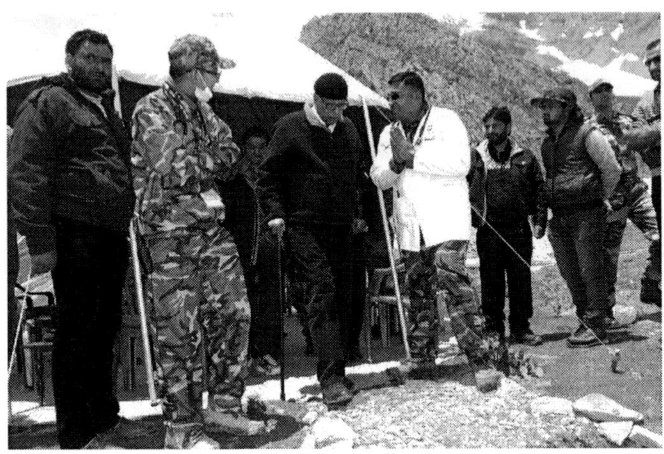

Public Health Professional work at Kashmir

Those interested in working for a nonprofit organization can find jobs in health advocacy, policy, or research for organizations such as the American Cancer Society, the Red Cross, or a local nonprofit that focuses on specific health issues.

Still other public health professionals will find work in the private sector —working in randomized control trials for pharmaceutical companies or for health insurance companies.

What kind of Job Title can I Expect after Graduating with a Degree in Public Health?

Job titles, position descriptions, and salary ranges of recent public health graduates will vary greatly based on their course of study and interests. Some sample career titles are listed below:

- Public Health Management Analyst
- Director of Programs and Services
- Health Communications Specialist
- Research Scientist
- Environmental Health Intelligence Analyst
- Manager, Breastfeeding Initiatives.

What is the Difference between the Different Degrees? How do I Choose the One that's Right for Me?

There are many different degree programs for those that interested in studying public health. Some of the programs include:

- Master of Public Health (MPH)
- Master of Hospital Administration (MHA)
- Master of Health Services Administration (MHSA)
- Master of Science in Public Health (MSPH)
- Doctor of Public Health (DrPH)
- Doctor of Philosophy (PhD)

In general, the MPH degree will include coursework in a number of public health disciplines, such as administration, epidemiology, environmental health, and behavioral health. Specialized degrees such as a Master of Health Administration will be more focused on a specific topic.

Another distinction between degrees is the professional degree versus the academic degrees. Professional degrees generally have a greater orientation towards practice in public health settings. The MPH, DrPH, and MHA are example of degrees which are geared towards those who want careers as practitioners of Public Health in Traditional Health Departments, managed care organizations, community-based organizations, hospitals, consulting firms, international agencies, state and federal agencies, among others.

Academic degrees are more oriented toward students wishing to seek a career in academics and research rather than public health practice. Examples of academic degrees are the MS, PhD, and ScD.

However, each school of public health can tailor their degree programs significantly. Student interested in getting a degree in public health should check with individual schools for more information on specific degree programs.

Why should I Consider a Dual Degrees in Public Health?

Dual degrees are available to those that are pursuing degrees or have degrees in fields such as nursing, law, social work, public policy, business, medicine, dentistry, and veterinary medicine. At many schools of public health, people with an advanced degree are eligible for an accelerated MPH program. A public health degree will help those in other fields understand the principles of public health and apply these principles to their practices.

Distinctions Between Public Health and Clinical Health Professions

In public health, the focus is on populations and communities rather than individual patients. Public health careers offer something for everyone. Epidemiology and biostatistics involve mathematics and modeling.

Environmental health includes a wide range of science skills. Health administration incorporates business and management skills. Health education involves skills required to develop community-wide prevention programs. Health policy includes an understanding of law-making processes.

Perhaps never has there been a more exciting time to pursue a career in public health. Why? Because...

- Most experts agree that major advances in improvement of health over the next decades will not come from new medical findings or cures, but rather the broader development and application of population-based prevention programs.
- Health services delivery systems are undergoing rapid change. Greater emphasis is being placed on health promotion and disease prevention as a means to reduce the costs of care by improving the health of our populations. These changes have created a broad array of new opportunities for professionals with advanced training in public health.
- As the public has become better informed about the effects of toxic wastes and pollutants on their health, greater emphasis is being placed on assuring the safety of our communities as well as worker health and safety. As a result, there is growing demand for experts in environmental health and industrial hygiene.
- Public health research is focusing more on women's health, and child and substance abuse, and an increased emphasis is being placed on behavioral change to prevent the risk of STDs, HIV/AIDS, tuberculosis, and unplanned pregnancies. Greater emphasis is also being placed on school health and the health of minority and disadvantaged populations.

Other Associate Options is Public Health Administrator

A Day in the Life of a Public Health Administrator

Public health administrators focus on community-wide disease prevention and health promotion. As the name of the profession shows, there are two parts to their jobs. Public health administrators try to improve the welfare of the community at large and run the organizations that disseminate information about health. The majority are employed by governmental health agencies, while others work for not-for-profit organizations and educational institutions. They assess community health issues and educate members about the prevention or alleviation of health problems. The public health administrator executes community outreach programs to make people aware of dangers such as lead poisoning and to address chronic problems afflicting the community, like sexually transmitted diseases.

The administrator's job calls for the management skills of a CEO. She creates budgets, hires staff, organizes the office, and obtains any necessary equipment. Writing grant proposals and fundraising take up more and more of the administrator's time as budget cuts flourish.

Whenever, she notices a health related trend or event, she must write a report on what she believes its effect on the community will be. The public health administrator must be prepared to delicately balance limited budgets with the compassion needed to provide basic care. Since she is often faced with contradictory information and demands, she must be able to make decisions. She also needs self-confidence when called on to defend her decisions to public officials or the press. The administrator attends community events frequently.

Usually she devotes five and a half days a week to her career, but some are on 24-hour call. In an era of shrinking healthcare budgets, officials are expected to complete projects faster and with less support staff than ever before. This has forced many administrators to exercise their creative juices in designing new ways to handle the issues they face.

Paying Your Dues

There is no one way to become a public health administrator, but most professionals have worked in related fields and acquired advanced degrees. Employers require at least a Bachelor's degree in Healthcare Administration or a related field, but the field is so competitive that master's degree holders have a significant advantage. While health-related courses, business administration, and finance are important parts of your academic background, make time for communications and English, too. You will need to write and present many reports professionally and confidently.

Many administrators receive their degrees after having worked in other areas in the field. They are often former health inspectors, who insure that consumer products meet federal health and safety standards, or regulatory inspectors, who enforce observation of public welfare laws and regulations. Those with keen entrepreneurial skills and backgrounds are encouraged to enter the field, bringing their efficiency to it. Some people gain their initial training in the Peace Corps before returning to school.

Many graduate programs offer specialized joint degrees, such as a combined healthcare management and law degree. While dozens of schools offer graduate and undergraduate degrees in public health administration, only twenty-six are accredited. Whether you choose an accredited school or not is largely dependent on your plan of study, career expectations, and financial situation. Public health administrators enjoy a combination of study and work throughout their careers. Most public health administration students enroll in internship programs to gain experience. Once they start working, they are expected to take continuing education courses every year to keep up with the latest in health care services. Beginning in school and continuing throughout their careers, public health administrators should read trade papers about healthcare and the literature supplied by its providers.

Associated Careers

The public health administrator works with a host of people in different professions, and can apply his skills, with some extra training, to these other fields if he wishes to change careers. Biostatisticians compile and study vital statistics. They determine the incidence of diseases in different populations and create life-expectancy tables.

Public health administrators turn to them for advice regarding issues such as which vaccines are better than others. Public health administrators can become health economists, who examine financing and organization of healthcare facilities, and advise them on running their businesses. The demand for health economists is growing due to the changing organization of the healthcare industry.

Job Prospects

Those successfully complete the MPH program are eligible to become healthcare professionals and managers or administrators in government, nongovernmental and public sector organizations and hospitals. Graduates can also occupy technical and leadership positions in the implementation of public health or community health programs of the State and Central governments and the World Health Organization.

Chapter 2

Emerging Trend in Healthcare

INTRODUCTION

India healthcare expenditure is still amongst the lowest globally and there are significant challenges to be addressed both in terms of accessibility of healthcare service and quality of patient care.

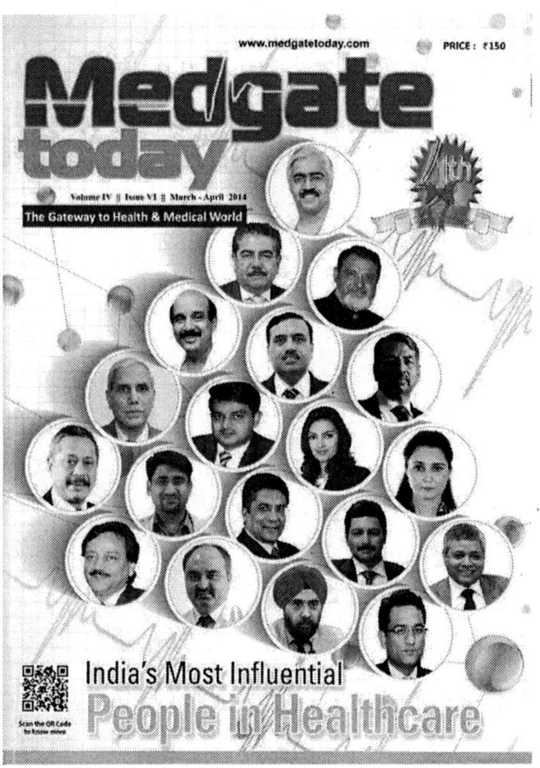

CURRENT STATE OF HEALTHCARE IN INDIA

The India healthcare sector currently represents a US$ 40 billion industry. A break-up of the sector as of 2009 is provided (Fig. 2.1).

India's healthcare spend is significantly low when compared to the global, developed and other similar emerging economies. To future illustrate this point, we have examined the Indian healthcare spend on various parameters.

The Indian healthcare spend is less than half the global average in percentage terms when compared on a 'percent a gross domestic product (GDP)' basis (Fig. 2.2).

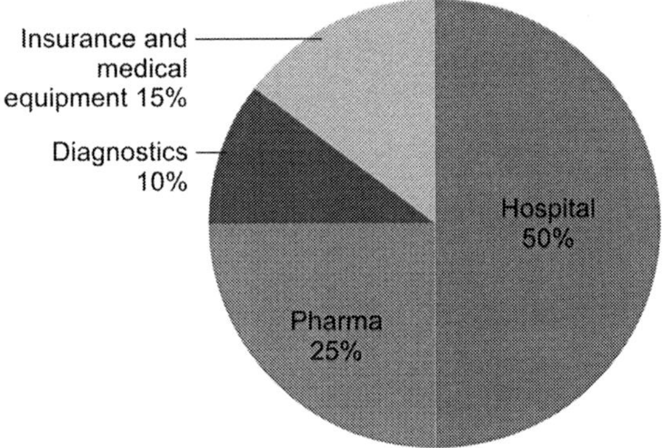

Fig. 2.1 Healthcare industry break-up
Source: IDFC Securities Hospital Sector November 2010.

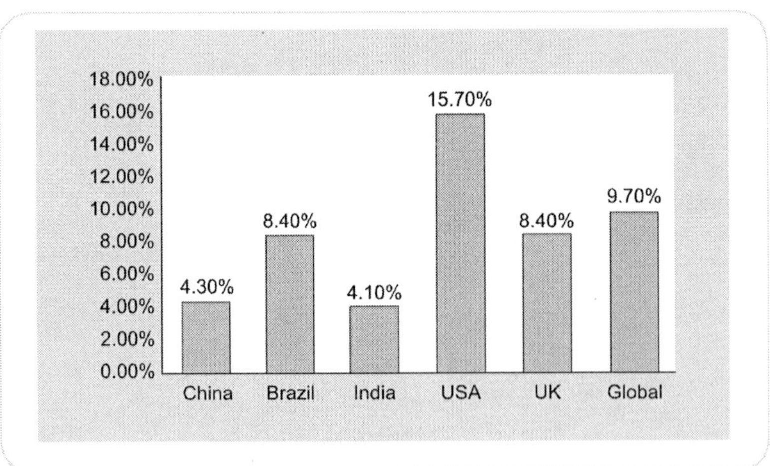

Fig. 2.2 Spending as a percent of GDP
Source: WHO World Health Statistics 2010.

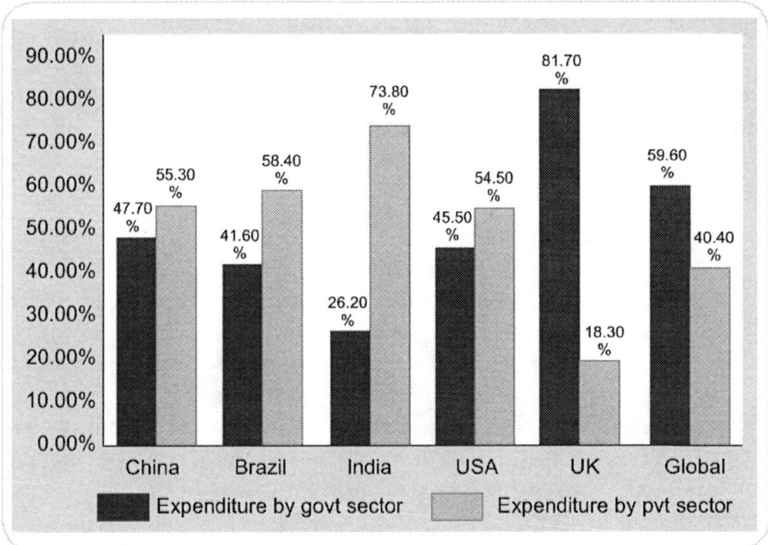

Fig. 2.3 Comparison of healthcare speed
Source: WHO World Health Statistics 2010.

The healthcare spend, when compared on the basis of public-private contribution, also depicts a skewed picture. As is noted from the comparison below, private sector contribution to the healthcare sector at ~75% is amongst the highest in the world in percentage terms. Public spending, on the other hand, is amongst the lowest in the world and is ~23% points lower than the global average. Figure 2.3 shows comparison of healthcare management.

Finally, the healthcare spend examined on a per capita basis, both in terms of US$ (at average exchange rate conversion) and in terms of purchasing power parity (PPP), is amongst the lowest globally. Further, when compared to the global average, the per capita India healthcare spend is ~95% lower on an average exchange rate basis and ~87% lower on a PPP basis.

GROWTH IN THE HEALTHCARE INDUSTRY

As stated earlier, the India healthcare industry is currently estimated at US$ 40 billion. The industry is expected to grow to ~US$ 79 billion by 2012 and ~US$ 280 billion by 2020. The average compound annual growth rate (CAGR) for the next 10 years, therefore, has been estimated at ~ 21%.

DRIVERS OF GROWTH FOR THE HEALTHCARE SECTOR

A combination of demographic and economic factors is expected to bring about increases healthcare coverage in India which is expected to drive the growth of the sector.

Demographic Factors

- *Increase in population*: Expected increase in population from about 1.1 billion in 2009–2010 to 1.4 billion by 2026.
- *Shift in demographics*: 60% of the population in the younger age bracket and an expected increase of geriatric population from current 96 million by 2026. This represents a huge patient base and creates a market for preventive, curative and geriatric care opportunities.
- *Rise in disposable income*: Households in the above INR 200,000 per annum bracket can benefit from an increase in disposable income from 14% in 2009–2010E to 26% in 2014–2015P making healthcare more affordable.
- *Increase in incidence of lifestyle-related diseases*: There is likely to be a marked increase in the incidence of lifestyle-related diseases, such as cardiovascular, oncology and diabetes, when compared to the communicable and infectious diseases.
- *Rising literacy*: Growing general awareness, patient preferences and better utilization of institutionalized care as a result of increase in literacy rates.

Economic Factors

- *Tax benefits*: Lower direct taxes, higher depreciation on medical equipment, income tax exemption for 5 years to hospitals in rural areas, etc. are being provided by the Government to the sector.
- *Medical tourism*: India emerging as a major medical tourist destination with medical tourism market expected to reach US$ 2 billion by 2012.
- *Insurance coverage*: Increase in health insurance coverage with a number of private players and foreign players entering the market to cater to increased demand. The sector is expected to see an increase in the penetration from the current 10–15% to almost 50% at a CAGR of 24%. At an institutional level, insurance penetration is likely to continue to increase from 5–20%. In tertiary care this is almost as high as 40–55% with the inclusion of employer paid coverage.

EMERGING TRENDS IN HEALTHCARE: CHALLENGERS AND INTERVENTIONS

While the Indian healthcare sector is poised for growth in the next decade, it is still plagued by various issues and challenges:

- *Dual disease burden*: Urban India is now on the threshold of becoming the disease capital of the world and facing an increased incidence of lifestyle related diseases such as cardiovascular diseases, diabetes. cancer, chronic obstructive pulmonary disease (COPD), etc. At the same time, the urban poor and rural India are struggling with communicable diseases such as tuberculosis, typhoid, dysentery, etc. Rural India is also seeing a higher occurrence of noncommunicable lifestyle related diseases. This represents a serious challenge that the India healthcare system would need to address.
- *Lack of infrastructure and manpower*: Accessibility to healthcare services is extremely limited to many rural areas of the country. In additional, existing healthcare infrastructure is unplanned and is irregularly distributed. Further, there is a severe lack of trained doctors and nurses to service the needs of the large India populous.

The private sector has evolved a multipronged approach to increase accessibility and penetration. It has tackled the issue of lifestyle related diseases with the development of high-end tertiary care facilities. Also new delivery models such as day-care centers, single specialty hospitals, end-of-life care centers, etc. are on the horizon to service larger sections of the population and address specific needs.

The public sector is keen to continue to encourage private investment in the healthcare sector and is now developing public-private partnerships, i.e. PPP models to improve availability of healthcare services and provide healthcare financing.

Both sectors have also undertaken initiatives to improve functional efficiencies in the form of accreditations, clinical research, outsourcing of noncare areas, increased penetration of healthcare insurance and third party payers.

CHANGING DISEASE TRENDS

India rates poorly on even the basic healthcare indicators when benchmarked against not only the developed economics, but also the other Brazil, Russia, India and China (BRIC) nations. This is evidence of the fact that a significant portion of the Indian population is unable to access healthcare services (Table 2.1). This is a consequence of:

- Lack of healthcare infrastructure
- Lack of trained and qualified manpower.

Table 2.1 Disease indicators

Indicator	Year	India	Developed economies			Emerging economies		
			US	UK	Japan	Brazil	Russia	China
Life expectancy at birth (years)	2008	64	80	80	83	73	68	74
Infant mortality rate (probability of dying by age 1 per 1000 livebirths)	2008	52	7	5	3	18	9	18
Maternal mortality rate (per 100000 births)	2000–09	254	13	7	3	77	24	34

Source: WHO, World Health Statistics, 2010.

BURDEN OF NONCOMMUNICABLE DISEASES

Table 2.2 shows burden of noncommunicable diseases.

Table 2.2 Burden of noncommunicable diseases

Disease	Number of cases	Deaths 2005*	Projected number of cases 2015*	Projected deaths 2015**
Cardiovascular	3,80,41,090	20,89,508	6,40,71,981	34,20,752
Diabetes	3,10,39,932	N/A	4,58,09,149	N/A
COPD	1,70,20,000	N/A	2,22,10,000	N/A
Cancer	20,16,700	5,38,858	24,96,133	6,66,563

*CVD/diabetes data from 2005; COPD from 2004.

**Projected data for CVD/diabetes is for 2015; COPD is 2016; cancer is 2014.

Source: World Health Organization, World Health Statistics 2010.

CURRENT INFRASTRUCTURE

The healthcare infrastructure in India is inadequate compared with the global standards. It lags behind the global average in terms of healthcare infrastructure and manpower. India has an average 0.6 doctors per 1000 population against the global average of 1.23 which suggest an evident manpower gap (Tables 2.3 to 2.6).

Table 2.3 Hospital and doctors bed density

Indicators	Year	India	USA	UK	Brazil	China
Hospital bed density (per 10000 population)	2000–2009	12	31	39	24	30
Doctor density (per 10000 population)	2000–2009	6	27	21	17	14

Table 2.4 Evident manpower gap

Indicators	Year	India	USA	UK	Brazil	China
Births attended by skilled health personnel (percent)	2000–2009	47	99	NA	97	98
No. of doctors	2009	6,43,520	7,93,648	1,26,126	3,20,013	18,62,630
No. of nurses	2009	13,72,059	29,27,000	37,200	5,49,423	1,22,59,240
No. of dentists	2009	55,344	4,63,663	25,914	2,17,217	1,36,520
Average no. of doctors per bed	2009	0.6	0.81	0.53	0.69	0.46
Average no. of nurses per bed	2009	1.27	3	0.16	1.18	3.02
No. of doctors per 1000 population	2009	0.6	2.7	2.1	1.7	1.4
No. of nurses per 1000 population	2009	1.3	9.8	0.6	2.9	1

Source: www.oecd.org, www.whoindia.org.

Table 2.5 Forecast of bed required

	2008	2018	2028
Additional beds required	1.1 million	3.1 million	2 million
Bed/1000 population ratio	0.7–1.7	4	5

Source: CLL Technopak.

At six doctors per 10,000 people, the number of qualified doctors in the country is not sufficient for the growing requirements of Indian healthcare. Moreover, rural 'doctors to population' ratio is lower by 6 times as compared to urban areas.

Table 2.6 Doctors and nurses gap

Parameter	Current annual production	To fill the gap
Physicians	30,558	9,93,500
Nurses	1,14,218	2,510,250

Source: CLL Technopak.

EMERGING TRENDS IN HEALTHCARE DELIVERY

Investment Trends

Driven by increased domestic demand for high-end investment services as well as medical tourism, the healthcare sector has attracted huge investments lately. The healthcare sector is likely to see an increase in investment from US$ 34.2bn in 2012E (CAGR of 15%), with ~80% of investments from private players. The investments to this scale are expected to increase the bed ratio from 0.9 beds per 1000 people to 1.85 beds per 1000 people.

Moreover, large scale investments in infrastructure are required to make healthcare facilities on par with developed countries.

Foreign Direct Investment

The foreign direct investment (FDI) inflows in the hospital sector have not been significantly high despite government incentives to attract FDI investments (including 100% FDI in most health-related services). There are currently limited number of '100% foreign-owned healthcare' players in the Indian market. However, this scenario is expected to change given the attractiveness of the sector. Many foreign players are making a foray into the market through joint ventures with local healthcare units. For example, Singapore's Pacific Healthcare made its first foray into the Indian market, opening an international medical center, which is a joint venture with Indian's Vitae Healthcare, in the Indian city of Hyderabad. Singapore-based Parkway Group Healthcare PTE Ltd has entered the Indian healthcare market in 2003 through a joint venture with the Apollo group to build the Apollo Gleneagles hospital, a 325-bed multispecialty hospital at a cost of US$ 29 million and is looking at a joint venture for another tertiary care hospital in Mumbai. Many international diagnostic care players have entered India and others including medical education players are looking keenly at sectoral entry points.

Hospital and Research

In India, many corporate hospitals and major public hospitals are actively involved in conducting clinical trials of various drugs.

Private corporate hospitals such as Apollo Care, Narayana Hrudayalaya, Usha Cardiac Institute, Sankara Nethralaya, Indraprastha, Breach Candy, and Bayer diagnostics as well as public hospitals such as All India Institute of Medical Sciences, Nizam Institute of Medical Sciences and many of the Medical colleges and teaching hospitals are actively involved in various stages of clinical trials.

Many of them have state-of-the-art infrastructure facilities for conducting clinical trials and treating patients. These have not only helped in improving patient outcomes but also helped in tackling increased volume of patients suffering from debilitating diseases.

DEVELOPMENTS IN PRIVATE HEALTHCARE

Evolving Delivery Models

Day-care Centers

Need: The concepts of outpatient surgeries is growing worldwide as inpatient facilities can be expensive and inconvenient in some cases. A large number of surgeries can be performed without the patient having to be admitted at all with the help of Day-care Surgery Centers. This delivery model is advantageous for both healthcare providers and consumers. It is estimated that by 2020, 75% model is surgical operations will be carried out in ambulatory surgery centers/units. Today over a quarter of the surgeries are contributed by ophthalmic procedures. The cost advantage of day surgery is best achieved in free-standing centers or free-functioning units within hospitals.

In India, the concept of stand-alone day-care surgery centers is currently in its infancy. Many of the major hospitals have a separate day-care surgery center which caters to the management of ambulatory (also commonly referred to as 'same day surgery') procedure. In India, about 20% of all surgical procedures are performed on outpatients.

Studies reveal that treatment in these centers would cost about 47% less than in hospitals. This model can be economically efficient for the Indian healthcare which is scarce in resources.

Potential Benefits

The range of services provided and the cost are the prime benefits of the day-care services.

Nova Day-care Center: **Case Study**

The promoters and the US-based private investment firm, plan to set-up around 100 day-care surgery centers in the next three to four years with an investment of over INR 800 crore. The company executives' claim that the patients could save about 15–20% in surgery costs at Nova's day-care centers compared to the corporate hospitals rates.

The low-cost model and the high efficiency rates of 450 surgeries per month per center would make it a befitting model for India, which has a bed to population ration of 0.7 per thousand persons compared to the word average of 3.3. Overnight room costs and related overhead costs are eliminated and the model enables surgeons to attend to more patients in less time.

It essentially aspires to focus on minimally invasive surgeries, which use the technological advances in most optimum manner. The day-care surgery model has a market potential of INR 42,000 crore in the country. (Suresh Soni, chairman and co-founder, Nova told FE.) In the first phase, the group plans to build 25 centers in 10 major cities in the next two years. They plan to build around 125 operation theaters.

In a hospital with the day-care services the surgery department provides services for eye surgery, including removal of foreign bodies, providing the patient with plethora of services in a small the frame.

An average corporate hospital on the other hand takes a minimum of 18 months in the making and a minimum of three to five years to break even. Company executives point out that even in a hospital set-up around 75% of revenue is finally made from the surgeries. This fact further supports the growth of day-care centers.

Capex and EBIDTA: Due to the dependency on the specialty and level of care that a Day-care Center would cater to it is difficult to pen down an industry on the Capex but a fair indicator would be INR 3.5–4.5 million /bed for an international standard day-care center. EBIDTA margins for day-care centers range between 25% and 30% with a pay back of ~3–4 years.

DEVELOPMENTS IN PUBLIC HEALTHCARE

Initiatives by the Government

To tackle the challenges mentioned, the Government has taken various initiatives to improve the public healthcare system in India. The Government launched the National Rural Health Mission (NRHM) in 2005 which aims to provide quality healthcare for all and increase the expenditure on healthcare from 0.9% of GPD to 2–3% of GDP by 2012–11.

According to Union Budget 2010–11, the plan allocation for Ministry of Health and Family Welfare has increased from US$ 4.2 billion in 2009–10 to US$ 4.8 billion in 2010–11.

Moreover, in order to meet revised cost of construction, in March 2010 the government allocated an additional US$ 4.2 billion for six upcoming AIIMS-like institutes and up-gradation of 13 existing Government Medical Colleges.

The Union Cabinet on October 20, 2010 approved the proposal of the Ministry of Health and Family Welfare to declare National Institute of Mental Health and Neurosciences (NIMHANS), Bengaluru as an Institute of National Importance on the lines of All India Institute of Medical Sciences, New Delhi, Postgraduate Institute of Medical Education and Research, Chandigarh and Jawaharlal Institute of Postgraduate Medical Education and Research, Puducherry.

Private-Public Partnerships

The Indian Government is focused on developing the PPP model to cover the demand-supply gap prevalent in the healthcare sector. Private sector expertise coupled with efficiencies in operation and maintenance would lead to improved healthcare services delivery to the masses. This model can act as a catalyst in the creation of new capacity and improvement of efficiency in the existing infrastructure established. The Government also embraced PPP model to counter epidemics like H1N1 swine flu, HIV, etc. However, it is evident that this model be far more beneficial.

Few successful PPP projects are mentioned below.

- Karnataka Karuna Trust; Yashaswini Scheme
- Tamil Nadu Mobile Health Services
- Andhra Pradesh Aarogyasri
- Andhra Pradesh Diagnostic Services for 4 Medical Colleges
- West Bengal Mobile Health Services
- Madhya Pradesh Community Outreach Program
- Rajasthan Contracting in Public Hospitals
- Gujarat Chiranjeevi Project.

Emerging Role of TPAs

The TPAs (Third Party Administrators) have added to the changing scenario of health insurance in India. Their role is gradually changing from green field ventures to an established system. Their wide spread networking with hospitals and other healthcare providers have certainly strengthened the health insurance structure in India. There are more then 45 TPAs.

OPPORTUNITIES WITHIN INDIA'S HEALTHCARE SECTOR

Medical Tourism on the Rise

Medical tourism is one of the major external drivers of growth of the Indian healthcare sector. A Google search of 'Indian medical tourism' turns up more than 2 two million results.

The emergence of India as a destination for medical tourism leverages the country's well educated, english-speaking medical staff, state-of-the-art private hospitals and diagnostic facilities, and relatively low cost to address the spiraling healthcare costs of the western world. India provides best-in-class treatment, in some cases at less than one-tenth the cost incurred in the US (Table 2.7). India's private hospitals excel fields such as cardiology, joint replacement, orthopedic surgery, gastroenterology, ophthalmology, transplants and urology.

Table 2.7 Cost of key healthcare procedures

			India HC	
Currency: US$	US	Thailand	India	Cost-x of US
Cardiac surgery	50,000	14,250	4,000	12.5
Bone marrow transplant	62,500	62,500	30,000	13.33
Liver transplant	500,000	75,000	45,000	11.11
Orthopedic surgery	16,000	6,900	4,500	3.56

Source: India Brand Foundation Report, IBEF Research.

Emerging Health Insurance Market

The Insurance Regulatory and Development Authority (IRDA) eliminated tariffs on general insurance as of January 1, 2007, and this move is expected to drive additional growth of private insurance products. In the wake of liberalization, health insurance is projected to grow to $5.75 billion by 2010, according to a study by the New Delhi-based PHD Chamber of Commerce and Industry. The IRDA believes that eliminating tariffs will encourage scientific rating and adoption of better risk management practices, and lead to independent pricing for each line of business, so that premiums will be based on actual risks and costs. The implementation of the new policy also will encourage the development of innovative practices and customer-friendly options for policyholders, boosting penetration.

In the postliberalization era, some companies have been licensed to act as third party administrators of health services. The objective is to strengthen the health insurance industry and increase its penetration by bringing more professionalism to claims management, facilitating cashless services to policyholders, and reducing the claims ratio. Currently there are 25 licensed third party administrators in the Indian health insurance industry.

Growth of Telemedicine

Only 25% of India's specialist physicians reside in semiurban areas, and a mere 3% live in rural areas. As a result, rural areas, with a population approaching 700 million, continue to be deprived of proper healthcare facilities.

Clinical Trials

India historically lacked the expertise to perform clinical trials, because most companies only tested different processes for producing copycat versions of Western products, and the rules were quite lenient. Several drug makers have also been caught behaving unethically or even illegally.

However, in recent years, India has become a more attractive market for clinical testing. One reason is that in November 2004, the federal government amended Schedule Y of the Drugs and Cosmetics Act to make the rules on clinical trials more consistent with international practice. In addition, in January 2005 India became compliant with the Trade-Related Aspects of Intellectual Property Rights (TRIPS) Agreement and formally recognized product patents. This triggered growth in Indian clinical trial activity by contract research organizations, such as Quintiles, Omnicare, PharmaNet and Pharma-Olam, and by multinational corporations such as Novo Nordisk, Sanofi-Aventis, Novartis and GSK. Some multinationals, such as Pfizer and Eli Lilly, have been conducting tests locally for a while. Government taxation incentives are further boosting R&D in India.

As a market for clinical testing, India holds other attractions as well. According to a study by Rabo India Finance, a subsidiary of the Netherlands-based Rabo Bank, the huge patient population offers vast genetic diversity, making the country 'an idea site for clinical trials'. It has the largest pool of diabetic patients, the population is relatively easy to access, and many people are 'treatment-naïve'; they have not been treated with medications being tested, which potentially could distort test results.

EMERGING TREND IN HEALTHCARE 2015

New research highlights leading industry trends for healthcare and what to expect more of in 2015. Consumers are increasingly seeking to take a more active role in their own care. To that end, providers and payers are working together to harness technology to enable an integrated approach to healthcare.

MOBILE HEALTH

As consumers are becoming more dependent on their smartphones, there is great opportunity for health care professionals, retailers and brands to develop innovative strategies to reach and engage with consumers when they are on the go. Analysts note a shift from stand-alone 'unsponsored' mobile apps to more meaningful 'sponsored' apps supported by insurance companies, healthcare providers and other institutions, which will result in higher patient adoption and engagement. It addition, integrated mobile health apps will be created that can connect with other devices, apps and data for more holistic healthcare, where information is safely shared across platforms regardless of the vendor.

CONSUMERS' ONLINE AND OFFLINE WORLD'S MERGE

Marketers need to be thinking about the complete consumer experience across all touch points. Take, for instance, CEO of National Retail Federation Matt Shay's comment in USA Today: "What we're going to see is that the two (online/offline) become further and further indistinguishable from one another. Everyone is playing everywhere now."

Advertisers, of course, need individual strategies for mobile, retail and other platforms, but they must start to integrate all those consumer touch points for a better, more holistic consumer experience.

SOCIAL MEDIA'S GROWING IMPORTANCE

Facebook has more than 1 billion users, Twitter has 500 million, and platforms like Pinterest and Instagram are growing in popularity. Social is here to stay and is where consumers are increasingly spending their time interacting, learning and being influenced. Healthcare marketers need to create vibrant, engaging and real-time social identities.

PERSONALIZATION DRIVERS CONSUMER EXPERIENCE

The rise of digital, social and mobile—along with the empowerment of consumers—is directly tied to the growing trend of consumes wanting personalized communications from brands. No more cookie-cutter approach. Consumers know advertisers have a wealth of data about them and they expect it to be used to customize consumer preferences and needs.

Other healthcare trends that are expected to move from pilots to large-scale implementation in 2013 include:

- Hospitals and other healthcare institutions will begin to move more and healthcare data into the cloud, with data analytics to better manage healthcare costs by finding and addressing patient needs earlier.

  Remove patient monitoring will move from pilots to large-scale adoption as more hospitals adopt the accountable care organization model to reduce hospital readmission costs associated with chronic conditions.
- Upswing on telehealth to bridge the significant gap between physician resources and patient demand.

Source: Foster, Bart. "Top 10 Trends for 2013." MediaPost's Marketing: Health blog. 4 Dec. 2012. Web. 19 Dec. 2012; AT&T Forhealth. AT&T. 3 Dec. 2012. Web. 19 Dec. 2012.

MOVING BEYOND CLINICAL EXPERTISE

Rising costs, expanding demand, and increasing customer expectations characterize healthcare today and are redefining the roles of patients, providers and payers. This is especially true as health facilities across the chain (primary, secondary, tertiary) are increasingly being run by corporate and funded through private equality—which demands better management practices and accountability mechanisms. The need for efficiently managed health systems, while containing costs and increasing access and profitability, has brought about a shift in focus from just medical expertise to principles of business and management. A part from clinical specialization, corporate hospitals are focusing on internal business functions such as inventory, asset, financial and human resource management, as well sales and marketing and customer relationship management (CRM). This trend will continue and create a demand for a specialized resources base.

The striking feature of the healthcare sector is its potential to grow at an exponential rate in the foreseeable future and present new opportunities within related industries, which will emerge as growth drivers. There is immense potential for each stakeholder (e.g. government, entrepreneurs, healthcare service providers, pharmaceutical companies, medical equipment manufactures) to invest in and grow with the sector. However, given the complex and interdependent nature of the sector there is a need for a cohesive and collaborative and interdependent nature of the sector there is a need for a cohesive and collaborative approach, where all stakeholders effectively work synergistically and leverage the opportunities to create a lasting impact.

Chapter 3

Nursing Stations Design

Nursing is the backbone of hospital and healthcare sector. It is estimated that by the year 2015, $200 billion will have been spent on hospital design and construction across the United States (Ulrich, Quan, Zimring, Joseph, and Choudhary, 2004). Current healthcare design trends include an emphasis on patient- and family-centered care, improvements in the quality and cost-effectiveness of care delivery, the integration of new technologies, and adherence to new design guidelines intended to promote safe, sustainable, and healing environments for patients and staff (Agency for Healthcare Research and Quality, 2005).

With the growth in the healthcare design market, opportunities come to create innovative design solutions to address current as well as long-standing healthcare delivery issues. Improving the work environment of staff, specifically nurses, is an important component of the healthcare delivery equation.

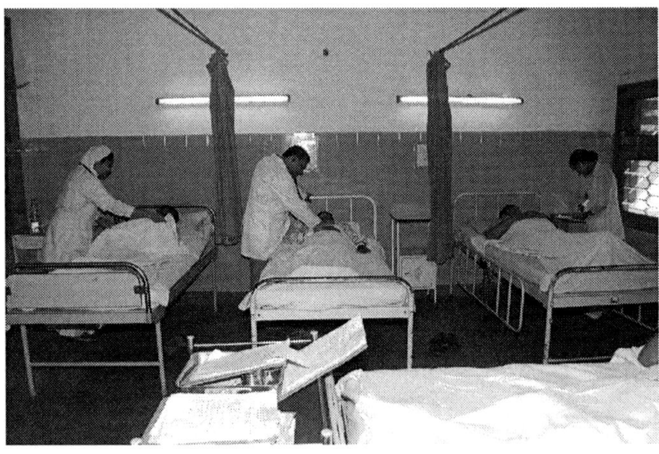

Quality Nursing Care Improves Bed Turnover

THE WORK ENVIRONMENT OF NURSES

As a profession, nursing has become better able to accommodate high turnover volumes, increased patient acuity, and variable staffing requirements. However, a shortage of qualified nurses is a growing concern in the United States. Although the demand for nurses is expected to grow by 40% between 2000 and 2020, the number of new nurses entering the field is expected to increase by only 6%. The resulting shortage of nurses, combined with an increased turnover rate of approximately 20% per year among the aging nursing workforce (Joint Commission, 2002), will result in an alarming situation that must be addressed by hospitals within the next 10 years (Hendrich, Fay, and Sorrells, 2004).

There is growing awareness of the importance of improving the work environment of nurses. According to a Peter D Hart Research Associates (2001) survey of registered nurses, the primary reason nurses leave healthcare, other than retirement, is to find a job that is less stressful and physically demanding. This issue was directly addressed in the Institute of Medicine report, *Keeping Patients Safe: Transforming the Work Environment of Nurses* (2004). The report notes, "It is also essential to foster collaboration of nursing staff with other healthcare personnel in identifying high-risk and inefficient work processes and workspaces and (re)designing them for patient safety and efficiency". Providing a work environment that supports both the physical (functional) and psychological needs of nursing staff is crucial to improving patient care and nursing efficiency.

A growing body of research suggests a relationship between characteristics of the physical environment and the reduction of stress and fatigue among healthcare staff (Berry and Parish, 2008; Joseph, 2006; Ulrich et al., 2004). Evidence suggests that a supportive physical work environment, along with factors such as high autonomy, low work pressure, and supervisor support, may increase job satisfaction and reduce burnout among nurses (Mroczek, Mikitarian, Vieira, and Rotarius, 2005; Tyson, Lambert and Beattie, 2002). It would logically follow that increased job satisfaction and decreased burnout may improve nursing staff retention, reduce turnover, and increase patient satisfaction.

THE NURSING STATION

The nursing station is the heart and soul of nursing care activities in a hospital or long-term care facility. It is typically the primary work area assigned to a specific unit. The nursing station usually includes unit reception along with records storage and charting work areas (Office of Space Analysis, 2006). Walking distances, accessibility, visibility, and ease of supervision have been identified as crucial issues in nursing station design (Hamilton, 1993).

Advances in information technology have enabled nurses to move away from traditional centralized paper-charting stations to smaller, decentralized workstations and charting substations located closer to or inside patient rooms. Nursing units of the past were designed with one centralized nursing station. Advances in information technology have enabled nurses to move away from traditional centralized paper-charting stations to smaller, decentralized work stations and charting substations located closer to or inside patient rooms. Coupled with mandated private rooms in new hospital construction, these changes create longer patient care units and therefore longer distances for nurses to walk.

Healthcare is a multidisciplinary practice in which nurses, doctors, respiratory therapists, pharmacists, and other support staff need a place to interact. A centralized nursing station can provide space for collaboration among caregivers. Wakefield (2002) identified a number of other social functions that may be facilitated by the centralized nursing station. The results suggested that centralized nursing stations represent a symbolic barrier separating the public and private spaces of a unit and that they operate as a mechanism of social control where individuals are expected to formally seek permission to enter the unit before proceeding to patient rooms. From a pivotal location within the unit, the nursing station also serves to maintain workflow and is the setting for frequent social interaction and formal and informal teaching and learning activities. Research suggests that some of these important social functions may be affected in decentralized nursing station designs (Tyson et al., 2002).

More nursing unit designs are incorporating decentralized nurses' stations outside patient rooms so that staff members are distributed around the unit closer to the point of care. This can improve visibility of the patient and reduce time spent walking. Ulrich and colleagues (2004) concluded that decentralized nursing stations allow nurses to interact more closely with patients. Hendrich, Fay, and Sorrells (2004) demonstrated that decentralized nursing stations reduced staff walking and increased patient care time, especially when supply spaces were also decentralized and placed near the nursing stations.

Although decentralized nursing stations may improve patient visibility and reduce walking distance, nurses report feeling more isolated from their colleagues and losing the sense of team connection in comparison to centralized nursing stations (Tyson et al., 2002). This implies that there are important social behavior components of nursing station design that should be considered.

Chapter 4 Laws Applicable to Medical Practices

HEALTHCARE IN INDIA

Healthcare in India features a universal healthcare system run by the constituent States and Territories. Law is an obligation on the part of society imposed by the competent authority, and noncompliance may lead to punishment in the form of monetary fine of imprisonment or both. The earliest known code of laws called the code of Hammurabi governed the various aspects of health practices including the fees payable to physician for satisfactory services. The first ever code of medical ethics called the Hippocratic oath was laid down 2500 years ago, in the 5th century BC, by Hippocrates—the Greek Physician. The modern version of Hippocratic Oath (called the declaration of Geneva), devised by the WHO after the Second World War and is accepted by international medical fraternity. The process of establishment of healthcare system during the colonial rule also necessitated creation of legislative framework for practitioners of medicine. As the number of doctors qualified in Indian medical colleges increased,

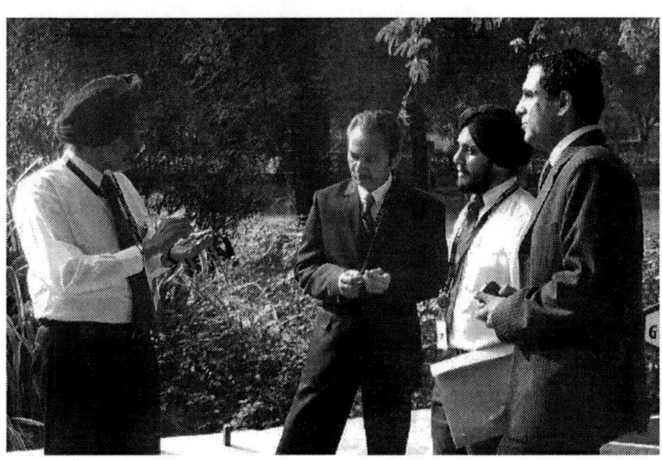

Medical Director and Doctors Practising Modern Medicine with Ethics and Law Applicable

creation of laws for them became necessary. The medical council of India, a national level statutory body for the doctors of modern medicine, was constituted after the enactment of Indian Medical Council Act 1993. The first legal recognition and registration for the Indian systems of medicine came when the Bombay Medical Practitioner Act was passed in 1938.

Laws governing the commissioning of hospital are the laws to ensure that the hospital facilities are created after due process of registration, the facilities created are safe for the public using them, have at least the minimum essential infrastructure for the type and volume of workload anticipated and are subject to periodic inspections to ensure compliance. There are other laws pertaining to governing to the qualification/practice and conduct of professionals, sale, storage of drugs and safe medication, management of patients, environmental safety, employment and management of manpower, medicolegal aspects and laws pertaining to safety of patient, public and staff within the hospital premises. There are laws governing professional training and research, business aspects, licences/certifications required for hospital, etc. A hospital administrator should be aware about all these laws, regulations, policies, procedure, reports and returns and keep abreast with the latest amendments to be on the safe side of law and provide quality care to the patients.

HUMAN CULTURE

Human culture is built upon the formulation of values that from the basis of an ethical society, honesty, integrity, respect, pursuit of excellence, civic duty, accountability and loyalty. Since the dawn of civilization, by trial or error, it has become established that a society and more so it is medical profession, a public oriented and noble profession, can survive and thrive only by observance and practice of certain rules of conduct guided by ethical, moral, legal and social values of land.

Healthcare in India features a universal healthcare system run by the constituent States and Territories. The Constitution charges every state with raising the level of nutrition and the standard of living of its people and improvement of public health as among its primary duties. Law is an obligation on the part of society imposed by the competent authority, and noncompliance may lead to punishment in the form of monetary fine or imprisonment or both.

In a survey conduction at Mumbai, eight out of ten doctors feel that the laws that govern the practice of healthcare in India are outdated and even higher majority feels that there are too many laws and licences that are required to keep their practice going. A survey among 297 doctors across specialization says that there are about 50 different laws that govern the practice of healthcare in India. The study conducted by Medscape India, a nonprofit trust of doctors, revealed that 78% of doctors feel that many of the laws that govern medical practice are outdated. Licences have to be procured by doctors running a hospital every year.

MEDICAL LAWS IN INDIA

The earliest civilization known to us is the Indus urban culture of 3000 to 2000 BC. The renowned medical historian Henry Sigerist believed that public health facilities of Mohenjo Daro were superior to those of any other community of the ancient orient. Since the ancient times, certain duties and responsibilities have been cast on persons who adopt this sacred profession. This is exemplified by Charaka's oath (1000 BC) and Hippocratic Oath (460 BC). The written evidence of the state's involvement and regulatory function is available from the *Kautilya's Arthashastra.* Kautilya considered famine as a bigger calamity than pestilence and epidemics, as the remedies can be found for the diseases. He believed that the king should order the physician to use medicine to counter epidemics.

The earliest known code of laws of health practices were the laws formulated around 2000 BC by Hammurabi, the great king of Babylon. There laws, also called the code of Hammurabi governed the various aspects of health practices, including the fees payable to physician for satisfactory services. The laws were drastic and penalties for harmful therapy stringent. Doctors whose proposed therapy proved wrong ran the risk of being killed. This was the first codification of medical practice.

The first ever code of medical ethics called the Hippocratic Oath was laid down 2500 years ago, in the 5th century BC, by Hippocrates—the Greek physician. He is remembered till today as the 'Father of Western Medicine' Hippocratic oath has been guiding and regulating the conduct of doctors for centuries. The modern version of Hippocratic Oath (called the declaration of Geneva), devised by the WHO after the Second World War and accepted by international medical fraternity as the international code of medical ethics, draws heavily upon the ancient oath.

During the Ashoka period (270 BC), the state showed interest in the public works and provision of medical care and as a law. He founded hospital all over his empire with medical attendance at state expense. Ethics is described in the *Charaka Samhita,* in details and Ayurvedic physicians of ancient India has a well-defined medical ethics.

The process of establishment of healthcare system also necessitated creation of legislative framework for practitioners of medicine. In the earlier period of rule, the physicians and surgeons brought by the East Indian Company and after 1857 by the British Government, needed some discipline and regulations. Lt Colonel DG. Crawfords 'A history of Indian medical services, 1600–1913' narrates several instances of in-discipline, insubordination, malpractice, etc. by such doctors and the punishments (including deportation) meted out to them. It also narrates the regulation devised by the East India Company for the hospital established by them.

After the enactment of the law, establishing General Medical Council in 1857 in England, the British doctors employed in India were registered with the GMC and came under its disciplinary registered. As the number of doctors qualified in Indian medical colleges increased, creation of laws for them became necessary.

As a part of criminal procedures and for other purposes, the colonial government had, in 1871, enacted coroner's act applicable to Bombay and Calcutta. It defined the role of medical professionals in the work of conducting autopsy and inquests. However, the laws for the creation of indigenous medical councils took many more years for enactment. Meanwhile, the laws were enacted for the prevention of the spread of dangerous epidemic disease, for the segregation and medical treatment of pauper, etc. The Epidemic Disease Act was first enacted in 1807 and is still in force with amendments, while the Lepers Act 1898 was repealed and substituted by another law in early 1980s.

Grant Medical College Society in 1880 passed a Bombay Medical Act and established the medical council. The draft rule of this Act included the appointment of a Registrar, maintenance of name in register and penalty for doing wrong things. The Bombay Presidency enacted Bombay Medical Act in 1912. Medical Acts in some other provinces soon followed. The Bengal Medical Act and Madras Medical Registration Act enacted in 1914.

These provincial Acts were immediately followed by the Indian Medical Degree Act, passed by the Indian Legislative Council and approved by the Governor General in 1916.

The first legal recognition and registration for the Indian system of medicine came when the Bombay Medical Practitioner Act was passed in 1938.

Post-independence Development

The independence in 1947 inaugurated a new phase of development of organized healthcare services creating more entitlement for the people. Along with that, the state also embarked on enactment of new laws, modification of the colonial laws and judiciary developed care laws to consolidate people's entitlement of healthcare and to extent the right.

At the time of independence and the first few years of planning, the task confronting the country was to create physical and institutional infrastructure for the rapid development or modernization if Indian.

With time, the Parliament has passed a large number of Bills and Acts to strengthen the healthcare delivery in India.

Prerequisites of Medical Practice

A duly qualified medical professional, i.e. a doctor has a right to seek to practice medicine, surgery and dentistry by registering himself with the Medical Council of the State of which he is resident, by following the procedure as prescribed under the Medical Act of the State.

The State Medical Council has the power to warn, refuse to register/ remove from the name of doctor who has been sentenced by any court for any nonbailable offence or found to be guilty of infamous conduct in any professional respect. The State Medical Council has also the power to re-enter the name of the doctor of the register.

The provision regarding offences and professional misconduct which may be brought before the appropriate Medical Council (State/ Medical Council of India) have been stated in the Indian Medical council (Professional conduct, etiquette and ethics) Regulation 2002. No action against a medical practitioner can be taken unless an opportunity has been given to him to be heard in person or through an advocate.

Emergency Healthcare and Laws

The Supreme Court has been emphatic in declaring that the fundamental right to life covered within its scope the right to emergency healthcare. The landmark judgment that marked this momentous event is that of Parmanand Katara versus Union of India (Supreme Court 1989). In this case, a scooterist severely injured in a road accident was refused for admission when taken to nearest hospital on the excuse that hospital was not competent to handle medicolegal cases. The Supreme Court, in its judgment, pronounced that the obligation of medical professionals to provide treatment in cases of emergencies overrode the professional freedom to refuse patients. Accounting to the right to emergency treatment, the status of a fundamental right under Article 21 (Fundamental Right of Life), the court categorically stated that Article 21 of Constitution casts the obligation on the State to preserve life. Interestingly, the Supreme Court went on to say that not only government hospital but also every doctor whether at a government hospital or otherwise has the professional obligation to extend his/her service with due expertise for protecting life.

In another case (Paschim Banga Khet Majdoor Samity vs State of West Bengal, Supreme Court,1996) a person suffering from head injuries from a train accident was refused treatment at various hospital on excuse that they lacked the adequate facilities and infrastructure to provide treatment. In this case, Supreme Court further developed the right to emergency treatment, and went on to state that the failure on the part of government hospital to provide timely medical treatment to a person in need of such treatment result is violation of his/her right to life guaranteed under Article 21.

Latest Amendment to the PC and PNDT Rules

1. Vide Gazette notification dated 4-6-2012, the PNDT (Amendment) Rules, 2012, have been notified, the effect of which is as follows:
   A. Sub-rule (3) has been added to Rule 3 as follows:
      (3) "Each medical practitioner qualified under the Act to conduct ultrasonography in a genetic clinic/ultrasound clinic/imaging center shall be permitted to be registered with a maximum of two such clinics/centers within a district. The consulting hours for such medical practitioner shall be clearly specified by each clinic/center,"
   B. Application fee as per Rule 5(a) and 5(b) has been enhanced from ₹ 3000 and 4000 to ₹ 25000 and 35000 respectively.
2. The effect of sub-rule (3) above is as follows:
   a. An ultrasonologist under the Act shall be permitted to be registered with a maximum of two such clinics/centers within a district.
   b. The consulting hours for such medical practitioner shall be clearly specified by each clinic/center.
3. The first question that arises is this—"Can an ultrasonologist register himself in more than one district"? This is particularly relevant to those living near district boundaries. For example, Delhi has nine districts. A doctor living in one district can reach any other district in 15–60 minutes. Will it be illegal for him to practice in a center each in two different districts?
4. The legal answer to the above question is that this should be possible. There is nothing in the PC and PNDT Act or Rules that bars one from working in two districts.
5. The second question that arises is this—Is it legally correct that—"The consulting hours for such medical practitioner shall be clearly specified by each clinic/center"?
6. The legal answer to the above question is that:
   a. Let the center try to get registered by submitting an application in terms of section 18(2) of the Act, specifying therein the consulting

hours as follows: "The doctor will be on call duty and will be available as and when he is called".

b. If the registering authority refuses to accept this as a proper answer and rejects the application in terms of section 19(2), the applicant would be entitled to file a WP in the HC against such rejection.
c. The ground taken in the WP will be that the rule is violative of Article 19(1)(g) and places an unreasonable restriction on carrying out the profession, occupation, trade or business. My hunch is that if argued properly, the HC will decide in favor of the petitioner.

7. The third question that arises is this—"Can the increase in application fee be challenged?"
8. The answer to the above question is:
   a. Yes, it can and should be challenged.
   b. The first step—IMA or a radiologists' association or a nursing home owners' association should send a legally drafted representation to the Ministry of Health, GOI, against such increase.
   c. The second step—If the MOH does not take action, file a WP.
   d. The grounds taken in the WP will be:
      i. The increase in fee has to have a rational basis. There is no rational reason for the increase from 3000–4000 to 25000–35000.
      ii. The fee is nonrefundable in terms of Rule 5(1). The government cannot be allowed to loot the public in this manner.
      iii. This will lead to an increase in charges to consumers and will thus be an antipeople Act.

Laws applicable in Hospital and Healthdare

Tables 14.1 to 14.11 show for further details of law applicable in hospital and healthcare.

- Laws related to governing the commissioning of hospital (Table 4.1)
- Laws governing the qualifications/practice and conduct of professionals (Table 4.2)
- Laws governing storage/sale of drugs and safe medication (Table 4.3)
- Laws governing biomedical research (Table 4.4)
- Laws governing to management of patients (Table 4.5)
- Laws governing medicolegal aspects (Table 4.6)
- Laws governing the safety of patients, public and staff within the hospital premises and environmental protection (Table 4.7)
- Laws governing the safety of patients, public and staff within the hospital premises (Table 4.8)

- Laws governing the employment of manpower (Table 4.9)
- Laws governing to professional training and research (Table 4.10)
- Regulations governing the business aspects of hospital (Table 4.11)

Table 4.1 Laws related to governing the commissioning of hospital

S. No	Name of Act/Rule	Year
1.	Society Registration Act	1960
2.	Companies Act	1956
3.	Municipality to Local Authority	
4.	Delhi Fire Service Act	2007
5.	Delhi Fire Prevention and Fire Safety Act	1986
6.	Fire Safety Rules	1987
7.	Electricity Rules	1956
8.	Delhi Lift Act	1942
9.	Bombay Lifts Act	1939
10.	Delhi Nursing Home Registration Act	1953
11.	Bombay Nursing Homes Registration (Amendment) Act	2005
12.	Bombay Nursing Homes Registration (Extension and Amendment) Act	1959
13.	Bombay Nursing Homes Registration Act	1949
14.	Radiation protection Certificate for Radiology Department from BARC	
15.	Atomic Energy Regulatory Body Approval for Radiology/Nuclear Medicine Services under the Atomic Energy Act	1962
16.	Atomic Energy (Safe Disposal of Radioactive Waste) Rules	1987
17.	Indian Telegraph Act	1885
18.	Clinical Establishments Bill	2010
19.	Building and Other Construction Workers (Regulation of Employment and Conditions of Service) Act	1908
20.	The Registration Act	1908
21.	The National Capital Territory of Delhi Laws (Special Provisions) Second Bill	2007
22.	Government Buildings Act	1899
23.	Karnataka Medical Registration (Amendment) Act	2003
24.	Red Cross Society (Allocation of Property) Act	1936
25.	St John Ambulance Association (India) Transfer of Funds Act	1956

Table 4.2 Laws governing the qualifications/practice and conduct of professionals

S. No	Name of Act/Rule	Year
1.	Indian Medical Council Act	1956
2.	Indian Medical Council (Professional Conduct, Etiquette and Ethics) Regulations	2002
3.	Indian Medical Degrees Act	1916
4.	Registration of Medical Practitioners with State Medical Councils	1956
5.	Indian Nursing Council Act	1947
6.	Delhi Nursing Council Act	1997
7.	The ICN Code of Ethics for Nurses	1948
8.	The Dentists Act	1948
9.	The Dentists (Code of Ethics Regulation)	1976
10.	Dental Council of India Regulations	2006
11.	AICTE Rules of Physiotherapy	
12.	All India Council for Technical Education Act	1987
13.	The Apprenticeship Act	1961
14.	Rehabilitation Council of India Act	1992
15.	Rehabilitation Council of India (Amendment) Act	2000
16.	Kerala Anatomy Act	1957
17.	Kerala Co-operative Hospital Complex and the Academy of Medical Sciences (Taking over the Management) Act	1997
18.	Kerala Professional Colleges or Institutions (Prohibition of Capitation Fee, Regulation of Admission, Fixation of Nonexploitative Fee and Other Measures to Ensure Equity and Excellence in Professional Education) Amendment Act	2007
19.	Karnataka Anatomy Act	1957

Table 4.3 Laws governing storage/sale of drugs and safe medication

S. No	Name of Act/Rule	Year
1.	Drugs and Cosmetic Act	1940
2.	Drug and Cosmetic Act Amendment	1982
3.	The Drug and Cosmetics Rules (Amendment 2005)	1945
4.	The Drugs Control Act	1950
5.	Pharmacy Act	1948
6.	License for Possession and Use of Rectified/Denatured Spirit	
7.	Narcotics and Psychotropic Substances Act	1985
8.	Central Excise Act (for permit to use and store sprit)	1944
9.	Retail Drug License	

Contd....

Contd....

S. No	Name of Act/Rule	Year
10.	VAT Act	
11.	Central Sales Tax Act	1956
12.	Sales of Good Act	1930
13.	Adulteration of Drugs (IPC Sec 274)	
14.	Sales of Adulterated Drugs (IPC Sec 275)	
15.	Sales of Drug as Different Drug or Preparation (IPC Sec 276)	
16.	Negligent Conduct with Regard to Poisonous Substances (IPC Sec 284)	
17.	Blood Bank Regulations under Drugs and Cosmetic (2nd Amendment) Rules	1999
18.	Homeopathy Central Council (Amendment) Act	2002
19.	Homeopathy Central Council Act	1973

Table 4.4 Laws governing biomedical research

S. No	Name of Act/Rule	Year
1.	Breeding of and Experiments on Animals (Control and Supervision) Amendment Rules	2005
2.	Reconstitution of Committee for the Purpose of Control and Supervision of Experiments on Animals (CPCSEA)	

Table 4.5 Laws governing to management of patients

S. No	Name of Act/Rule	Year
1.	Drugs and Magic Remedies (Objectionable) Advertisements Act 1954	1954
2.	PNDT Act	1994
3.	Preconception and Prenatal Diagnostic Techniques (Prohibition of Sex Selection) Rules	1996
4.	MTP Act	1997
5.	MTP Rules	1971
6.	Transplantation of Human Organ Act	1994
7.	Transplantation of Human Organ Rule	1995
8.	Rules for Insurance Cover for the Sterilization Cases	
9.	Laws of Contract Section 13 (Consent required)	
10.	Birth and Death and Marriage Registration Act	1886
11.	Delhi Registration of Birth and Deaths Act	1969
12.	Indian Lunacy Act	1912
13.	The Epidemic Disease Act	1897
14.	Delhi Municipal Corporation (Malaria and Other Mosquito Borne disease) Bye Law	1975

Contd....

Contd....

S. No	Name of Act/Rule	Year
15.	Lepers Act	1898
16.	Guardians and Wards Act	1890
17.	National Guidelines for Clinical Management of HIV/AIDS , NACO, Govt Of India	
18.	Manual for Control of Hospital Associated Infections : SOPs, NACO, Govt of India	
19.	The Mental Health Act	1987
20.	Ear Drums and Ear Bones (Authority for Use for Therapeutic Purposes) Act	1982
21.	Eyes (Authority for Use for Therapeutic Purposes) Act	1982

Table 4.6 Laws governing medicolegal aspects

S. No	Name of Act/Rule	Year
1.	Law of Privileged Communications	
2.	Indian Evidence Act (Disclosure of Privileged/Confidential Patient Related Information before a Court of Law – Under Protest)	
3.	Law of Torts	
4.	Consumer Protection Act	1986
5.	Protection of Human Rights Act	
6.	IPC Section 52	
7.	IPC Section 80	
8.	IPC Section 89	
9.	IPC Section 92	
10.	IPC Section 93	
11.	IPC Section 269	

Table 4.7 Laws governing the safety of patients, public and staff within the hospital premises and environmental protection

S. No	Name of Act/Rule	Year/Amendment
1.	Biomedical Medical Waste Management Handling Rules	1998/2000
2.	Water (Prevention and Control of Pollution) Act	1974
3.	The Water (Prevention and Control of Pollution) Cess (Amendment) Act	2003
4.	The Water (Prevention and Control of Pollution) Act	1974/1988
5.	The Water (Prevention and Control of Pollution) Cess Rules	1978
6.	The Water (Prevention and Control of Pollution) Rules	1975
7.	The Noise Pollution (Regulation and Control) (Amendment) Rules	2010
8.	The Noise Pollution (Regulation and Control)(Amendment) Rules	2006
9.	The Noise Pollution (Regulation and Control) (Amendment) Rules	2002

Contd....

Contd....

S. No	Name of Act/Rule	Year
10.	The Noise Pollution (Regulation and Control) (Amendment) Rules	2000
11.	Business Rules	1975/1976
12.	Rules Regarding the Safe Discharge of Effluents in the Public Sewers/Drains	
13.	DMC Sanitation and Public Health Bye Laws	1959
14.	Air (Prevention and Control of Pollution) Act	1981/1987
15.	The Air (Prevention and Control of Pollution) (Union Territories) Rules	1983
16.	The Air (Prevention and Control of Pollution) Rules	1982
17.	Environment Protection Act	1986
18.	Environment Protection Rule	1986
19.	Noise Pollution Control Rules	2000
20.	IPC Sec 269 (Negligent Act Likely to Spread Infection or Disease Dangerous to Life, Unlawfully or Negligently)	
21.	IPC Sec 278 (Making Atmosphere Noxious to Health)	

Table 4.8 Laws governing the safety of patients, public and staff within the hospital premises

S. No	Name of Act/Rule	Year
1.	Indian Boilers Act	1923
2.	Explosive Act 1884 (For Diesel Storage)	1884
3.	Petroleum Act + Storage Rules	2002
4.	Gas Cylinder Rules	2004
5.	Rules for Provision of Safe Drinking Water	
6.	Rules for Provision of Uninterrupted Power Supply	
7.	Prevention of Food Adulteration Act	1954
8.	The Radiation Surveillance Procedures for the Medical Application of Radiation	1989
9.	Radiation Protection Rules	1971
10.	AERB Safety Code No. AERB/SC/Med -2 (REV -1)	2001
11.	Insecticide Act	1968
12.	Arms Act	1950
13.	IPC Sec 336 (Act Endangering Life and Personal Safety of Others)	
14.	IPC Sec 337 (Causing Hurt by Act Endangering Life and Personal Safety of Others)	
15.	IPC Sec 338 (Causing Grievous Hurt by Act Endangering the Life and Personal Safety of Others)	
16.	The Indian Fatal Accidents Act	1955

Contd....

Contd....

S. No	Name of Act/Rule	Year
17.	The Cigarettes and other Tobacco Products (Prohibition of Advertisement and Regulation of Trade and Commerce, Production, Supply and Distribution) Bill	2003
18.	Prohibition of Smoking in Public Places Rules	2008
19.	The Tamil Nadu Medicare Service Persons and Medicare Service Institutions (Prevention of Violence and Damage or Loss to Property) Act	2008
20.	The Tamil Nadu Medicare Service Persons and Medicare Service Institutions (Prevention of Violence and Damage or Loss to Property) Act	2008
21.	Vaccination Act	1880
22.	Vaccination (Repeal) Act	2001
23.	Disaster Management Act	2005
24.	Protection of Human Rights Act	1993

Table 4.9 Laws governing the employment of manpower

S. No	Name of Act / Rule	Year
1.	Child Labour Act	
2.	Citizenship Act	1955
3.	Employees Provident Fund and Misc Provision Act	1952
4.	ESI Act	1948
5.	ESI (Central) Rules	1950
6.	Employment Exchange (Compulsory Notification of Vacancies) Act	1959
7.	Equal Remuneration Act	1976
8.	Minimum Wedge Act	1948
9.	Payment of Bonus Act	1965
10.	Payment of Gratuity Act	1972
11.	Payment of Wages Act	1936
12.	PPF Act	1968
13.	TDS Act	
14.	Maternity Benefit (Amendment) Act	2008
15.	Workmen's Compensation Act	1923
16.	Workmen's Compensation (Amendment) Act	2009
17.	Indian Trade Union Act	1926
18.	Industrial Disputes Act	1947
19.	Shops and Factories Act (for National Holidays)	
20.	Negotiable Instrument Act	1881

Contd....

Contd....

S. No	Name of Act/Rule	Year
21.	Persons with Disabilities Act	1995
22.	SC and ST Act	1989
23.	Weekly Holidays Act	1942
24.	Official Secrets Act	1923
25.	Persons With Disabilities (Equal Opportunities, Protection of Rights and Full Participation) Act	1995
26.	Karnataka Prohibition of Violence against Medicare Service Personnel and Damageto Property in Medicare Service Institutions Act	2009
27.	Information Technology (Amendment) Act	2008
28.	Information Technology Act	2000

Table 4.10 Laws governing to professional training and research

S. No	Name of Act/Rule	Year
1.	MCI Rules for Internship Training	
2.	National Board of Examinations Rules for DNB Training	
3.	Nursing Council of India Rules for Staring School/College of Nursing	
4.	ICMR Rules Governing Medical Research	

Table 4.11 Regulations governing the business aspects of hospital

S. No	Name of Act/Rule	Year/Amendment
1.	Charitable and religious Trust Act	1920
2.	Contract Act	1982
3.	Income Tax Act	1961
4.	Customs Act	1962
5.	Foreign Exchange Management Act	1999
6.	Insurance Act	1938
7.	Rules for Display of Red Cross Insignia	
8.	Sales of Good Act	1930
9.	Vehicle Registration Certificate	
10.	Wireless Operation Certificate from Post and Telegraphs	
11.	Cable Television Network Act	1995
12.	Gift Tax Act	1958
13.	Copyright Act	1982
14.	The Public Liability Insurance Act	1991/1992
15.	The Public Liability Insurance Rules	1991/1993

CLINICAL ESTABLISHMENT ACT (2010)

1. Every institution and individual run establishment (including GP clinic) will have to compulsorily register with the body established by State government.
2. The minimum criteria for every establishment both in instrumentation and personnel will be prescribed by the government body.
3. A certain fee shall be charged for registration and this registration will be valid for 5 years only.
4. Monetary penalties for nonregistration and noncompliance shall range from ₹ 10,000 to 25,000 for first offence, ₹ 50,000 to 2,00,000 for second offence and ₹ 5,00,000 for third offence.
5. Inspectors can visit your clinic anytime for ensuring that you comply with all rules and regulations laid down. Thus in effect, even a SDM can threaten you with a fine of ₹ 5,00,000 on any pretext under CI 42 (1&2) This opens up unlimited avenues for undue extortion.
6. Doctors practicing in polyclinics or hospital as visiting faculty shall be liable for monetary punishment if said institution does not confirm to the rules.
7. Cl. 46 provides for recovery of the fine as arrears of land revenue from clinical establishment owners.
8. All clinical establishments will be expected to intervene to "stabilize" the patient with an emergency medical condition—whether myocardial infarction or appendicitis—before transferring them. This imposes too much responsibility on clinical establishments.

Chapter 5

Cost of Medical Education

INTRODUCTION

Medicine has been a noble profession since ages. From *hakims* to *vaidyas,* the field of medicine has come a long way to specialized areas which are intense, exhaustive and crucial to the understanding of the human body. Being a doctor is not only a job of extreme responsibility, but it also requires intense hard work and dedication coupled with the desire to help the sick and unwell to heal in the best possible way.

Profession of a doctor was considered to be one of the noblest professions for the right reasons. A doctor treated everybody without discrimination on any ground. He would even do his best to save the life of his enemy. But, of late, this profession has taken the shape of a commercial business establishment where monetary returns over rule all other considerations. We often hear of reports that private clinics are more interested in conducting tests than in diagnosing the disease. Some hospitals have gone to the extent of enquiring about the amount of patient's mediclaim so that they inflate the

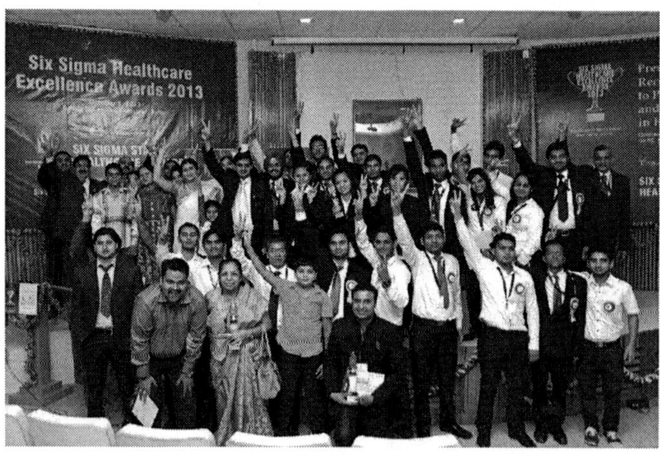

Medical Professionals in a Medical Education Program

bill round about to that limit. Sometimes operations have been conducted when there was need for none. These are the practices which are bringing into disrepute this noble profession. It is time the private practitioners and hospitals shed their greed for money and concentrate on helping the ailing humanity.

INCREASE IN DEMAND

The role of a doctor is even more important and multifarious today due to an increase in the diseases and ailments affecting the large population of India, due to changing lifestyles and high-stress levels.

The growing demand for doctors is reflected in the amplified number of diseases as well as growth of healthcare sector which currently stands strong as a $34 billion industry. By end 2012–13, it is estimated to grow to nearly $40 billion. India's increasing life expectancy and an ever growing population also demand that healthcare professionals are pitched in to take care of the old and the newborns of the country. Besides this, with a projected figure of 73.5 million diabetes patients in India by 2025, and several millions suffering from lifestyle diseases like hypertension and cancer, communicable diseases like AIDS, dengue, tuberculosis and malaria, India is set to fight a battle against these diseases for which it will require a strong army of doctors.

The availability of doctors including specialists, therefore, needs to be planned accordingly. At present there is a large gap in the requirement and the turnout from the established agencies. According to a Planning Commission study released in 2012, the country is facing a shortage of 6 lakh doctors, 10 lakh nurses and 2 lakh dental surgeons.

With a boom in the healthcare sector, there are other areas too where medicine professionals are highly in demand. MBBS doctors can find placements in hospitals which promote medical tourism. Besides this, the emerging health insurance market, growing pharmaceutical industry, telemedicine sector, clinical research, pharmacovigilance, etc. hold great charm and promise for doctors.

The cost of studying medicine can be more expensive than one can imagine but student educational loans and scholarships help students cover the costs. One needs to also be aware of the choice of college whether in India or abroad to ensure that the institute one joins is not a fake. Medical education is heavily subsidized in India with almost 31,000 doctors graduating from 269 medical colleges each year according to a press information bureau report.

Padded with a degree of MD, and a couple of years of work experience, a doctor could well be earning ₹ 1–12 lakh per month depending upon his area of specialization. There is no upper ceiling to the earnings of a competent and capable doctor. One can also be a visiting doctor at several hospitals and charge by the hour.

COST OF PRODUCING AN MBBS DOCTOR

According to *Dr Tatyarao Lahane*, the Dean of JJ Hospital and the Grant Medical College, Mumbai, Maharashtra, India, it costs the government anywhere between ₹ 25 and ₹ 35 lakh for creating a doctor over five-and-a-half years. The student, however, pays a fee of about ₹ 40,000 per year.

Further, the fees vary from state to state. In Government Medical Colleges in West Bengal, the fees are about ₹ 9,000 per semester with an additional ₹ 750–1000 per paper while at Jawaharlal Institute of Postgraduate Medical Education and Research in Puducherry (JIPMER), it would cost about ₹ 2,500 per year to become a doctor.

The country's premiere medical institution, AIIMS, spends ₹ 1.7 crore to produce a single MBBS doctor. This is the finding of a first-of-its-kind study submitted by AIIMS' Department of Hospital Administration to the dean recently. The figure includes both direct (services of the faculty and stipend) and indirect (services of nonteaching personnel and furniture) costs incurred by the country's premier teaching hospital over the five-and-a-half year period.

According to the study 'determination of the cost of training of MBBS student at AIIMS' conducted under the supervision of Dr Shakti Gupta, Head, Department of Hospital Administration at AIIMS, if computed using a traditional costing method, AIIMS spends ₹ 31.31 lakh on every undergraduate student per year per course. When calculated using the Time Driven Activity Based Costing method (TD-ABC), the study says that total costs incurred on one MBBS student is ₹ 98 lakh per course. "As against this, the annual fee of an MBBS student at AIIMS is ₹ 850 per year that includes hostel and tuition fee," Dr Gupta told TOI.

What's worse, an earlier study by the Media Study Group found that over 53% of students who pass out as doctors from AIIMS leave India to work abroad. Of the 2,129 students who passed out in the first 42 batches of the MBBS program at AIIMS—from its inception in 1956 to 1997—the study team tracked down 1,477 doctors. Of them, 780 or 52.81% were found to be working abroad.

Dr Gupta gave a solution to curb such brain drain. "Medical students who graduate from the Armed Forces Medical College in Pune have to serve in the Army for a minimum of five years or else they pay ₹ 15 lakh to be allowed to practice in the private sector. Similarly, AIIMS too should think of imposing such a clause where students have to sign a bond agreeing to work in India for a certain period of time after graduating from AIIMS". The planning commission should make the doctors accountable as a first step to make a compulsory bond for at least 5 years like AFMC so that the number of doctors attending per 10,000 is at least increased for the period they are accounted for. It can make a huge difference to the health and safety of Indian masses.

PRESENT SCENARIO

A recent Planning Commission report said India is short of six lakh doctors, 10 lakh nurses and two lakh dental surgeons. Indian doctors, however, form 5% of the medical workforce in developed countries. Almost 60,000 Indian physicians are working in countries like US, UK, Canada and Australia alone. One can, therefore, suggest that Indian tax payer is paying for education of doctors in its Medical Colleges for serving the people abroad.

India has a dismal patient-doctor ratio. For every 10,000 Indians, there is one doctor. In contrast, Australia has 249 doctors for every 10,000 people, Canada has 209, UK has 166 and US has 548.

The situation is a creation of the faulty policies. At one end you have the government colleges, gaining entry into which is becoming increasingly difficult due to allocation of seats for higher education for service candidates and caste-based reservations. A deserving student then has either an option to go in for higher education in a private medical college which will financially exploit his/her predicament or to look for avenues in a university abroad. During the medical training, the concept of social training is ingrained into the psyche of a medico. And every person does help in his or her small way. Every doctor during the course of training realizes that the knowledge which is gained is suitable mostly for the Indian scenario. All those who emigrate outside are not people who did not want to settle in India but are people who have given up trying after facing a system that can just not accommodate their aspirations. And the comparison with IIT and IIM is plainly unfair. A person graduating from IIT/IIM is assured of 6 figure salary while most of the medicos continue to be students till mid 30s and do not earn more than 3,5000 till the age of 40. And lastly, the onus of social responsibility need not lie solely on the shoulders of doctors. The onus is also on lawyers, engineers, businessmen, sportsmen and lastly our good and very old politicians.

STUDYING MEDICINE ABROAD

With so many aspirants and so few seats, a lot of contenders prefer to do their MBBS from abroad. The favourite destinations include US, UK and Australia. The degrees abroad are competitive and the infrastructure and facilities are excellent yet, students have to clear a lot of tests and hurdles before they get admission.

First of all they have to obtain an eligibility certificate from the Medical Council of India (MCI). After returning from the completion of the course too, students have to undergo a screening test and get registered with the MCI.

There is also an important concern about reducing the cost of medical education. Many middle-class families are forced to mortgage or sell a lifetime's hard-gained assets to pay for their children's medical education. By severely restricting the number of postgraduate medical seats, especially when there is such a huge demand for doctors, we have created an artificial demand-supply imbalance.

The cost of one postgraduate seat often goes up to ₹ 1–2 crore, depending on the specialization. After putting in more than a decade of hard work, doctors begin to earn when they are well into their 30s. Their peers in other professions usually start earning almost a decade earlier!

What Needs to be Done?

One has to think "Out of the Hat" to improve the situation post-haste. The important thing is to make medical education less expensive. Public investment in new medical colleges and liberalizing infrastructure norms for setting new medical colleges will certainly help in this regard. However, this is not such an easy task.

Further, there should be a concerted effort to improve the terms and conditions of Doctors to lure them into the profession and retain them. For example, a better pay package will enhance the quality of not only the teaching faculty but be an incentive for more to join the profession. With better pay scales, no one would hear comments like, "what's the big deal in being a doctor, even our local gym has a doctor working on daily wages". The salaries at the corporate hospitals are also very less. A 22 years old software engineer earns more than a 35 years MD doctor. Rules like "In order to do postgraduation, one has to be under 30 years of age", are definitely against the constitutional rights. Improving the working hours and abolishing 24 or 36 hour duty roster is another important area for consideration. Spending more on improvement of the sanitation in the hospital, and crackdown on corruption in equipment and drug purchase would be necessary.

India needs generalist doctors who can look after the primary health care centers. Besides, most of these doctors in India are overworked and underpaid. Those who want to do superspecialty programs or medical research will find them at loss in India.

Scrap reservation—most of us are not against giving additional liberal facilities (extra tutoring hours to students finding difficult to understand a topic, more monetary support, increase the age limit for entrance) to students who are slow learners. Solution could be rather simple...serve the tax payers for at least 5 years or pay back to the government. If you want to go out for study or superspecialization, only 3–5 years mandatory service in India may be enough. However, if one decides to settle down abroad, then paying full fee with 100% interest may be considered.

Doctors should, however, pay for the expense on their education—why should any government give charity? The students should be given loans for the fee. In Western countries this was implemented long back, why we are not adopting the model? Politicians make issues if the fee is hiked as they get another reason to lure popular vote banks. There should be a mechanism to recover the money spent on making doctors, in case they decide not to serve their society. Other alternative to retain the local talent is to direct the Indian Medical Council not to issue 'Certificate of good standing' unless they have served in India for at least 10 years before planning to leave the country.

POSTGRADUATE MEDICAL EDUCATION

The postgraduate entrance exam for medicine in India is so hard to crack. Even if you manage to, it is highly unlikely that you will get through the stream of your choice. I know cases where the student wanted to pursue specialization in anesthesia but was offered pathology instead. In such cases, students would prefer to do their PG abroad than risk taking up a specialization they are least interested in. After all it's a matter of their career.

One reason for going abroad is that postgraduation and superspecialization courses are very less in India. According to one report, there are currently 'less than 5,000 seats for an MD degree across the country' and this remains of the largest bone of contention amongst young doctors. With caste reservations taking up most of the seats in government colleges, deserving candidates are left with the option of either going to a private medical college in India or go overseas. One often comes across students who narrate how they tried for two years to get into the merit category for a PG seat in surgery course in India, and finally resolved to pay the fee and get the seat as they were losing time. The sum is as high as whopping ₹ 1-2 crore. The cost of getting a postgraduate seat in India is still higher than what they would have to pay in the US.

Postgraduate medical education needs to be liberalized and the number of seats increased by allowing large public and private hospitals to impart postgraduate education. This will help lower the cost of medical education. There is an imperative need to eliminate the practice of making undercover payments for postgraduate medical seats. We should encourage existing hospitals to become teaching institutes by liberal accreditations from the National Board which would the most cost-effective method of making higher medical education liberal and cheap.

The present scope of postgraduate medical education in some hospitals could be liberalized to encompass more hospitals (even smaller in size). This would ensure that a substantial number of MBBS students who go abroad in search of avenues for higher learning stay back and their services are available to our people. This could be done by the National Board of Education if it ensures that its existing policies are more pragmatic and realistic rather than making them more stringent by the year. Yes, one learns with experience—but such learning to bring in improvements does not imply squeezing this avenue or window to the maximum extent. This hospitals should be encouraged to apply for accreditation by the National Board of Education and to start postgraduate courses in their respective areas of core competence. It should be understood that these hospitals do not earn any money while imparting training to the students. They could, therefore, be given incentives by way of soft loans, deferred payments, tax exemptions, and allotment of land at subsidized price for starting medical/paramedical/nursing institute. Even the burden of paying stipends by these hospitals to the students should be taken away from them. The students undergoing training there should be made to pay more than the presently stipulated annual fee of ₹ 50,000. The thrust, on the other hand, probably to ensure a better quality of education, is to make the criteria stringent after every batch/year (if one goes by the past experience). Such an approach, if not modified immediately, would ultimately throttle this avenue of higher medical education.

One simple step, if implemented, would almost double the availability of postgraduate seats in these colleges. The ratio of professor to student was liberalized in the Medical Colleges a few years ago—from one student per professor to two students per professor—to ensure more seats for PG students in these colleges. Why the authorities shy away to apply the same criterion to the hospitals running similar courses. Further, application of age limits to the Professors in the hospitals running these courses is also a step beyond any comprehension. Professors, Lawyers and Doctors grow professionally with age and experience. All hospitals crave to avail the services of the Head of the Departments and Professors in Medical Colleges, who generally after their superannuation, join them. This experienced class of professionals is made to superannuate in Medical Colleges at a predetermined age not because they suddenly lose their acumen on the midnight of the date of their superannuation but because of the constraints of creating promotional avenues to those junior to them. Rather than taking advantage of these experienced professionals, the Board follows the same principals of age for "employment as PG Teachers" as in the Government set-up. If autonomous bodies also have to follow the same rules as the Central Government, why have them. Who will "think out of the Box"?

The healthcare needs to be treated as an industry and granted infrastructure status, with tax incentives at par with other infrastructure service sectors, with parallel subsidies on power, water and other utilities to reduce the overall costs.

In one of the recent 'Satyameva Jayate' TV program on medicos, the IMA President admitted there are serious problems with healthcare in India. What about reservations and donation colleges which dole out degrees without quality and release them into the healthcare market? There are many such problems but our Politicians/Ministers are also responsible for serious acts of maladministration that contributes to poor health care outcomes. Not so long ago a DMK-party Health Minister in the UPA Government sacked an eminent Cardiologist as Director of AIIMS and when the Doctor won his case on appeal to Supreme Court, the Minister changed the legislation retrospectively to terminate the Director. When all this was being carried out, the MPs, Ministers and the PM watched as mute helpless spectators. If the highest office in the country turns a deaf ear to blatant violation of ethics/ principles, is there any hope for the country to fix its medical profession?.

To address the shortage of doctors in rural areas, Australia reserves seats in medicine for Rural Bonded Scheme. The students have to work in rural area for five/six years after graduating from the university studying there for five/six years. If they do not work in rural areas, they have to pay equivalent full fee which is about $50,000 per year. May be India can follow a similar policy. Of course, it is very important that the scheme be realistic, and enforced accordingly.

According to Dr Devi Shetty, "The system is jacking up the price of doctors—the way we go about it has made education expensive. MCI does not allow existing hospitals to become teaching institutions. So, a nonprofit organization has to get land, like a football ground, and build a college and a hospital. Naturally, the burden of the cost shifts to students. It costs ₹ 2 crore for a seat for MD in radiology, in Bengaluru, today".

He further adds, "Though diabetes is widespread and, as a result, people suffer from kidney diseases, the country produces only 60 Nephrologists a year. The system is jacking up the price of doctors by creating such shortages. This would have to change. It is time for the world to come together and tackle this problem. We are proposing a medical education system outside India, using the best from curricula across the world, and trying for recognition from global universities. There is no Indian way of removing pain and a French way of removing pain. There is only one way. So, there is no conflict".

He concludes very aptly by stating that in India, students pay hospitals to learn, while in the West, the hospitals make you work while you learn. So, you do not need to pay. It is like an apprenticeship.

It is high time that organizations like the IMA/MCI/NBE do some introspection to realize why people have lost faith in the medical profession. No technology can replace the bond of faith between a doctor and patient, a vital ingredient of patient care. This bond of faith is solely dependent on ethical values. The use of hi-tech medicine without ethical standards can be detrimental to patient care as well as to society at large.

■■Chapter 6

Hospital Project Management Victory

Engineers bring a unique perspective to problem-solving. Understanding how to manage and/or work with the unique engineer psyche can help your team achieve victory everytime.

PLAN FOR CONTINGENCIES

Engineers have an innate sense of optimism and confidence that our solutions will work. We study the fundamental laws of engineering and enter the workforce eager to put them into practice. We are thrilled to deliver solutions that work. As we do, our confidence grows. We *expect* our plans will succeed.

One such confident engineer had a tendency to submit budgets that were too low. Time and again, his budget did not allow for any adjustments or contingencies. Even when confronted with this, he was uncomfortable increasing his budget.

As engineers, we need to be mindful of such overconfidence. With the engineer's propensity toward optimism in mind, project managers (PMs)

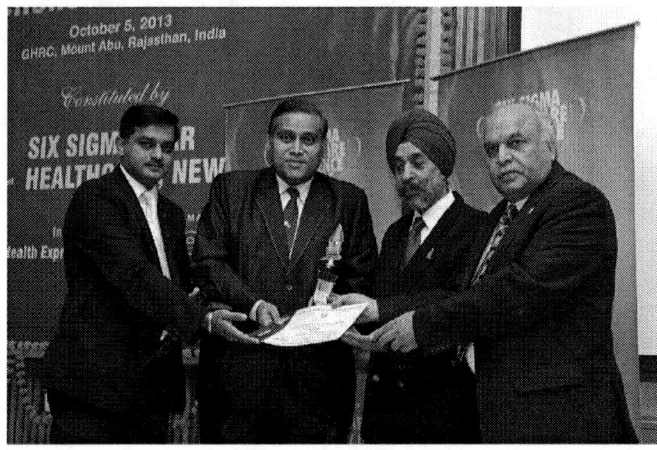

Hospital Management Victory

need to be objective in identifying potential pitfalls and be sure that plans allow for contingencies.

GET EVERYONE TALKING

Engineers respect precision. We work with precise measurements. We offer definitive solutions with firm parameters. We do not like the word "may be." We are not likely to speak up unless we can back up what we say with facts and figures.

While this certainly seems logical, it confines the engineer's input to the "what is" and eliminates the "what if"—and, in fact, may limit the engineer's overall contribution.

On one project, I watched an animated purchasing manager openly share his vision. He spoke up often during meetings, making grand statements based on projections. The engineer, however, only stated what he knew at each stage of the project. As a result, the purchasing manager commanded more of the group's attention, respect, and confidence.

As engineers, we need to have more confidence in our own knowledge and abilities—and trust that our instincts are based on our many prior successes. We also need to speak up so our clients will have confidence in us—even if we need to qualify our statements.

Likewise, effective team leaders need to understand the natural reticence of the engineer and encourage participation from all, not just a few. It is important to draw others out to determine the best course of action and ensure that nothing is overlooked.

This type of communication tends to be easier and more effective in face-to-face meetings, which are sometimes viewed as luxuries in our 160-character e-communications.

BREAKDOWN THE SILOS

Meetings are a fact of life during construction. These gatherings bring together the many professionals involved—from the PM and general contractor to architects, engineers, subcontractors, and more.

Many meetings follow a tight agenda, asking for contributions from each team member as appropriate. Unfortunately, this regimented approach may not bring out the wealth of experience and resources in the room.

As participants in this process, engineers need to have the confidence to speak up, ask questions, and offer opinions—even if it means stepping out of our comfort zones.

Likewise, PMs need to embrace flexibility and be willing to go off of the agenda. Often the best solutions are the result of a multidisciplinary free flow of ideas.

DIG DEEP—DO NOT TAKE "NO" OR "I DO NOT KNOW" FOR AN ANSWER

The famous Greek philosopher Plato defined knowledge as "justified true belief." I believe that engineers embrace this view of knowledge, forever analyzing and proving that our plans and solutions will work.

Therefore, when we say we "know" something, it is a serious assertion. Conversely, when we do not know something, we simply may mean that it has not been rigorously vetted.

I once observed, an engineering team deliver a presentation on heating, ventilating and air conditioning (HVAC) design and emergency power generation. Following the presentation, the client asked a question regarding a conceptual aspect of the HVAC design. As the engineer had not yet fully analyzed this, he responded, "I do not know," eroding the team's confidence in his proposal.

Therefore, as engineers, we need to avoid saying, "I do not know." Instead, we need to define what it is we do know and explain what we need to get a complete answer. Conversely, when we "know" that our solution is correct, we need to be tenacious in supporting it.

Likewise, team leaders should not accept "I do not know" as an answer. Dig deeper—find out specifically what information is needed and allow time for analysis and discovery. When the discovery process is complete, have the confidence to rally the team behind the solution and stand strong together.

RESPECT EACH OTHER'S STRENGTHS

There are many misconceptions about engineers. Some people equate engineers with mechanics and assume that we can fix anything and everything. Many confuse the different engineering disciplines—civil, mechanical, and structural engineering. All too often, we are called upon to field questions that are outside of our area of expertise.

Consider this example in which a new retaining wall showed signs of failure. The PM repeatedly questioned the structural engineer, who insisted the wall was sound. Eventually, it was the civil engineer, not the structural engineer, who solved the real problem—improper water drainage.

As engineers, we need to take time to educate our fellow team members regarding our areas of expertise when these situations arise. PMs also have responsibility to clearly understand the proficiencies of their team members.

Chapter 7

Furniture Design Features and Healthcare Outcomes

Quality care delivery continues to challenge healthcare leaders. The Society of Actuaries (2010) commissioned a medical claims-based study revealing that 1.5 million avoidable medical errors added $19.5 billion to the healthcare bill nationwide. In spite of intense efforts to improve patient safety and care outcomes since the Institute of Medicine published its report on medical errors over a decade ago (IOM, 1999), many chronic problems remain stubbornly unsolved, such as the failure to reduce postoperative bloodstream and urinary tract infections (AHRQ, 2010). Landrigan and colleagues (2010) found 25.1 harms per 100 admissions at 10 North Carolina hospitals over six years, 63% of which were thought to be preventable. The Department of Health and Human Services' Inspector-General found that 13.5% of hospitalized medicare patients experienced adverse events, and another 13.5% experienced temporary harm, 44% of which were thought by physician reviewers to be preventable (Levinson, 2010). These results continue to occur despite a vast array of patient safety improvement interventions during the past decade (Watcher, 2010).

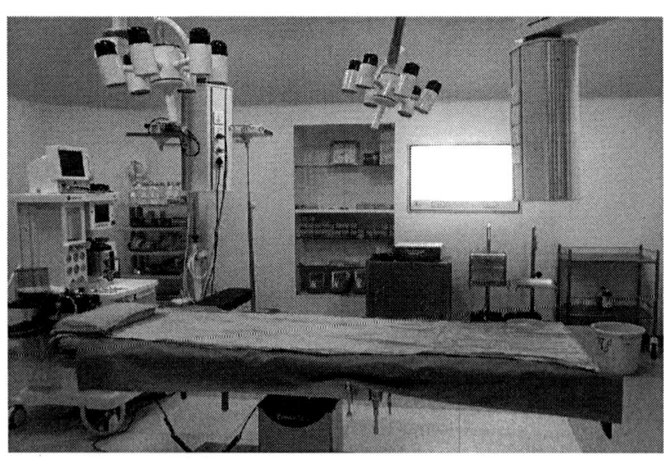

Modern Furniture Design in Operation Theater

One of the many reasons for the slow progress in performance improvement may reflect the lack of complete scrutiny and consequent understanding of all the variables and their inter-relatedness that shape the complex systems of healthcare delivery. James Reason (2000) hypothesized that healthcare accidents and errors occur as a result of organizational vulnerabilities. A combination of active failures (unsafe acts by those providing care) and latent conditions (termed, resident pathogens) or contributing dormant system conditions (such as chronic understaffing, inexperience, physical environment, and inadequate equipment and furniture), when combined under the right circumstances, can enable a hazard to slip through an organization's flawed defenses.

Complete understanding of these system vulnerabilities requires human factors engineering—an approach that examines human capabilities and limitations with regard to products, processes, systems, and work environments—to maximize safety, reliable performance, and effectiveness and to reduce operational errors, operator stress, fatigue, and training and product liability (Henricksen, et al, 2009; Center for Systems Reliability, 2010). High-risk industries like aviation have long understood the role that the physical environment plays in supporting preferred human responses.

In the past quarter century, the healthcare industry has begun to embrace a growing body of work that examined the relationship between the physical environment, human responses and consequent healthcare outcomes. Evidence-based design (EBD)—or the process of basing decisions about the built environment on credible research to achieve the best possible outcomes (Goetz, et al, 2010)—is being used by a growing field of healthcare architects, practitioners, researchers, and administrators to better understand the impacts of the healthcare environment on healthcare outcomes, including patient safety outcomes (Malone, 2010). Maximizing infrastructure investments like the building, technology, equipment, and furniture to achieve strategic outcomes requires an internal synergy of effort between leaders who can transform organizational culture and a staff that can reengineer clinical and administrative processes.

Using a multidisciplinary team to execute and institutionalize the work, all of which is based on evidence-based research, pre- and postoccupancy measures are used to track desired outcomes, the results of which ultimately further EBD science. Additional information about the evidence-based design model can be found in *The Center for Health Design's Evidence-Based Design Study Guide 1*, page 76 (Goetz, et al, 2010) athttp://edac.healthdesign.org/EDAC_StudyGuide1.pdf.

Objects, such as furniture, also require careful EBD research to fully understand the role those objects play in realizing desired patient and staff outcomes. Furniture will be bought and replaced multiple times during the 30-year-plus-lifetime of most healthcare facilities. A typical new 200,000 square foot, 120-bed inpatient hospital may have over 1,600 individual pieces of furniture. Healthcare administrators often consider furniture a sunk cost, similar to walls, lighting, and heat; a facility must have furniture in order to serve patients, families, and the healthcare team. The high- risk healthcare industry demands much from these common objects, ranging from embodying an organization's brand, providing patient comfort and support during stressful times, enabling staff to work efficiently and safely as a team, and perhaps most importantly, not contributing to patient and staff and organizational harm.

Facility managers, designers, and others charged with the responsibility of recommending furniture purchase options for c-suite approval face a dizzying assortment of choices, complicating the furniture evaluation and selection process. First-time costs frequently dictate furniture selection that overlooks facility life cycle costs and organizational performance improvement goals. The purpose of this chapter is to describe the creation of an evidence-based design furniture checklist, based on current EBD research findings and industry standards. Healthcare leaders can use the list to make informed furniture investment decisions to improve healthcare outcomes across the furniture life cycle. We conclude the paper with recommendations for future EBD furniture research, government and industry standards development, and further checklist development.

Chapter 8

Ignite Healthcare Management Excellence and Passion by NLP Technology

Become an outstanding performer by applying neurolinguistic programming (NLP) in healthcare management.

IMPROVE PERSONAL, PROFESSIONAL AND HEALTHCARE SUCCESS BY NEUROLINGUISTIC PROGRAMMING (NLP)

By implementing NLP, clinicians can save valuable amounts of time without foregoing tremendous amounts of energy. An additional benefit of NLP is increased patient safety.

The asset of any hospital is its human beings. When these human resources become productive they become invaluable resources of the hospital.

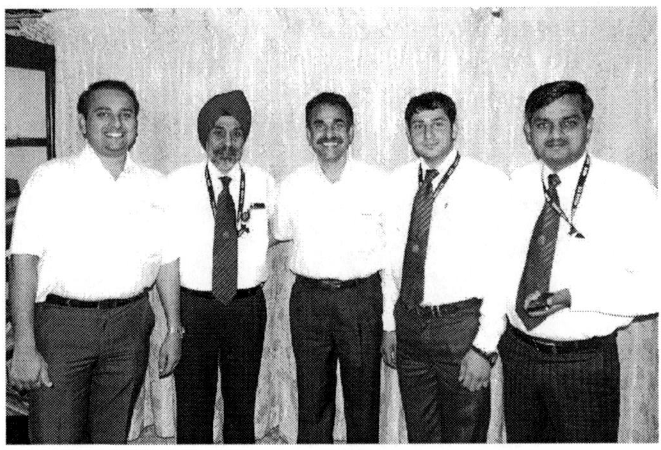

Human Resources Management Team

WHY USE NEUROLINGUISTIC PROGRAMMING IN HEALTHCARE?

Healthcare management is one of the toughest management on earth. Since healthcare professionals are dealing with the question of life and death, Stress-related illness is a growing issue in our working environments (Fig. 8.1). In USA, *45 million working days were lost due to stress and depression in 2008*. Estimated cost to society is over *£3 billion* a year. What is the cost in your Organization?

Neurolinguistic programming (NLP) represents an investment in ensuring a healthy workforce equipped with effective tools to become more powerful champion of changes.

Have you ever wondered why you do not get along with particular employees, why some members of your hospital team do not follow to your instructions, or why, when you think you are approaching something correctly, it just does not have the desired effect? Neurolinguistic programming, is fundamentally about making sense of how we do things and how we can affect change to make things better.

Oftentimes in healthcare when things go badly, we believe something is wrong with the people we are dealing with; it does not occur to us to change our own attitudes and behavior. Even if we realize we could handle a situation better, it can be difficult to know how to make effective changes—changes that can endure. The NLP can provide a framework for making the desired changes. By following its techniques, you have an excellent chance of fundamentally changing the way you think and behave, and therefore how you interact with others.

The NLP is not about what to do; it is about how to do it. It can help you improve how you manage people, how you communicate with others, and how you lead your team. According to NLP, leadership is action, not position.

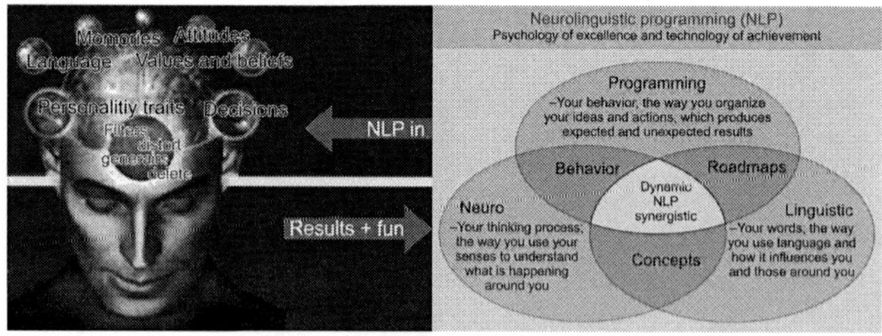

Fig. 8.1 Neurolinguistic programming outcome in management practices

NEUROLINGUISTIC PROGRAMMING CONCEPT

Neurolinguistic programming (NLP) was developed in the late 70s by Dr Richard Bandler a mathematician and John Grinder, a linguist. They became interested in study of people who were excellent performers, effective communicators and catalyst of change in others. They asked themselves a fundamental question. How someone who excels in a field, is different from the one who is merely an average or poor performer? This question led them to the discovery of "How we create a model of perceived world and organize our thinking that influences our skills and capabilities."

Neurolinguistic programming is the study of human excellence. NLP is the new technology of achievement and can be called as the 'Software of Mind' which brings out the best in every person, inspite of many barrier in the society. It is a practical methodology for improved performance, HR development and well-being of the organization. Originally developed by Dr. Richard Bandler (USA) in the 1970.

WHAT IS NEUROLINGUISTIC PROGRAMMING?

- It is the study of human excellence
- It is the powerful and practical approach to change anything
- It has many powerful concepts that can be utilized in various learning program.

Neuro refer to our nervous system and five senses—see, hear, feel, taste and smell.

- 'N' stands for 'Neuro' the 'Brain'
- 'L' stands for 'Linguistic' the 'Communicative Language'
- 'P' stands for 'Psychological Programming of a new behavior'

The *NLP* is one of the most advanced personal change and growth technologies. World over it has also been hailed as one of the most effective science of brief therapy.

Neuro relates to our nervous system and the way our brain works.

Linguistic relates to language and how we communicate with ourselves and others.

Programming relates to using the power of language and nervous system to create appropriate changes in behaviors and the results we want.

According to the NLP, all human beings can be classified into three types of society:

1. Audio type.
2. Video type.
3. Feeling type.

NLP is about

- Correcting perceptions
- Aligning goals
- Powerful persuasion
- Consistency and focus
- Lifting team spirit
- Modeling excellence
- Emotional freedom
- Keeping high esteem
- Team working and team building
- Interpersonal effectiveness and relationships
- Leadership and empowerment
- Customer orientation and relations management
- Negotiation skills
- Stress and emotional management
- Emotional intelligence and management
- Achieving personal excellence
- Coaching and counseling
- Assertiveness skills.

The NLP is increasingly being applied in personal development, counseling, education and business:

Correcting perceptions

- You are absolutely right in your terms
- Others make mental and natural errors while perceiving you
- You can catch and correct them.

Aligning goals

- You keep on enhancing personal and business goals
- Yet find there is misalignment. You can balance your life.

Powerful persuasion

- You try your best to communicate with positive intentions
- Others still seems to take wrong meaning. You can change their stand.

Consistency and focus

- You know what you want
- Still you lack focus. You can learn to be consistent.

Lifting team spirit

- Your people are good individually
- Yet collectively they create conflicts. You can be an inspiring anchor.

Modeling excellence

- Someone around you is excelling despite competition
- You work hard yet it is difficult to create impact. You can develop strategies.

Emotional freedom

- You try to keep cool but somehow
- Disturbing elements puts you off-track. You can be a light hearted person.

Keeping high esteem

- You manage to keep your head high in front of others
- Inside may be feel low. You can improve self-image.

Being whole

- Professionally you are skillful
- Yet your family and personal front is getting ignored. You can be more practical.

HOW TO USE NEUROLINGUISTIC PROGRAMMING?

The NLP and getting the best out of people:

- It enables you to attract and nurture the best of talent
- Productive terms and efficient organizations depends on developing talents and co-operational attitude of members
- This results in an organization that is greater than the sum of its parts. NLP practitioners can use vital skill sets to crate cohesive, united and powerful organization. Initiatives that reflect values, culture and intention of organization can be design and implemented.
- Using powerful modeling methodologies of NLP, natural abilities of high performers and great leaders can be calibrated and then passed on to those who need it. Innovative base of excellence is continuously widened creating an ocean of NLP tools
- Thus NLP is a sure way to transform an average performer into a peak performer and making a peak performer to continuously give the best performance.

SET OF SKILLS THAT YOU WILL LEARN AND APPLY

Analysing perceptions, language of brain, setting anchors, creating field of commitment, breaking mental patterns, dissolving past blocks, nonverbal cues, linguistic models meta programs, new behavior generator, mental maps, swish pattern, stacking resources, outcome conditions, utilizing strategies, modeling framework, tracking time lines, etc.

PERSONAL BENEFITS

- You will be able to quickly connect internal resources and exercise a better control on your approach

- You will enjoy far greater control and freedom over your own state of mind, responses, and interaction with others
- You will find it much easier to turn your dreams in realistic goals and devise a strategy to achieve them
- You will be able to consciously identify barriers that may be unconsciously holding you back
- You will be able to change the unwanted habits and behavioral patterns that are coming in your way
- You will understand your team members and other people's needs and hidden communication styles
- You will be able to enter into strong rapport with seniors as well as down the line
- You will recognize how others style of language they use to influence you
- You will find your personal and professional goals can be magically achieved in less time.

PROFESSIONAL BENEFITS

- The NLP enabled professionals to create new approach to deliver values at work
- High-end professionals develop the capability to answer tough questions in meetings without loosing focus
- Some customer care professionals reported that they revived their so called lost customers
- The NLP helps you to become an outstanding performer in your field as you come to know your unique style of success
- This results in opening doors to new possibilities
- Core decision makers learned a solid way of making rewarding decisions
- Team heads could make certain irresponsible members to make higher level of commitment
- Many professionals have reported that they could coach and mentor people; effectively align them to business strategies
- This has led people to live a balanced life at work
- Many professionals are able to formulate a future vision and align whole team with their objectives
- Some professionals became very good facilitators to conduct high level negotiations and collaborations
- Team heads found it easier to align people with business strategies.

As with all new systems, a whole new vocabulary has come-up around NLP. Here are some of the words used to describe NLP skills:

VOCABULARIES IN NEUROLINGUISTIC PROGRAMMING

Anchoring

The process of forming an association between one thing and another. Anything that reminds us of something, which triggers off a physiological response, can be called an anchor. It can be based on any of the five senses, but the visual, auditory and kinesthetic (feeling) are best used for the NLP approach. The anchor helps bring about some positive associated images, thereby changing a person's attitude. An auditory anchor, for example, could be a word that best fits the state you desire, such as confidence, or calmness.

Chunking

Any subject can be viewed in larger or smaller parts or chunks. By adding new associations, chunking lets you see the matter differently. Chunking up puts the issue in perspective, chunking down gives it a new, narrower focus. Top business negotiators use this NLP technique, probably unwittingly, to find a common ground and thereby close the deal in a manner satisfactory to both sides.

Mirroring

You can create a better sense of rapport by mirroring the body language of the person with whom you are trying to communicate. This is a skill used by expert communicators. A salesperson would use this technique to make his client appear more receptive.
Modeling: NLP is against reinventing the wheel. Instead, it teaches you copying, or modeling, human excellence. Skills, abilities and even so-called thinking strategies can be transferred from one person to another.

Pacing and Leading

By gradually making the other person unconsciously mirror you, pacing and leading help in better communication. Future pacing is mentally rehearsing new skills, knowledge or attitudes in an imaginary future where they will be needed.

Reframing

The context or frame of any event can be changed to get another meaning. This process is called reframing and helps you become aware of alternatives. You can reframe your over two-hour-long daily commuting time by spending it profitably, say, learning a new language.

The NLP skills briefly introduced here can easily lead you to what NLP really is—an approach that gets you whatever you want.

KEY PRESUPPOSITIONS IN NLP: BELIEFS OF EXCELLENCE

- Communication is more than what you are saying
- No one is wrong or broken
- People already have all the resources they need
- Behind every behavior is a positive intention
- Every behavior is useful in some context
- The meaning of a communication is the response you get
- If you are not getting the response you want, try something different
- There is no such thing as failure. There is only feedback
- Choice is better than no choice
- In any system, the element with the most flexibility exerts the most influence
- The map is not the territory
- If someone can do something, anyone can learn it
- You cannot fail to communicate.

APPLICATIONS OF NLP IN ADMINISTRATION

- Able to build more fruitful business relationships with a wider variety of people
- To achieve greater success rates in both the planning and achievement of defined objectives
- They are able to lead their people through periods of change by taking with them, thus reducing resistance
- Enhance the performance of their team
- Make their trainings come alive and memorable by using sensory based language
- Improved questioning techniques.

CORE BENEFITS OF LEARNING NLP IN HEALTHCARE

The NLP takes you on a journey of self-discovery. It allows you to generate your own learnings and comc to your own realizations and awareness from working through the processes taught and you will benefit from the acquisition of models of excellence in human behavior. This will provide you with a true leading edge in understanding yourself and others in any context—business, career, social, competitive and leisure. Once having learnt for self, NLP then can be used to help others.

PRODUCTIVITY BENEFITS

- The NLP will give you the skills and techniques required to become a superlative communicator
- Clarity of outcome for self, organization and client in order to increase productivity and enhance relationships
- Understand business strategies which will bring clients to a quicker decision point
- Minimize unproductive maintenance time
- Be perceived as a person who gets down to business and makes it a pleasurable experience
- Remember events in your personal history as useful and leading you to a successful and powerful present with a compelling future
- Respond to challenging situations with a positive attitude for a successful outcome
- Develop decision making strategies which are aligned with your values
- Develop flexibility, focus and purpose.

ORGANIZATIONAL BENEFITS

- Gain tools which accelerate learning for faster response time in structural changes
- Increase your ability to accommodate a stressful environment with calmness and equanimity
- Develop the ability to give concise reports with clarity of expression to enable management to allocate resources in a timely and appropriate manner
- Discover how to dissolve conflict
- Adjust quickly to changes in structure, organization and product
- Spend less time in preparing for a client
- NLP will allow you to increase your perception of customer service
- Gain a more comprehensive and sophisticated level of questioning skills using different language models
- Stay more 'present' without distraction from either within or outside of the business environment
- Personal, mental, emotional and physical alignment
- Self-motivation and enthusiasm

- Learn to transform fear into action
- Gain clarity of outcomes
- Increase your self-esteem and self-image
- Overcome the blocks and resistance within your unconscious, releasing purposeful energy
- Experience all emotions as useful
- Choose your emotions instead of being run by them
- Lose limiting beliefs and learn empowering ones
- Choose to release bad habits and replace them with useful habits
- Align your own conscious and unconscious minds to access all your resources and gain maximum personal power
- Learn the skills of building the rapport that allow others to 'see eye to eye' with you and allows you to get your message across
- Understand the difference between goals and outcomes, realizing that becoming 'outcome conscious' allows you to determine and control your life
- Create your own ideal self by learning to master your internal feelings and emotions
- Learn how you create your reality and how others create theirs and learn the differences and similarities
- Be the creator and controller of your feelings and the pictures, sounds and voices inside your head
- Choose different ways to understand the meaning of events
- Understand exactly what are your core values and how these determine your behavior and shape your life.

SENSORY AWARENESS BENEFITS

- Learn how our senses such as eyes, ears, skin and emotions—take in and process information
- Learn all the various 'languages' of human communication so that you can 'read' what is really being communicated to you and ensure that you are communicating clearly with others
- Understand how we link ideas, memories and feelings by using triggers and learn to dissociate from those which are negative and disempowering and enhance or create links which enable us to be resourceful
- Create your own ideal self by learning to master your internal feelings and emotions.

BENEFITS SPECIFICALLY FOR BUSINESS

- NLP will allow you to increase your perception of customer service
- Gain a more comprehensive and sophisticated level of questioning skills using different language models
- Learn and model strategies of leadership excellence
- Learn the language skills which give you clarity, precision and success in business
- Model the behaviors of excellence you have observed in your mentors and desire for yourself
- Learn the skills and strategies of top negotiators
- Maximize your business potential and gain a competitive edge
- Achieve the goals you have set faster and with greater effect
- Gain the results you have wished for in every area of business.

LANGUAGE OF INFLUENCE BENEFITS

- Spoken language cannot influence the listener. The same is true for nonverbal or 'physiological language'—sometimes called 'body language' and the language of metaphor. Body language and metaphor influence the listener at the unconscious level and are therefore extremely effective. Learn the skills to develop conscious awareness and control over your unconscious communication
- Learn to understand the power to influence positively and ecologically
- Learn the skills to present your ideas in a way that the audience—be they few or many—can observe and respond to appropriately.

NEUROLINGUISTIC PROGRAMMING IN HEALTHCARE EDUCATION

Learning and applying NLP in healthcare is a new concept. NLP is an emerging market with tremendous growth potential in the healthcare vertical. By implementing NLP, clinicians can save valuable amounts of time without foregoing tremendous amounts of energy. An additional benefit of NLP is increased patient safety.

The asset of any hospital is its human beings. When these human resources become productive they become an invaluable resources of the hospital.

Certified Neurolinguistic Programming Courses

- NLP premier practitioner
- NLP master practitioner
- NLP trainers certification.

Neurolinguistic Programming Learning Centers

New Delhi

Alphastars Tap New Age Foundation
[Only Authorized NLP Institute of Dr Richard Bandler (USA) in India]
215-Vinoba Puri, Lajpat Nagar-II, New Delhi, India
Contact : 9811379590, 9313613547
E-mail: info@achievethebest.com or mail@indianlptraining.com
Web: www.indianlptraining.com

Global Institute of Healthcare Management
10A, Sai Baba Enclave, Tehsil Road
Near SDM Office, Najafgarh, Delhi
Contact: 9818868727, 011-25324000
E-mail: gihmdelhi@gmail.com
Web: www.gihmdelhi.com

Useful NLP Websites

- NLP World: www.nlp-world.com
- NLPInfo.com: www.nlpinfo.com
- www.indianlptraining.com.

Books Recommended to learn NLP

- **Neuro-Linguistic Programming, vol. 1** by Dilts, Grinder, Bandler, DeLozier, and Cameron-Bandler (Meta Publications, 1979).
- **Using your Brain—for a Change** (1985) by Bandler, and **Change Your Mind and Keep the Change** (1987) by Steve and Connirae Andreas.
- **Introducing Neuro-linguistic Programming** by Joseph C'Connor and John Seymour.
- **Beliefs Pathways to Health & Well Being**, by Robert Dilts, Tim Hallbom & Suzi Smith.
- **Time for a Change**. This is Richard Bandler's latest book.

Chapter 9

Principles of Medical Ethics

ORIGINS OF MEDICAL ETHICS

The Hippocratic Oath may be the oldest and most well-known system of medical ethics, but it is not alone. China and India began to incorporate ethics into medical practices about a hundred years after Hippocrates. They specified guidelines that encouraged humility of doctors, and concern and compassion for patients. Early church teachings focused on medical ethics. Thomas Aquinas, the Roman Catholic scholar, wrote about issues in medicine and religion in the early 1200s. And doctors from all nations contributed to the field. For instance, the Muslim doctor Ishaq bin Ali Rahawi wrote *The Conduct of a Physician* in the ninth century, the first text dedicated to medical ethics. Physician Thomas Percival wrote an expanded version of the Code of Medical Ethics in Britain in 1803 where he coined the expression *medical ethics.* (It was first published as a pamphlet in 1794). Dr Percival's code gave moral authority to doctors, along with independence

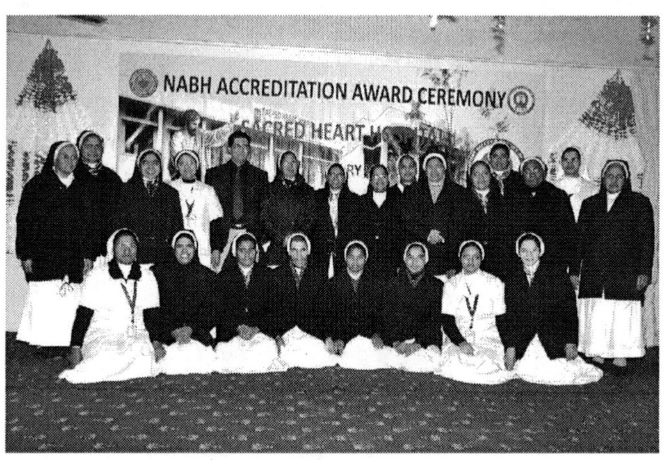

Healthcare Provider known for Good Ethics Management

and individual honor. At about the same time, Dr Benjamin Rush at the University of Pennsylvania began teaching ethics to its medical students.

Life in today's society is complicated, and there are not many professions as complicated or challenging as medicine. Furthermore, because doctors and healthcare providers have been so highly educated and the decisions they make may mean the difference between life and death, they are held to a higher standard of behavior and conduct. And because patients are so vulnerable when they are sick, the conduct of providers must be of the highest moral quality. Doctors and healthcare professionals are usually regarded as upright and moral. But doctors, like anyone else, have the potential to be unethical. Throughout history, codes of ethics have been developed to help guide physicians. So where did morality in medicine come from? Who decides what is ethical and what is not? Is there a time when lying to a patient or helping someone die is ethically acceptable?

Ethical behavior in the hospital and the influence of religion on ethical judgment are important part of medical ethics. We have to decide how personal morals can affect clinical judgment, and when a conflict of interest is unethical. Doctors study life as a biological function, but the emotional, spiritual, and psychological parts of human beings must be considered as well. When we treat the whole person, morality and ethics become paramount.

Applying the principles of medical ethics and the theories of morality help healthcare providers decide what course of action to take. Basically, ethics is all about asking the question, "What is the right thing to do?" What is *morality?* Most people define it as choosing the right beliefs or behavior in a difficult situation. *Ethics* is then reflecting on those moral standards and acting upon them. Ethics sets moral standards for behavior in many professions. With the four principles of medical ethics, providers often must weigh and balance one against another. When these principles seem to contradict, deciding which one has more moral weight, based on moral arguments, is the task of medical ethics.

At first, many scholars thought that ethics belonged solely to the study of religion or philosophy, but as medicine advanced, ethics became part of the practice of medicine through interdisciplinary studies. Although many laws are derived from ethical or moral precepts, ethics and morality are not the same as the law. For instance:

- Some laws uphold ethical standards. For example, its illegal for a doctor to have a sexual relationship with a young patient. And that behavior is highly unethical.
- Some ethical standards are stricter than the law. For instance, the case of the doctor who posted a sign on his door stating that anyone who voted

for President Obama should seek care elsewhere. Although it was legal for this doctor to state this, the action was not ethical.

- Sometimes ethics partially conflict with laws. Some physicians are ethically opposed to abortions and will not perform them. The law in many states restricts abortion in the second and third trimesters. However, abortions are legal in the first trimester, and doctors are ethically required to tell this to their patients, even if they are morally opposed to abortion.
- And some laws are directly opposed to ethical standards. For instance, lethal injection is, in many countries, used as a means of capital punishment. But the Code of Medical Ethics states that participating in this activity is a violation of ethical standards.

Some have said that good ethics take over where legal sanctions end. These ethical standards are not enforceable by law, but act as approved guidelines for healthcare provider behavior. Every country in the world has a different code of medical ethics, although most have similar basic principles. For example, access to healthcare for all is an important ethical issue around the world. Patient autonomy, nonmaleficence, beneficence, and justice are usually embraced in most societies, but there are some exceptions. In some cultures, doctors do not tell the truth to terminally ill patients, because tradition states that doing so will undermine the patient's will to live. Unfortunately, there have been times when ethical standards in medicine have been disregarded, both here and in other countries. Terrible and unethical experimentation on human beings prompted the Nuremberg Code, the Declaration of Helsinki, and the Belmont Report that guide modern medicine today. Institutional review boards and government agencies that oversee research are founded on these codes and declarations.

Because humanitarian goals are the point of medical ethics, they were codified. Some speculate that the first medical ethics codes were written in response to behavior that many doctors thought was unacceptable and outrageous. The codes of medical ethics are guide to the doctor in his ability and authority to self-regulate. Most ethicists think that whenever you are in an ethically tricky situation, it helps to ask yourself some questions. These questions might include:

- Is there a published standard of behavior about this issue?
- Would I want a member of my family to be treated this way?
- How will this action or treatment affect the patient?
- How will my conscience feel after I take this action?

Ethical codes and standards are, of course, much more complicated than these simple questions. But stopping to think about an action or behavior before you do, it is an important step in developing an internal ethical formula.

The codes of medical ethics were framed because there were no overarching government regulations or ethical standards. The code has been modified through the years; the first version of the code specified physician behavior and manners. These codes were not enforceable, but still serve as the standard of behavior for medical professionals with moral integrity.

The Code of Medical Ethics has eight basic principles:

1. Provide competent and compassionate medical care
2. Maintain the highest professional standards
3. Respect the law
4. Keep the confidence of patients and colleagues
5. Advance scientific and medical education
6. Do not discriminate among peers and patients
7. Improve public health
8. Honor responsibilities to patients and support access to care.

These Codes were made to promote and measure high ethical standards and expectations for healthcare providers. They test the ethical issues and standards, and create questions that doctors and patients can ask themselves and develop criteria for performance and policies. As the basic duty of healthcare providers is to assist the patient and their families however they can, with dignity, respect, care, and compassion. The Code places the patient as the center of a healthcare provider's responsibility, but acknowledges that as a professional, they have an obligation to act with responsibility and dignity in society.

Therefore practice of medicine is an art and a science. The art comes from dealing with human beings, who can be fragile and unpredictable when they are sick and need your help. The science comes from years of research and study. Medical ethics puts the art and science together in practical applications to tricky problems. Here we will examine the basics of medical ethics, its principles, and some controversies. Everyone makes mistakes, but it is possible to learn from medical errors and design your practice so that they are caught and fixed before they become serious problems or affect patients. Everyone is a patient at some point in their life, so understanding the philosophical side of medicine can only make the process smoother. And the more providers understand about the ethics of their profession, the more satisfying their professional lives will be.

Medical ethics, also called bioethics, are the underpinning of any medical practice. Doing the right thing sounds simple, but can be difficult in practice. The four main principles of medical ethics, are the basics of running an ethical practice, examine the doctor-patient relationship, and discover what to do when mistakes are made. Every time a story is written about any medical issue, whether it is abortion, end-of-life care, or multiple births, everyone has an opinion about what is right and what is wrong. We are bombarded with two or more opposing viewpoints, and each one sound reasonable. But which one is right? And that is medical ethics in a nutshell. What is the right thing to do? How do we structure clinics, hospitals, and government so the most people benefit and patients are treated with respect and compassion? What should you, as the provider, do in certain situations? There are guidelines and principles in place to help us make decisions, but sometimes those come into direct conflict with each other. When that happens, we need to use logical reasoning skills, ethical theories, and some tools of philosophy to balance and weigh our options. Even after all of that is done, there are still questions. Medical ethics gets into the gray areas of life. As you look at these issues in more depth, you realize there are not many that are truly black and white.

We look at the differences between ethical and legal behaviors, and explain the difference between patient rights and provider responsibilities. We need to understand the guidelines and guideposts to follow while treating patients in all stages of life. We look at some of the common and hot-button controversies and take a peek at the ethics of medical research, which is on the forefront of medicine. Healthcare providers have always been respected and even revered. As societies were formed, ethical principles were developed by physicians and scholars from all walks of life. As a result, Code of Medical Ethics that covers most situations healthcare providers faces in their careers. These guidelines and opinions written by ethical scholars and physicians.

The four principles of medical ethics help us to look at the differences between ethics and the law, and how you should reconcile patient care with ethical standards. One of the most important facts in medical ethics is that they are not static. Medical ethics have changed over the years and will continue to evolve as medicine advances. What are ethics? Ethics and morality mean the same thing to many people, and they are similar. Morals are used to describe personal character, whereas ethics defines behavior in different situations. Morality refers to personal character, beliefs, and behavior; ethics is about the reflection on morality and deciding how to act as a person or a professional. An ethical person and a moral person are usually one and the same. We use *medical ethics* to refer to those guidelines and behaviors that we expect a medical professional with moral integrity to exhibit.

Ethics has developed over the centuries as a code of conduct, especially for professionals. Healthcare providers have so much knowledge about the human body, so much potential power over patients, and the ability to change and save lives. Because of these factors, the ethical bar is set very high, and providers have moral obligations to their patients. The field of medical ethics is really about reflection on how to behave as a medical professional as well as the morality of particular medical interventions. Medical ethics are simply some key ethical principles applied to the practice of medicine. These principles are the bedrock of good clinical practice, and they are autonomy, nonmaleficence, beneficence, and justice. But they often come in conflict with each other as they are applied to a case. By using these principles in each individual case, it can be easier to make difficult decisions with your patients as you guide them through their care.

PRINCIPLES OF MEDICAL ETHICS

There are four major principles of medical ethics:

1. *Autonomy*: This principle is focused on the patient's independence or liberty. A competent adult has the right to make decisions about what happens to his body. The person must be capable of rational thought and not be manipulated into any decision. An adult can refuse medical care or treatment or accept treatment when his provider suggests it. That person then lives with the consequences of his decision.
2. *Beneficence*: This principle states that a physician must act in the best interest of the patient. Providers are required to promote their patient's health and well-being. Most doctors agree that healing is the main purpose of modern medicine. Beneficence means providers must help their patients.
3. *Nonmaleficence*: First, do no harm. Physicians must not harm a patient through carelessness, malice, vengeance, or dislike, or even through treatments intended to help the patient. This principle is balanced with beneficence in that any risks of a treatment or procedure to a patient must be outweighed by benefit. Some treatments always carry a risk of harm. But when the treatment is very risky, the benefit must be great, or the risk of not performing the procedure must be great.

   Double effect is an offshoot of nonmaleficence. A treatment that is normally used to help someone may have an unintended negative effect. For instance, a vaccine used to prevent disease can, in rare cases, actually because the infection it is intended to prevent. This principle provides specific guidance when determining when unintended effects are justified and when they are not.
4. *Justice*: Justice refers to fairness with respect to the distribution of medical resources. This principle draws upon ethics, the law, and public policy. Who should receive scarce medical resources, and how should we distribute them in order to realize the best outcomes? Making the

- *Abortion and birth control*: Countries and states have different laws regarding access to abortion and birth control. Doctors and providers must follow these laws depending on where they live.
- *Euthanasia*: Some countries allow physician-assisted suicide. Those laws state specifically what providers are and are not allowed to do for a patient.
- *Privacy and confidentiality*: Confidentiality laws and regulations are strictly enforced to protect the privacy of the patient at all times.
- *Access to medical care*: State-sponsored medical care, provides access to people who usually could not afford the care. Universal healthcare is provided in most of the countries around the world.

Medical ethics standards do have an effect upon the law. Many laws are devised and written based on the ethical codes of doctors and nurses. It is important that you, as a provider, know the laws in your state as well as understand the ethics guidelines that apply in different situations. If you are in the medical profession, you do your best to become the kind of provider who is trusted by your patients. You want your patients to know that you have their best interests at heart, and you want to build relationships with your patients so you can give them the best care possible. Medical ethics provide guidelines to becoming a better provider. Ethics can help you communicate better, be a better partner to your fellow doctors and nurses, reduce risk of errors, and increase job satisfaction. When you embrace ethics as simply doing the right thing, there will be few conflicts between medical ethics and good patient care. In many cases, it may help to put yourself in your patient's shoes (or hospital slippers). What would you want if you were the patient? Would you want your doctor to be compassionate and caring? Would you want test results delivered to you quickly? Treating patients with a sense of courtesy comes first. The Golden Rule applies in medical ethics. If you treat your patients as you would want to be treated, or as you would want someone to treat a cherished family member, you will provide good medical care.

TURNING TO ETHICAL GUIDEPOSTS AND GUIDELINES

For a healthcare organization, your employer may have a code of ethics as well. It is a good idea to read over an ethics code every now and then, not just when you have questions about issues. These codes are not perfect or even enforceable, but taking the time to learn their principles and following the basic rules will help you enjoy your practice more, will result in more satisfying patient relationships, and will help make you a more effective provider.

Medical ethics can be divided into five main areas of discussion: individual rights or privacy; beginning-of-life issues; end-of-life issues; access to healthcare; and ethics in research are the main overarching areas that can generate the most need for medical ethics guidelines. We will look at each of the first four of these areas of ethics and talk a bit about how the four ethical principles can clash and intersect as people make decisions about their lives and providers make decisions about how to best help their patients. All four ethical principles apply to situations in these areas of ethics, and how a dilemma is resolved depends on which ethical principles you follow.

Privacy and Confidentiality Concerns

Privacy and confidentiality go hand in hand with the principle of autonomy. In fact, because privacy upholds all four medical principles, it can be considered the cornerstone of your practice. Patient autonomy rules this issue because competent, informed patients can legally and ethically make all decisions about their care. It can be frustrating when a patient refuses treatment you know will help, but respecting his decisions, whether those decisions are made on personal, religious, or cultural grounds, is paramount.

Complying with regulations and putting safeguards in place in your office and clinic are important. It is also important to train your staff about privacy and confidentiality. Running an ethical practice means respecting patient privacy at all times. If a patient does not trust that you will keep their information private, he will be less likely to confide in you about matters that may be important in making the correct diagnosis. Patient confidentiality demonstrates all of the medical ethics principles. Confidentiality is crucial to respecting autonomy because patients need to know that their decisions about their health and any diagnoses are being kept in a personal space. Nonmaleficence is important because if that information falls into the wrong hands, the patient can be hurt. Doing the best for your patient, or beneficence, means honoring the trust he places in you. And justice demands that confidential information be kept private because when others can learn information about intimate matters, patients can feel violated. Manage paperwork, deal with managed care situations, and handle sharing information with third parties, particularly insurance companies. But complying with these standards is the bare minimum of keeping patient information confidential. It is important that you pay attention to what you are discussing with others and where, and what you communicate through the written and spoken word.

Most information about a patient, including test results, diagnoses, treatments, and vital statistics, can be shared only with others when the patient has given express permission for that release. That permission, when at all possible, should be in the written form. Honoring confidentiality and learning to not discuss patient information with anyone except other providers who are involved in the case or whom you are consulting is important. Practice it until it becomes second nature and it is important to remember that in medical ethics, the law really is the lowest common denominator. Ethics goes above and beyond the law, from what is legal to what is right. So complying with the law is important, but to be the best healthcare provider, go beyond the law and add compassion, respect, and honesty to your practice. And speaking of honesty, medical errors do occur, and the best practice is to report them to your patient. We look at the best ways of disclosing medical errors. Reproduction and beginning-of-life issues reproduction includes access to birth control, abortion, the right of a woman to choose or refuse care, the rights of the fetus, reproductive technologies, and access to care. Autonomy often comes into conflict with the other principles in reproductive issues simply because these matters are so personal.

For instance, a pregnant woman is allowed to refuse healthcare for her and her fetus up until the moment of birth. Respecting the woman's autonomy means that she is allowed to decide for herself what happens to her body, even when pregnant. How to weigh the rights of a mother versus the rights of her fetus and pro-choice and pro-life stances on abortion. The definition of personhood also is explored as it relates to the rights of the fetus. Access to birth control becomes an issue when minors request it. Because the law has decided that mature minors can have access to prescribed birth control, how do we respect a minor's privacy and autonomy while not interfering with the parent-child relationship? We take a look at adolescent patient's rights, emancipated minors, mature minors, and how to balance privacy with your obligations to your patient and her parents.

Finally, assisted reproduction can raise many ethical issues. We look at the ethics of artificial insemination, *in vitro* fertilization, surrogacy, and sterilization. How do we balance risk and harm to the mother and fetus? Who should receive genetic screening, and how do you prepare your patient for the results? What are your responsibilities toward your patient as you try to provide the best care?

End-of-life Issues

As at the beginning of life, the end-of-life raises many difficult ethical issues. With the advent of medical technology that is capable of supporting life far beyond what had once been possible, we need to understand when life ends. Death is defined, and the rights of dying patients are discussed by looking at some landmark ethics cases. The physician's role in end-of-life cases is discussed, including the ethics of physician-assisted suicide. We then look at honoring a patient's wishes at the time of death. Healthcare directives, or living wills, are addressed as vehicles for patient autonomy. How can we help patients die with dignity and as little suffering as possible? The rule of double effect 'The four principles of medical ethics' is pertinent in this issue. Giving a patient drug with the intent to make them comfortable can hasten death. Is that an ethical move? Euthanasia and terminal sedation are hot-button topics. Who decides when it is someone's time to die? When it becomes obvious that life is ending, how much help should we offer someone who is suffering? One of medical science's advances is the ability to help relieve suffering. That is one of the greatest opportunities for beneficence. When someone is at the end of life, however, balancing beneficence and nonmaleficence can become tricky.

Access to Care

Universal healthcare has been in the news and passionate supporters of this concept and equally passionate opponents have made their voices heard. But what is the reality of the situation? And what does a medical ethic have to say about access to care? The principle of justice takes center stage with this topic. Because this act will take years to implement, there are still millions of who are uninsured and underinsured, and no real guarantee that provisions of the act will ever be put into place. Thousands of people die every year because they do not have access to medical care, and thousands more go bankrupt because of the prohibitive cost of medicine. The principle of justice is most applicable to this issue. In providing the basic minimum of care to the most people possible, while not reducing the standard of care enjoyed by others, is the balancing act. This fulfills a utilitarian approach to ethics by maximizing benefit to the greatest number of people. As a provider, you can help your patients by volunteering at free clinics, by prescribing generic drugs and less invasive and expensive procedures first, and by encouraging people to live healthy lifestyles. Respecting patient autonomy, guarding against harm (including financial harm), trying to do the best for your patient, and treating all patients equally is challenging but necessary in the current healthcare climate and looking at integrating your patient's spiritual and cultural beliefs into their care as a way of enhancing treatment as well.

MOVING MEDICINE FORWARD

Ethics of Research

Medical research has brought great advances in the 20th and 21st centuries. With the progress has come some dark days. Patients have been abused, hurt, and killed in the name of medical research before standards were put into place. Even now, some researchers fail to follow guidelines and end up harming patients. For example, in July 2010, media sources revealed that the drug manufacturer SmithKline Beecham hid results that showed Avandia, their successful diabetes medication, was harmful to the heart. Patients in the clinical trial had serious heart issues, including a significant risk of increased myocardial infarction, that were not recorded in the tally of adverse events. The FDA is now deciding whether the drug should be withdrawn from the market. Clearly, if SmithKline Beecham knew about adverse side effects from this drug, they should have been made public. If true, this was a clear violation of nonmaleficence.

Whether you are a researcher or a caregiver of patients in the trials, research in some special populations, such as animals, children, and psychiatric patients needs to be given to protect research subjects who cannot give full informed consent.

Ethics in a Hospital

Healthcare providers are constantly trying to balance the social and scientific parts of their brains. Emotion and compassion have to be balanced with medical knowledge and the ability to reason and diagnose. The bedside manner is where these two parts come together in an ethical dance. In this section, we look at ethics inside the hospital, including what a hospital ethics panel does. Most hospitals have a patient bill of rights; we look at what purpose these documents serve. And we look at ethics in the emergency room, where different rules prevail. We have all heard stories about doctors who lack good bedside manner. Although it is true that doctors and providers must be at least somewhat removed from emotion while treating a patient, there is a balance between diagnostic excellence and caring for the whole patient.

Understanding the Hospital Ethics Panel

Most hospitals have ethics panels, composed of doctors, nurses, and other providers, administrators, social workers, lawyers, chaplains and other clergy, and some laypersons. All of these members are volunteers. These panels convene to discuss ethics situations, advise providers and patients about making healthcare choices, review hospital policies, and help educate hospital staff about ethical issues. The ethics panel can be convened at the request of a provider or patient or a patient's family when there is some disagreement about the course of treatment. The panel can also convene at the request of other hospital staff, such as nurses or administrators, if there are conflicts in care. What is best for the patient is at the center of every discussion, and the patient's family values play a big role in the decisions made by the ethics panel.

Some of these topics addressed by ethics panels include:

- Disagreements between providers and patients, within families, or within hospital staff about the best course of treatment for a patient.
- Clarification of ethical issues in a particular situation for providers and families.
- Review of criteria for waiting lists for treatments or transplants.
- Appropriate course of action when medical errors are committed.
- Whether or not to continue life-sustaining treatment.
- The need for informed consent and how this is best communicated with the patient.
- Proxies and decision-making, such as living wills and advance directives.
- Equity of care for minorities, the poor, or those with different religious beliefs.
- Review of hospital policies involving ethical issues such as end-of-life care or abortion.

When discussing and deciding on these dilemmas, the ethics panel will consider:

- What the patient really wants for the best outcome.
- What the proxy, or designated representative, thinks the patient would want.
- What doctors and other providers believe is the best course of treatment.
- What to do when care is futile.
- When lifesaving treatments should be withdrawn.
- Whether to approve or deny cutting-edge medical treatments.
- How cultural or religious beliefs factor into healthcare.

Hospital ethics committees facilitate an open discussion and bring out the ethical issues involved in a case. They may or may not make a recommendation, but it remains the role of the provider and patient or patient's family to make the final decisions about the care given to the patient.

Hospital ethics panels do not:

- Sanction or discipline doctors or other providers.
- Publicize their decisions.
- Issue binding legal judgments.

It is important to remember that using a hospital ethics panel to help decide course of treatment is often a last resort. When a conflict about care cannot be resolved, this panel is a great and underutilized resource. Some of the panel's additional responsibilities are to guide hospital administrators on policies involving ethical issues, and to educate staff about medical ethics and decision-making.

PATIENT RIGHTS

Most hospitals and clinics publish patient's rights and these documents set forth the type of treatment and care a patient and his family can expect to receive in that hospital or clinic. Physicians and Surgeons published a list of patient freedoms and rights for different hospitals which might be slightly different, but all have the same basic principles:

- To choose a physician freely.
- To agree on terms with their provider.
- To be treated with respect and consideration.
- To have an advance directive on their chart.
- To expect confidentiality and privacy.
- To be fully informed about their condition and any treatments or drugs.
- To receive responses to questions or requests in a reasonable time frame.
- To be informed about business relationships among providers, the hospital, payers, and other entities.
- To make choices about their care.
- To refuse medical treatment.
- To full disclosure of their condition, insurance plans, and treatment plans.
- To expect continuity of care.

Along with rights, patients also have responsibilities, which are discussed in patients must fully disclose information about their condition, and should ask questions if they do not fully understand their diagnoses or course of treatment.

EMERGENCY ROOM ETHICS

Emergency medicine has special ethical rules. The patients and providers usually do not have a longstanding relationship, and decisions about life and death can sometimes be made in seconds. So what are the ethical standards that should exist in emergency rooms? Doctors must quickly evaluate a situation, think about available options and treatments, and then take action. When considering decision-making in the ER, providers should first look for a policy or precedent that may apply to the situation, and then look for an option that can be found while the patient is stabilized, and use logical reasoning skills to reach a decision. Providers should also consider these questions:

- What would you want, if you were the patient?
- Could you defend this action to others?
- And would this decision work in other situations?

Some of the unique situations in emergency room ethics include:

- *Triage*: Doctors and providers must make quick decisions about whom to treat first, who can wait for treatment, and who is so severely injured or sick that treatment is futile. This is one of the first considerations in an ER, especially when there is a community-wide emergency.
- *Quick action*: In an emergency situation, providers have to make split in second decisions about treatment and care, sometimes with little or no information about patient history.
- *Implied informed consent*: In an emergency situation, informed consent is implied when a patient is unable to provide consent. That is, providers assume that the patient would want treatment to save his life, even if he is unable to consent. Aggressive care is expected until the situation is futile.
- *Staff teamwork*: Patients are often very sick with life-threatening conditions. A team of staff with defined roles must work quickly and efficiently to care for the patient. Because medical treatment may sometimes be given with little or no discussion and under unpredictable conditions, ER providers must be ready to help each other at a moment's notice.
- *Respect for the law*: From domestic violence issues to child abuse to attempted murder, emergency room providers can face many situations where law enforcement is involved.
- *Impartiality*: Because many patients present to the emergency room from poor socioeconomic conditions, they must all be treated with respect no matter what their living situation is. Even those charged with violent crimes must be treated fairly and with the same standards as every other patient.
- *Resilience*: The emergency room can often be chaotic with many very sick patients being managed at the same time, and providers must remain as calm and flexible as possible in the face of trauma.

Adaptability is an important virtue for emergency room staff. All of the other ethical considerations in medicine, such as beneficence, respect for autonomy, nonmaleficence, and justice apply to the emergency room, of course, but these additional values and skills are important additions to the provider's toolbox.

Bioethics as a Field of Study

Medical ethicists commonly work at colleges and universities, teaching and publishing papers. Some hospitals and clinics have medical ethicists as consultants to help them navigate the often difficult maze of ethical situations. They often serve on hospital ethics committees. These professionals can help providers by rendering decisions about ending life-sustaining treatments or judging the capacity of patients. Medical ethicists help providers keep the ethics of every situation in mind as they do their jobs. Bioethics has existed only since the 1960s, prompted by advances in traditional medicine that included dialysis, intensive care units (ICUs), transplants, and respirators. These advances forced doctors to address complicated moral issues such as when to remove life-sustaining treatment, or when to admit or remove someone from an ICU. Medical advances continue to drive new ethical issues, such as advances in genetics that may raise questions about genetic testing.

The Institute of Society, Ethics, and Life Sciences, now called the Hastings Center, was founded in 1970 in New York. The Institute began as a way to bring together scholars in religion, philosophy, law, science, and medicine to tackle the issue of bioethics. And the Kennedy Institute of Ethics was founded at Georgetown University in 1971. Now there are more than 50 universities in the United States alone that have departments in medical ethics. Several publications focus on this field, including the Journal of Clinical Ethics, the Hastings Center Report, the Cambridge Quarterly of Healthcare Ethics, and the American Society for Bioethics and Humanities. The American Society for Bioethics and Humanities has tried to codify core competencies and critical areas of knowledge for medical ethicists. They stated that medical ethicists should be familiar with healthcare, moral reasoning, laws affecting healthcare, and be able to listen and communicate well when asked to participate in ethics consultations.

Chapter 10

Medical Tourism: India the Global Healthcare Destination

INTRODUCTION

Medical Tourism India/Health Tourism India is a developing concept whereby people from worldwide visit India for their medical and relaxation needs. The most common treatments are heart surgery, knee transplant, cosmetic surgery and dental care. The reason why India is a favorable destination, is because of its infrastructure and technology in which it is in par with those in USA, UK and Europe. India has some of the best hospitals and treatment centers in the world with the best facilities. Since it is also one of the most favorable tourist destinations in the world, medication combines with tourism has come into effect, from which the concept of Medical Tourism is derived.

India is promoting the 'high-tech healing' of its private healthcare sector as a tourist attraction.

India to become a 'global health destination'.

Medical Tourism in India, also known as Health Tourism India, is a growing concept whereby people from all over the world visit India for their medication accompanied with a short holiday. The healthcare sector in India has witnessed an enormous growth in infrastructure in the private and voluntary sector. The private sector, which was very modest in the early stages, has now become a flourishing industry equipped with the most modern, state-of-the-art technology at its disposal.

INDIA: UNTAPPED POTENTIAL IN THE MEDICAL TOURISM MARKET

The Indian healthcare market is ₹ 15 billion and growing at over 30% every year. Indian private hospitals are increasingly finding a mention in the travel itineraries of foreigners, with the trend of medical tourism catching up in the country. If industry estimates are to be believed, the size of the medical tourism industry stands at ₹ 1,200–1,500 crore (₹ 12–15 billion).

A recent CII-McKinsey study on healthcare says medical tourism alone can contribute ₹ 5,000–10,000 crore (₹ 50–100 billion) additional revenue for upmarket tertiary hospitals by 2012, and will account for 3–5% of the total healthcare delivery market. Compared to countries like the UK or the US, procedures like heart bypass surgery or angioplasty come at a fraction of the cost in India, even though the quality of doctors and medical equipment is comparable to the best in the world.

A heart bypass surgery in India costs US$ 3,000–6,000, while in the US it costs between US$ 15,000 and US$ 40,000. The Indian Health Care Federation (IHCF), an association of the healthcare delivery sector that includes the Escorts Heart Institute, Apollo Hospitals Group, Fortis Healthcare among others and CII, under the leadership of Dr Naresh Trehan, executive director, Escorts Heart Institute and Research Center (EHIRC), New Delhi have also decided to project India as a major healthcare destination. Even travel agents are aggressively promoting India as a destination for medical tourism. This is a huge, untapped market, not just for therapeutic medical tourism like *Ayurveda*, but also for curative treatment.

The benefit to tourism industry could be of the order of ₹ 1,000 crore (₹ 10 billion). Indian NRIs, Asians and tourists from around the world are beginning to realise the potential of modern and traditional Indian medicine. Health and medical tourism is perceived to be one of the fastest growing segments in marketing 'Destination Incredible India' today. While this area has so far been relatively unexplored, we now find that not only the Ministry of Tourism, Government of India, but also the various state tourism boards are all promoting health and medical tourism as a segment with tremendous potential for future growth.

Indian hospitals have also realized the potential of this niche market and have begun to tailor their services for foreign visitors. Visitors, especially from the West and the Middle-East, find Indian hospitals as an affordable and a viable option rather than grappling with health insurance and national medical systems in their native lands.

Areas where Indian healthcare excels:

- Clinical outcomes being on par with the world's best centers
- Internationally qualified and experienced doctors
- Technology edge
- Competitive costs—one-fifth to one-tenth of costs in the West
- Quality of service
- No waiting time
- Patient-centric care
- Exotic experience, increasing popularity as a tourist destination
- Eastern healthcare wisdom along with the expertise of Western medicine

Areas where Indian healthcare has to focus:

- Accreditation norms to be adopted by all major hospitals
- Hospitals must conform to a code of ethics
- Provision of a uniform price band for major specialities especially for health insurance majors
- Handling of medicolegal issues.

Working with Indian Tourism Ministry and tour operators to promote medical tourism overseas. Cross-border travel for healthcare reasons is still a highly disorganized movement, but countries are slowly waking up to its potential. In some places, the governments have taken a lead. In others, travel agents specializing in medical tourism are driving the trend.

In India, private hospitals are trying to attract patients on their own and by showcasing Indian healthcare overseas through CII-IHCF led overseas missions. Developed nations will benefit majorly as costs and waiting time come down for a significant chunk of their population. Developing countries benefit through medical tourism as it brings in revenues and provides the right spur to improve their overall healthcare sector, apart from reducing brain drain in their medical fraternities. Least developed countries, too, benefit as they lack facilities for cutting-edge treatment.

The situation was so dismal that in 2002, the National Health Services (NHS) in the UK started a pilot scheme for 'overseas treatment' to see if surgery services abroad could be bought to shorten the waiting lists. The project focused mainly on facilities available in the European Union.

Meanwhile, many British patients take the initiative to seek their own treatment abroad without waiting for the NHS to sort out its problems.

A ₹ 15-billion-plus market growing at over 30% per year throws up huge opportunities for anyone smart enough to tap it. Thus, India not only offers world class cardiac bypass surgery, hip replacements, organ transplants, but also cosmetic, dental surgery and vision correction, etc. and alternative healthcare, which is a significant niche opportunity.

Healthcare insurers in the developed countries are aware of the fact that the option of medical treatment in countries like India could help them reduce premiums and offer options to people who are currently uninsured. Over the next few years, insurance firms are expected to provide a fillip to the medical tourism business in India.

MEDICAL TOURISM ADVANTAGE IN INDIA

Medicare is the latest reason to visit India. Is it because of the low costs? Is it the quality of treatment? Or is there something more? It is a combination of several factors that make India a unique healthcare destination.

- Over 60,000 cardiac surgeries are done every year with outcomes at par with international standards.
- Multiorgan transplants are successfully performed at one-tenth of the cost in comparison to the West.
- Patients from over 55 countries are treated at Indian hospitals.

The Indian healthcare industry is undergoing a phenomenal expansion and India is now looked upon as the leading country in the promotion of medical tourism, with an annual growth rate estimated at 30%. While India's top-rated education system provides an estimated 30,000 doctors and nurses each year to meet this demand, the Indian government's spend on the healthcare sector is expected to be around 8% of its GDP by 2010.

CARE OF INDIA

Five-star facilities and international quality treatment mark medical care in India. Some of its highlights are:

- Internationally qualified and experienced specialists and super specialists
- Latest equipment and infrastructure like the da Vinci surgical system for robotic cardiac surgery, 64 slice CT scan, linear accelerators similar to sloan kettering, New York
- Strict blood safety and infection control process
- Medical professionals can now consult specialists anywhere across the globe, send images and have a videoconference to arrive at the best decision for complicated cases.

Cost of Life

India also has one of the largest pharmaceutical industries in the world, exporting drugs to more than 180 countries. This, along with the cost advantage, attracts over a million patients annually.

- The average cost of healthcare in India is about one-fifth that of the West.
- There's zero waiting time for major surgeries.
- Cost of advanced surgeries in India is 10–15 times lower than anywhere in the world.

For the sake of comparison:

- While a heart surgery costs $30,000 in US, it costs $6,000 (approx) in India.
- A bone marrow transplant costs $26,000 here compared to $250,000 (approx) in the US.

Patient First

A number of Indian hospitals get patients from overseas. These patients usually get a package deal that includes flights, transfers, hotels, treatment and often a postoperative vacation. Here are some aspects that turn the balance in India's favor.

- Personalized care and hospitality
- Doctors who are proficient in English. Most hospitals even provide interpreters to cut across language barriers
- While the patient stays at our hospitals, we take care to see that the visit becomes a pleasant experience
- Niggling works like a shuttle service to and from the airport, the acceptance of international credit cards and the availability of international cuisine are taken care of.

The Holistic Approach

India is a country that views a human being in totality. Here, treatment is based on the physio, psycho, socio, nutritional, ecological, environmental and spiritual needs of each individual. Our holistic therapy, integrates traditional medical systems like *Ayurveda* and homeopathy with complementary therapies like *Yoga* and acupuncture to hasten the healing process.

India has provided succour to the needful since the beginning of time. Some come in search of physical remedies. Others come in search of mental peace. But whatever the ailment, the cure is not too far. Such is the promise of this life-giving land.

INCREDIBLE INDIA

Cardiology and Cardiac Surgery

- Over the years, cardiac care has become a specialty in India.
- Replacement of heart valve cost less than half in India compared to USA.
- Indian hospitals combine the latest innovations in medical electronics with unmatched expertise of leading cardiologists and cardiothoracic surgeons.
- The success rate of our physiotherapists helping patients regain their physical fitness and prevent cardiac problems is at an average of 99.5% at par with leading cardiac centers around the world.

Minimally Invasive Surgery

- Minimal access surgery (MAS) introduced a sweeping revolution in surgical practice ever since its dramatic entry more than a decade ago.
- MAS in India is employed routinely in many surgical sub-specialties including general surgery, pediatric surgery, urology and colorectal surgery.
- India has about 200 major laparoscopic procedures being performed every month.

Oncology

- Today's India is equipped to address all aspects of cancer control, including prevention, early detection, diagnosis and treatment.
- Cancer diagnosis and treatment is costly all over the world, but comparatively, quite inexpensive in India.
- Survival rates in most cancers are today comparable with the Western world.

Orthopedics

- All types of primary knee replacement as well as complex post-replacement revision surgeries are performed in India.
- The quality of treatment is enhanced by well-maintained hospitals with high levels of hygiene, caring staff and an ambience.
- Cost can be as low as one-third of what one would pay for the same procedure in the USA.

Cosmetology

- In India, the cost of many cosmetic procedures is comparatively low, making it a realistic option for everyone.
- Surgeons can now treat a wider variety of problems, with results that are more natural looking and longer lasting. Procedures like abdominoplasty, dermabrasion, facial implants, laser face resurfacing, and many more are done in synch with international standards. And healing times are shorter too.
- Improved surgical techniques and state-of-the-art equipment enable patients to avail themselves of the benefits of cosmetic surgery that are highly specialized.

Wellness

- Indian hospitals look at a holistic approach to healing where the latest medical techniques are applied along side ancient methods of post-operative care.

- Techniques like acupuncture, a traditional Chinese medicine (TCM) system, regular saunas and massages, daily sessions of *Yoga* and meditation are used to alleviate pain.
- Stress is not just on physical well-being, but also on mental and spiritual health that might have suffered in the course of the ailment.

VISA INFORMATION

Conditions

A medical category visa may be issued with the following conditions:

- The Indian Missions/Posts abroad may scrutinize the medical documents very carefully and satisfy themselves about the bonafide purpose for which a medical treatment visa is being requested.
- Missions may satisfy that the applicant has sought preliminary medical advice from his country of origin/country of residence and he has been advised to go for specialized medical treatment.
  In case the foreign national desires to go for treatment under Indian System of Medicines, his case may also be considered.
- This type of visa should be granted for seeking medical attendance only in reputed/recognized specialized hospitals/treatment centers in the country.

Although not exhaustive, following illustrative list of ailments would be of primary consideration; serious ailments like neurosurgery, ophthalmic disorders, heart related problems, renal disorders, organ transplantation, congenital disorders, gene-therapy, radiotherapy, plastic surgery, joint replacement, etc. The basic idea would be that the mission may satisfy about the need of the foreign national to come to India for medical treatment/ health enhancement.

Validity of Visa and Extension of Visa

The initial period for such a visa may be up to a period of one year or the period of treatment, whichever is less, which can be extended for a further period of up to one year by the State Government/Foreigner Regional Registration Offices (FRROs) on production of medical certificate/advice from the reputed/recognized/specialized hospitals in the country. Any further extension will be granted by the Ministry of Home Affairs only on the recommendations of the State Governments/FRROs supported by appropriate medical documents. Such visas will be valid for maximum three entries during one year.

State Government/FRROs may permit one additional entry in emergent situations, if required.

Visa to Attendant/Family Members

Attendant/family members of the patients coming to India for medical treatment shall be granted miscellaneous visa co-terminus with the 'M Visa' of the patient. Such visas maybe granted to the spouse/children or those who have blood relations with the patients.

However, not more than two attendants may be allowed at a time for grant of miscellaneous visas. Such visa will be called 'MX visa.' Such foreigners are also required to get themselves registered with the local FRROs/FROs well within 14 days from the date of the arrival.

Registrations

Foreigners coming on 'M Visa' will be required to get themselves registered mandatorily well within the period of 14 days from the date of arrival with the concerned FRROs/FROs.

Registrations for Pakistani and Bangladeshi Nationals

It may be clarified that 'Medical Visa' will be available to all the foreign nationals including China, Pakistan, Bangladesh and Sri Lanka. However, registration formalities for Pakistani and Bangladeshi nationals will be as per the provisions contained in the para 106 of the Visa Manual in respect of Bangladeshi nationals and para 18 in respect of Pakistani nationals. Similarly entry and departure of these foreign nationals will also be governed as per the existing policy in respect of these nationals.

India, with its cocktail of cultures, languages, rituals and colors is a dynamic stage for the drama of life. Its landscapes such as mountains, deserts, torrential rivers and placid lakes provide the setting. Its people and their varies lives provide for a captivating script.

It is through of visitors who have a role to play too—that of God. For them, this is a country that upholds the spirit of "*Atithi Devo Bhava*", words that life of the guest to the stature of the almighty.

India is a journey of the mind and soul
India is a journey of the five senses
It is a journey of self-discovery
It is a journey of self-fulfillment.

Chapter 11 Third Party Administrator Management is Knowledge Management

INTRODUCTION

Third Party Administrators

Third party administrators (TPAs) are not technically managed care organizations but play an important role in health insurance markets. Neither insurance companies nor care providers, they are intermediaries who bring all components of healthcare such as physicians, hospitals, clinics, long-term facilities, and pharmacies together.

It is long overdue for the clinician to undergo performance scrutiny and objective assessment of one's treatment outcomes. Before a third party evaluates performance and decides the efficiency of a clinician based on cutting costs rather than quality, it would be prudent for the clinician to submit for continuous voluntary evaluation through clinical audits, update one's armory by continuous medical education and compete with each other on the quality criteria, to secure contracts with TPA. This would be possible if the clinicians lay down code of conduct and regulate themselves by an autonomous body of clinicians. This will suitably dissuade the TPA to demand cost-cutting measures causing poor treatment outcomes as a whole. The seal of quality care by the healthcare providers is going to be their bargaining power in long run, be it with the insurance companies or the managed care.

The clinicians would rather be rewarded for being part of an organized, 42 of 102 accountable faculty, by the patient. Further, the clinician will retain the supreme authority of the patient's treatment.

IMPLICATIONS OF THIRD PARTY ADMINISTRATOR

The existing ill-structured system is being replaced by a reformed but organized structure called the TPA. An individual doctor through his attachment to a nursing home or a hospital is able to offer his professional services via the provider network extending to almost majority of the nursing homes and hospitals. In an ideal situation, the clinician is assured of a steady stream of patients, the nursing home is assured of a steady revenue flow and so the upkeep and facilities of the nursing home and hospital tend to be upgraded. The clinician finds himself in a better equipped set-up, luxurious clinics (which satisfy one's patient also), and there is no constant need to prove one's capabilities by the number of patients one brings to the hospital nor is one obliged to bring sufficient business to the hospital. A favorable work atmosphere creates a healthy and quality practice, which gives better bargaining power to the provider with the TPA. This is the brighter but achievable picture of Third Party Administration of healthcare. The flip side is the managed care crisis occurring in US. The reasons for the crisis though have to be studied in context with the American system of healthcare. It surely cannot be applied to the Indian scenario. We have to wait and watch how many more years it will take for managed care to arrive just as Health Insurance for all (Health for all!) reforms has taken 50 years postindependence.

It is long overdue for the clinician to undergo performance scrutiny and objective assessment of one's treatment outcomes. Before a third party evaluates performance and decides the efficiency of a clinician based on cutting costs rather than quality, it would be prudent for the clinician to submit for continuous voluntary evaluation through clinical audits, update one's armory by continuous medical education and compete with each other on the quality criteria, to secure contracts with TPA. This would be possible if the clinicians lay down code of conduct and regulate themselves by an autonomous body of clinicians. This will suitably dissuade the TPA to demand cost-cutting measures causing poor treatment outcomes as a whole. The seal of quality care by the healthcare providers is going to be their bargaining power in long run, be it with the insurance companies or the managed care.

The clinicians would rather be rewarded for being part of an organized, accountable faculty, by the patient. Further, the clinician will retain the supreme authority of the patient's treatment.

In the reformed system, the provider (the treating doctor, hospitals, diagnostic laboratory, radiology and imaging centers, etc.), will always be the vital link of the healthcare chain.

It is the fact that the present clinician must utilize optimally. What one can do is accept the change occurring and utilize it to our benefit with collective efforts. The issues of concern, the doubts can be tackled if viewed with a common eye. The arrival of a third party since time immemorial has been constructive. So it shall be in our country with diverse practice of medicine and varying population density and their unique disease patterns.

FUNCTIONING OF THIRD PARTY ADMINISTRATOR

A healthcare provider is one who, by virtue of its credentials provides healthcare services to the consumer/purchaser/customer. It may be a nursing home/hospital diagnostic center, primary care, secondary care or tertiary care provider.

Third Party Administrator System has arrived finally to India with a clearly defined identity. It is an entity which liaisons with the insurance company, the customer (the patient) and the providers to deliver healthcare. To seek the reasons for the arrival of TPA, one would have to give thought to the health insurance status in India, so far.

A patient when comes as an outpatient in a hospital has to pay for the consultation of the doctor.

Now, if the doctor feels he has to be admitted then he writes on the OPD card, the line of treatment and the duration of stay.

The patient is now asked to go to the department, which handles insurance companies, etc.

A preauthorization card is then filled with all the details like name of doctor, diagnosis, line of treatment, expenditure involved, past history, duration of stay, etc. (Every TPA has its own format for these preauthorization forms, but the information required is the same). This form is then faxed to the TPA.

The TPA then sends in an authorization slip stating the amount till what the patient is covered and the list of items no covered under insurance.

Once the patient is discharged, his signatures are taken on the final bill and all other relevant papers and reports in original are send to the TPA for claim processing. To follow right billing procedures are very important for speedy recovery of the payments.

IRDA REGULATIONS

In excrete of the powers conferred by Sections 14 and 26 of the Insurance Regulatory and Development Authority Act, 1999 (41 of 1999), read with Section 1.14A of the Life Insurance Act, 1938 (4 of 1938), the Authority, in consultation with the Insurance Advisory Committee hereby makes the following regulations, namely:

CHAPTER 1

1. **Short title and commencement:**
   i. These regulations may be called the Insurance Regulatory and Development Authority (Third Party Administrators—Health Services) Regulations, 2001.

ii. They shall come into force from the date of their publication in the Official Gazette.

2. Definitions:

In these regulations, under the context otherwise requires:

a. 'Act' mens the Insurance Act, 1938 (4 of 1938);

b. 'Agreement' means an agreement entered into between a TPA and an insurance company registered under Section 3 of the Act, prescribing the terms and conditions of health services, which may be rendered to and/or received by each of the parties thereto;

c. 'Authority' means the Insurance Regulatory and Development Authority established under sub-section (1) of Section 3 of the Insurance Regulatory and Development Authority Act, 1999 (41 of 1999);

d. 'Health Services' means all the services to be rendered by a TPA under an agreement with an insurance company in connection with 'health insurance business' or health cover as defined in regulation 2(f) of the IRDA (Registration of Indian Insurance Companies) Regulations, 2000, but does not include the business of an insurance company or the soliciting, directly or through an insurance intermediary including an insurance agent, of insurance business;

e. 'TPA' means a Third Party Administrator who, for the time being, is licensed by the Authority, and is engaged, for a fee or remuneration, by whatever name called as may be specified in the agreement with an insurance company, for the provision of health services;

f. All words and expressions used herein but not defined in these regulations but defined in the Act, or the Insurance Regulatory and Development Authority Act, 1999 (41 of 1999), shnll have the meanings respectively assigned to them in those acts.

CHAPTER 2

3. Condition of and procedure for licensing of TPA:

(1) Only a company with a share capital and registered under the Companies Act, 1956 can function as a TPA.

(2) The main or primary object of the company shall be to carry on business in India as a TPA in the health services, and on being licensed by the Authority, the company shall not engage itself in any other business.

(3) The minimum paid-up capital of the company shall be in equity shares amounting to ₹ 1 crore (Rupees One crore only).

(4) At no point of time of its functioning the TPA shall have a working capital of less than ₹ 1 crore.

(5) At least one of the directors of the TPA shall be a qualified medical doc or registered with the Medical Council of India.

(6) The aggregate holdings of equity shares by a foreign company shall not at any time exceed 26% of the paid-up equity capital of a third party administrator.

(7) Any transfer of shares exceeding 5% of the paid up share capital shall be intimated by the TPA to the Authority within 15 days of the transfer indicating the names and particulars of the transferor and transferee. *Explanation*: For the purpose of this sub-regulation 'working capital' means the difference between the aggregate of the current assets and current liabilities as on the date of reckoning.

4. (1) The TPA shall obtain from the Authority a license to function as a TPA for rendering health services.

(2) The application for license shall be made in writing to the Authority in Form TPA-1, appended to these regulations and shall be accompanied by a nonrefundable processing fee of ₹ 20,000 (Rupees Twenty Thousand only) to the Authority by way of a crossed demand draft in favor of the Authority payable in Delhi.

(3) The Authority may, in the course of examination of the application, call for such information or ask for production of such documents, as it may deem fit, and it shall be incumbent upon the applicant to furnish the same within the specified time.

(4) The Authority, on examination of the application and details furnished by the applicant, may issue a license, if it is satisfied that the applicant TPA is eligible to function as a TPA.

(5) Every TPA approved by the Authority shall pay a further sum of ₹ 30,000 (Rupees Thirty Thousand only) to the Authority as license fee before the license is granted to it and the same shall be paid to the Authority in the manner as stated in subregulation (2) of this regulation.

(6) A TPA whose application has been rejected by the Authority shall not, for a period of 2 years from the date of such a rejction, apply once again to the Authority for a license.

5. A copy of the agreement entered into between the TPA and the insurance company or any modification thereof, shall be filed, within 15 days of its execution or modification, as the case may be, with the Authority.

6. More than one TPA may be engaged by an insurance company and, similarly, a TPA can serve more than one insurance company.

7. The parties to the agreement shall agree between themselves on the scope of the contract and the facilities that have to be provided. Such an agreement shall also prescribe the remuneration that may be payable to the TPA by the insurance company.

8. (1) Every TPA shall appoint, with due intimation to the Authority, from among its directors or senior employees, a Chief Administrative Officer (CAO) or Chief Executive Officer (CEO) who shall be responsible for the proper day-to-day administration of the activities of the TPA.

(2) Such a CAO or CEO shall possess the educational qualifications mentioned in sub-regulation (4) of this regulation and also undergo a specified period of training with any institution recognized by the Authority.

(3) He shall not be:

i. Person of unsound mind
ii. An undercharged insolvent
iii. A person who had been subjected to a term of imprisonment for a period of 3 months by a court of competent jurisdiction on grounds of misconduct, misfeasance, forgery, etc.

(4) The qualifications referred to in subregulation (2) are:

i. A degree in arts, science or commerce or management or health or hospital administration or medicine.
ii. A pass in the associateship examination conducted by the Insurance Institute of India or such equivalent examination as may be recognized by the Authority and notified from time to time.
iii. Completion of practical training, as may be specified by the Authority, not exceeding one hundred hours with an institution recognized by the Authority, for these purposes, from time to time.
iv. The Authority may grant, on an application made to it, by the CAO or CEO through the TPA, time not exceeding 24 months from the date of the coming into force of these regulations for fulfilling the qualification, requirements as stated in sub-clauses (ii) and (iii) of this subregulation.

9. (1) Every application received by the Authority pursuant to these Regulations shall be considered by it within a reasonable time and its decision thereon communicated to the applicant.

(2) On an examination of the material placed before it and on the basis of enquiries made by it, where the Authority is of the opinion that the application does not deserve acceptance, it shall communicate its opinion to the applicant, who shall be given a reasonable opportunity to represent against the proposed rejection of the application.

system as a whole more fair is one of the goals of justice. There are two other values of medical ethics: truthfulness (or honesty) and dignity. Although these are important qualities, they are more standards of conduct, not overarching ethical principles.

These ethical principles all have merit, but they are not absolute and they are often in conflict. *Deontology* states that some actions are, in and of themselves, good or bad, no matter if the end result is good. *Universality* is the concept that what is right or wrong for a person is right or wrong for all people in all places and at all times. *Consequentialism* holds that the consequences of any action determine whether that action is just or right. And *utilitarianism* holds that the worth of any action is determined by the amount of good it produces. Even with all of these principles and tools at our disposal, medical ethics can be complicated and messy. There will be times in your practice where you and your patient will simply not be able to decide on one course of action or agree about a treatment. Sometimes, all we can do is try to think clearly about what is ethical, then decide on a path, act, and hope for the best.

DIFFERENCES BETWEEN ETHICS AND LEGALITY

What is ethical is not necessarily legal, and vice versa. For instance, doctors have a fiduciary and ethical duty to their patents to do no harm, tell the truth, and treat patients with respect. The law does not demand that patients receive respect or compassion; it simply demands good medicine applied according to current standards. Some have said that good ethics begins where the law ends.

In fact, ethical obligations often exceed legal standards. The law is expressed in our society through court rulings and legislation. A statute sets a conduct standard that must be met, and a court ruling is binding on all relevant parties. Ethics, on the other hand, are guidelines. And breaches of ethics are usually not legally enforceable, although providers can be sanctioned by different medical institutions or boards if a serious breach occurs. The law does have some bearing on medical ethics in several different areas. For instance, laws, legal opinions, and court rulings affect.

- *Informed consent*: A consent form is a legal document, which states that the patient has been informed about his condition and treatments, and that he understands and agrees to them.
- *Advance directives*: Directions for end-of-life care or care when the patient is incapacitated are legally binding. Although the patient does not need a lawyer to create an advance directive, it should be notarized or witnessed.

(3) Where on a complete examination of the materials, documents, information, etc., available to it, the Authority finally comes to the conclusion that an application be rejected; it shall do so by making an order in writing, which shall be communicated to the applicant at the earliest.

(4) Where the Authority decides to issue a license to the applicant to act as TPA, it shall issue the same in Form TPA-2.

10. Every license granted by the Authority to a TPA or any renewal thereof, in terms of these regulations, shal remain in force for 3 years, unless the Authority decides, either to revoke or cancel it earlier, as provided in these regulations.

11. (1) A license granted to a TPA may be renewed for a further period of 3 years on submission of the prescribed renewal application in Form TPA-3 along with a renewal fee of ₹ 30,000/- (Rupees Thirty Thousand only), at least 30 days prior to the date of expiry of the license.

(2) Any failure on the part of the TPA to get its license renewed before its expiry has to be explained to the Authority. A delayed application shall state the reasons for the delay and be accompanied by a late fee of ₹ 100/- (Rupees One Hundred only).

(3) The Authority after examining the reasons given in the application by the TPA may renew the license, if it is satisfied that the TPA was prevented by sufficient cause from applying for the renewal of its license at least 30 days (Thirty days) before the date on which the license ceased to remain in force.

(4) The Authority may, if it is satisfied that undue hardship would be caused otherwise, accept any application after the license ceased to remain in force, on payment, by the applicant of a payment of ₹ 750/- (Rupees Seven Hundred Fifty only).

12. Where a license granted by the Authority is lost or mutilated, the Authority may issue a duplicate license on payment of a fee of ₹ 1,000/- (Rupees One Thousand only) accompanied by an application in writing made by the TPA.

CHAPTER 3

Revocation or Cancelation of a Licence

13. A license granted to a TPA may after due notice be revoked or canceled by the Auhority for one or more of the reasons as provided in regulation 14.

14. The Authority may initiate action under Regulation 13 for any of the following reasons:

(1) The Authority, on the basis of information received by it, or on the basis of its own enquiry or investigation, is of the opinion that the TPA is functioning improperly and/or against the interests of the insured/policyholder or insurance company.

(2) The Authority, on the basis of information in its possession, is of the opinion that the financial condition of the TPA has deteriorated and that the TPA cannot function effectively or that the TPA has committed a breach of Regulations (3), (4), (5) and (8) of these regulations.

(3) The Authority, after enquiry or upon information, is of the opinion that the character and ownership of the TPA has changed significantly since the grant of license.

(4) The Authority, finds that the license or any renewal thereof granted to the TPA was on the basis of fraud or misrepresentation of facts.

(5) There is a breach on the part of the TPA in following the procedure or acquiring the qualifications laid down by Regulation 8 of these regulations.

(6) The TPA is subject to winding up proceedings made under Companies Act, 1956 or any statutory modification thereof.

(7) There is a breach of code of conduct prescribed by Regulation 21 of these regulations.

(8) There is violation of any directions issued by the Authority under the Act or these regulations.

15. Before proceeding under Regulation 13 to revoke or cancel a license granted to a TPA, the Authority shall grant a reasonable opportunity of being heard to the TPA.

16. (1) Every order made by the Authority under Regulation 13 shall be in writing, stating clearly the reasons for the revocation or cancelation of the license and the order shall be served on the TPA as soon as same is made.

(2) The Authority shall also send copies thereof to the insurance company with whom the TPA has subsisting agreement(s).

17. The TPA on receipt of an order under Regulation 13 shall forthwith cease to carry on its functions as TPA in relation to the insurance company and the insurance company shall immediately take such alternative steps including appointment of another TPA, as may be necessary to continue to cater to the insured/policyholders served by the TPA whose license has been revoked or canceled.

18. A TPA whole license has been revoked or canceled in terms of these regulations may file a review application with the Authority within 30 days of the receipt of the order canceling or revoking the license.

19. Within reasonable period of the receipt of the application for review but no later than 90 days thereof, the Authority shall dispose of the application after affording the applicant a reasonable opportunity of being heard.

20. Nothing contained in these regulations may be deemed to prevent or prohibit an insurance company in canceling or modifying for good and sufficient reasons an agreement that has been entered into by it with a TPA.

CHAPTER 4

21. Code of conduct for TPA:

(1) A TPA licensed under these regulations shall as far as possible act in the best professional manner.

(2) In particular and without prejudice to the generality of the provisions contained above, it shall be the duty of every TPA, its Chief Administrative Officer or Chief Executive Officer and its employees or representatives to:

(a) Establish its or his or their identity to the public and the insured/policyholder and that of the insurance company with which it has entered into an agreement.

(b) Disclose its license to the insured/policyholder/prospect.

(c) Disclose the details of the services it is authorized to render in respect of health insurance products under an agreement with an insurance company.

(d) Bring to the notice of the insurance company with whom it has an agreement, any adverse report or inconsistencies or any material fact that is relevant for the insurance company's business.

(e) Obtain all the requisite documents pertaining to the examination of an insurance claim arising out of insurance contract concluded by the insurance company with the insured/policyholder.

(f) Render necessary assistance specified under the agreement and advice to policyholders or claimants or beneficiaries in complying with the requirements for settlement of claims with the insurance company.

(g) Conduct itself/himself in a courteous and professional manner.
(h) Refrain from acting in a manner, which may influence directly or indirectly insured/policyholder of a particular insurance company to shift the insurance portfolio from the existing insurance company to another insurance company.
(i) Refrain from trading on information and the records of its business.
(j) Maintain the confidentiality of the data collected by it in the course of its agreement.
(k) Refrain from resorting to advertisements of its business or the services carried out by it on behalf of a particular insurance company, without the prior written approval by the insurance company.
(l) Refrain from inducing an insured/policyholder to omit any material information, or submit wrong information.
(m) Refrain from demanding or receiving a share of the proceeds or indemnity from the claimant under an insurance contract.
(n) Follow the guidelines/directions that may be issued down by the Authority from time to time.

CHAPTER 5

22. Maintenance and confidentiality of information:

(1) A TPA shall maintain proper records, documents, evidence and books of all transactions carried out by it on behalf of an insurance company in terms of its agreement. These books and records shall be maintained by it in accordance with accepted professional standards of record keeping and for a period of not less than 3 years. Such records, documents, evidence, books, etc., and the information contained therein shall be available to the insurance company and the Authority and access to them shall not be denied by the TPA on any ground.

(2) Every TPA shall, in maintaining the records in terms of sub-regulation (1), follow strictly the professional confidentiality between the parties as required, but this does not prevent the TPA from parting with the relevant information to any Court of Law/Tribunal, the Government, or the Authority in the case of any investigation carried out or proposed to be carried out by the Authority against the insurance company, TPA or any other person or for any other reason.

(3) If the license granted to the TPA is either revoked or canceled in terms of these regulations, the data collected by the TPA and all the books, records or documents, etc., relating to the business carried on by it with regard to an insurance company, shall be handed over to that insurance company by the TPA forthwith, complete in all respects.

CHAPTER 6

Miscellaneous Provisions

23. The Authority may, from time to time, constitute Committees consisting of members drawn from various sources including the TPAs, insurance companies, Authority, or any other persons as may be decided by the Authority to look into the proper and efficient performance of the TPAs.

24. (1) Every TPA shall furnish to the insurance company and the Authority an annual report and any other return, as may be, required by the Authority on its activities.

(2) The Annual Report, duly verified by a director of TPA and the Chief Administrative Officer or the Chief Executive Officer shall be submitted in Form TPA-4 (No. 1 to 7) within a period of 60 days of the end of its financial year or within such extended time as the Authority may grant.

(3) The TPA shall also make available to the Authority for inspection, copies of all contracts with insurance company.

CHAPTER 7

25. General:

(1) Any changes made from time to time in the agreement entered into by an insurer and a TPA shall be filed with the Authority.

(2) A TPA shall not charge any separate fees from the policyholders which it serves under the terms of the agreement with the insurance company.

(3) If any person fails to furnish any document, statement, return, etc., to the Authority, the same shall be construed as a noncompliance of the Act.

Major TPAs are:

1. Paramount Healthcare.
2. Vipul Corporation.
3. Raksha TPA.

4. E-Meditek.
5. Medicare.
6. Universal Medi-Aid Services.
7. Genins India Ltd.

Note: There are more than 45 TPAs.

CONCLUSION

The Third Party Administrator is a concept in which a patient coming to the hospital for treatment will show his/her TPA plastic card. The people dealing with insurance will then fill up the preauthorization form and obtain an authorization from the TPA and the patient need not pay anything.

The concept of TPA is a useful concept both for the patient and the hospital. The patient's benefit by availing cashless facility that is they do not have to shell out money while taking treatment and the hospitals have increased their business volume.

These days hospitals have a list of empanelled TPAs and all hospitals treat patients carrying TPA plastic cards. But on the other hand, all the TPAs are not on the panels of all hospitals. Only some of the TPAs are on the panels of all hospitals reflecting that TPAs, which are good, regular in making payments, do not demand cuts or commissions are the ones which are sought by the network hospitals.

The awareness level of patients is found to be very low. Some of the salient points pertaining to this aspect are as follows:

- Agents, which shell out these insurance policies, portray a very glorified image and the consumer/patient buys without verifying it. The patient needs to be educated about the terms and conditions of Mediclaim Policy.
- Majority of patients have a mediclaim policy, which is forced upon them by their employer so they do not pay much heed to the terms and conditions and treat this policy as a perk or a bonus. The rest either take a mediclaim policy to claim tax exemptions or due to old age and very few actually take this policy to meet any eventualities in the form of medical emergencies.
- Patients are not aware that they need to obtain an authorization from a TPA before going ahead with the treatment except in case of emergency. They feel that since they have a plastic card with them, they own the hospital and can get whatever they want.
- They are not aware that they will have to pay for the consultation in the outpatient department.

- They are also not aware that they have to be admitted for more than 24 hours to avail cashless facility and should not insist on leaving the hospital or taking a discharge before that.
- The patients also hide certain facts while filling the preauthorization form and later have difficulties getting reimbursement.
- Patients insist on getting their complete health profile investigated as in executive health check-ups, not realizing that investigations are not covered under mediclaim. Investigations followed by active management, justifying admission are all that are covered, not otherwise.
- They insist on getting their hernias or cataracts operated and when they are told that these diseases are not covered during the first year, they rant and rave or threaten the hospital with legal action.
- Patients insist on getting their dentures fixed or getting a new par of spectacles, which again is not reimbursable by the mediclaim policy.
  - Patients do not want to wait in the hospital to obtain an authorization and insist on going ahead with the surgery, which again is denied by the TPA.
  - The waiting time on an average is 2–5 hours, which in certain instances has crossed 5–10 hours.
  - The majority of patients agree that the quality of services being offer by the hospital, whether cashless or cash paying patients remains the same. Hospital authorities do not.
  - Discriminate against patients on such accounts, this is a good sign showing that the market has matured.
  - Majority of patients are not satisfied with the working of TPAs and their working style needs to be improved and made norm transparent.
  - Awareness levels of patients needs to be improved and this can be achieved by verifying claims of agents while taking the policy, going through the various terms and condition mentioned in the policy and attending the HR induction classes attentively where the HR people elaborate the terms and conditions of the policy.

The hospital should display a list of TPAs on the panel so that them is no confusion for the patient. The hospital authorities should not hide any information, which may go against the patient or delay the issue of his or her authorization letter.

The hospitals need to employ an extra staff and should train them to various aspects of TPAs running. The hospital's need to be tolerant when dealing with dissatisfied customers/patients who have been asked to wait, till an authorization is sent by the TPA. Hospitals even can have a booklet, highlighting the terms and conditions of mediclaim policies, which could be used to educate the patient, before things go out of hand. The hospitals also should not insist on authorization ever time and should provide first aid to the patient and even should go ahead in doing a life-saving procedure in an emergency. The hospitals may or may not extend discount, commissions to the TPAs depending upon their policies and procedure but it should definitely not be unethical.

Hospital using satisfied with the concept of TPOA would like to further insured their own staff through a TPA, as they feel satisfied with the services provided to them.

TPAs feel that it is a good business and a profitable one. They feel that hospital authorities should not hide any facts from then and should inform them within 24 hours of admission. They should admit a patient on its on merit and not fake emergency and give unnecessary treatment. They try to make the payment to the network hospital but end up not doing so. They do feel that at times both patients and network hospital use legal influence to get work out of them, but they seldom do so. They also share our concern that the patients consumers are not aware of the various terms and conditions and it is a collective responsibility of all three to make it more transparent and educative. People have high expectations from TPAs and when an authorization is denied to them create a scene. They feel that they should be given discount/commission but seldom insist for it.

■■Chapter 12

Power of Six Sigma in Hospital and Healthcare Management

Six Sigma methodologies can change the face of modern hospitals and healthcare delivery systems.

Corporatization and competition in healthcare sector are forcing healthcare organizations to look for new ways and means for improving their processes. This is for improving quality of the hospital's products and services and reducing patient dissatisfaction. As healthcare sector is becoming more complex, the opportunities for errors abound.

To reduce the errors and to move towards perfection, most of the corporate hospitals are now functioning at Three Sigma or Four Sigma quality levels. There is a need to breakdown the traditional boundaries that separate physicians, hospital administrators, pharmacists, technicians and nurses by shifting away from a culture of blame and by working together to systematically design safer, more effective and efficient systems. Six Sigma methodologies can help in this and can change the face of modern hospital and healthcare delivery system. Six Sigma can reduce variability and waste, translating to fewer errors, improve customer satisfaction, provide better processes, greater patient satisfaction rates, and happier and more productive staff. The popularity of Six Sigma is growing in healthcare industry. Many companies worldwide have already successfully implemented Six Sigma.

WHAT IS SIX SIGMA?

Six Sigma simply means a measure of quality that strives for perfection. It is disciplined, has a data-driven approach and methodology for eliminating defect in any process. Six Sigma provides a methodology to continue our improvement in everything we do. It is an organizational philosophy in establishing the belief of 'doing things right, first time and every time'.

FEATURES

- The term Six Sigma means standard deviation.
- Standard deviation measures how much variation exists in a distribution of data.
- Standard deviation is the key factor in determining the acceptable number of defective units found in a population.
- The target for perfection is the achievement of no more than 3.4 defects per million opportunities.
- The principles can apply to a wide variety of processes and services.
- Six Sigma projects normally follow a five-phase improvement process called DMAIC (Define, Measure, Analyze, Improve and Control).
- Six Sigma requires commitment from the whole organization.
- Six Sigma healthcare organizations have the ability and willingness to adopt contrary objectives, like reducing medical errors and getting things done faster.
- It is customer focused and raises performance at breakthrough level. Flow chart 12.1 shows the structure of a Six Sigma organization.

Flow chart 12.1 Structure of a Six Sigma organization

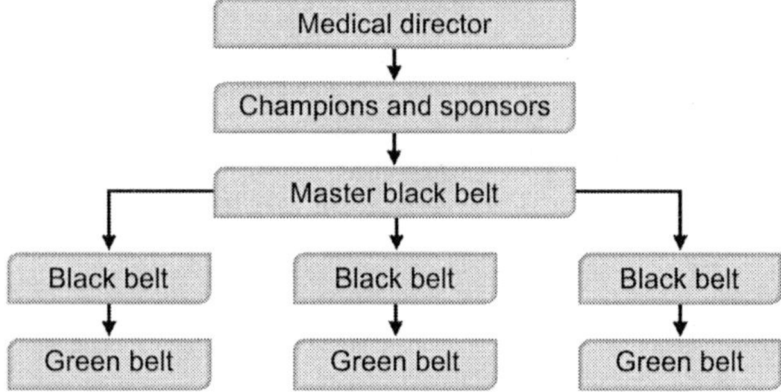

HOW AND WHEN TO USE IT?

First you need to determine your cost of poor quality. Six Sigma is complimentary to other initiatives such as ISO, JACHO, TQM, NABH, etc.

In a hospital, everything is built on integrity, trust and care. There is requirement for a fairly high level of understanding between hospital administrators, doctors, nurses, supportive staff and providers of services. Also, suppliers need to understand the sensitivities of the business. Clinches are not been discussed here, but these are life, death and every personal issue. First of all, hospital must develop new ways of doing business in order to achieve excellent clinical outcomes, patient safety and optimal financial results. The above can be achieved in the following ways:

- Understand who your consumers are and what your service is.
- Review consumer surveys, concession reports and other data.
- Screen and prioritize issues by severity, frequently/likelihood of occurrence, etc.
- Determine the internal processes causing the most dissatisfaction and pain.
- Find out why and where the defects are occurring.
- Devise ways to address these defects effectively.
- Set-up good metrics (Six Sigma places a lot of emphasis on measurement).

PHASES OF SIX SIGMA

There are six phases of Six Sigma:

1. Establish management commitment.
2. Business diagnostics.
3. Develop the management infrastructure.
4. Business process identification and metrics.
5. Project selection.
6. Deployment-training, project execution, and review.

TRAINING CENTERS FOR SIX SIGMA

Implementing Six Sigma within your healthcare organization is similar to implementing any other company-wide initiative. Six Sigma training is the most important factor that contributes to and helps modify and shape an organization's culture. Main training centers are:

1. GE Medical System delivers a Six Sigma Master Black Belt course designed exclusively for healthcare professionals.
2. Indian Statistical Institute 7, SJS Sansanwal Marg, New Delhi - 16; Phone : 011 - 51493967.
3. Quality Council of India, Institute of Engineers Building, BSZ Marg, New Delhi - 02; Phone : 011 - 23379321.

Steps in Six Sigma Methodology (DMAIC)

Define: Define the problem and improvement activity.

Measure: Measure the target metric and confirm that the measurement system is accurate. Measure the existing system. Establish valid and reliable metrics to help monitor progress towards the goals defined at the previous step.

Begin by determining the current baseline. Use exploratory and descriptive data analysis to help you understand the data.

Analyze: Analyze the system to identify ways to eliminate the gaps between the current performance of the system or process and desired goal. Use statistics to find the root cause of the problem and generate a prioritized listing of them.

Improve: Enhance the healthcare delivery system. Be creative in finding new ways to do things better, cheaper, or faster. Use project management and other operations, planning and management tools to implement new approach. Use facts and statistical methods to validate improvement.

Control: Monitor the new system. Institutionalize the improved system by modifying compensation and incentive systems, policies, procedures, services and other management systems.

MAIN PLAYERS

The key players in Six Sigma initiative are: Champions and Sponsors, Master Black Belt (MBB), Black Belt (BB) and Green Belt (GB).

Champion and sponsors: Six Sigma champions are high-level individuals who understand Six Sigma and are committed to its success. Sponsors are the owners of processes and systems who help initiate and coordinate Six Sigma improvement activities in their areas of responsibilities.

Master Black Belts (MBBs): He/she plays a vital role as a leader, project selector, coach, mentor, manager and strategic business planner. An MBB in healthcare needs a variety of skills and information in order to function effectively. An MBB teaches other sigma students and helps them achieve Green Belt and Black Belt Status.

Black Belt: He/she is a person that is part of the leadership structure for process improvement team called 'Black Belts'. They are highly-regarded personnel who have an ability to lead teams as well as to advise the management.

Green Belt: He/she is person trained in Six Sigma methodology and is a team member of a Six Sigma process improvement action team (Table 12.1).

Most Popular Outcomes from Six Sigma

Increased customer/patient satisfaction and care

- Higher satisfaction.
- Fewer complaints.
- Improved billing.
- Increased prescription accuracy.

Table 12.1 Six Sigma conversion table

Sigma	Yield	Defect per million opportunities (DPMO)
1	31.00%	6,90,000
2	69.20%	3,08,000
3	93.30%	66,800
4	99.40%	6,210
5	99.97%	230
6	99.99966%	3.4

- Reduced waiting time and variation.
- Safer and more efficient emergency services.
- Fewer medical errors and defects.
- Increased service orientation.
- Eliminate the 'I don't know' factor.

Increased physician satisfaction

- Reduced scheduling delays.
- Fewer physician complaints.
- Improved working condition of clinician and staff.

Reduced cost and savings

- Better financial and higher annual savings.
- Optimized materials management chain.
- Less rework and waste.
- Better recruiting and retention power.
- Stronger growth.

If you make Six Sigma a strategy in your hospital, the end result will get reflected in sustainable bottom line improvement. The average time taken to develop a plan and improve a process takes 3–12 months, depending on the scope and goals of the organization. Successful Six Sigma project requires cross-functional teams.

FORMULA OF SIX SIGMA

Quality (Q) × Acceptance (A) = Effectiveness (E)

Hence, the effectiveness of the result is equal to the quality of the solution time and acceptance of the idea.

Example: Six Sigma Problem Handling Strategy

Ask six questions (before solving any problem)

1. Before they walk, ask it is a problem or inconvenience?
   (If they distinguish they can solve it).

2. If, it is a problem? Write it down, if we write, we criticize the problem. (Most people are not able to do that).
3. Please write down possible causes of the problem.
4. Please write down possible solution of the problem.
5. What solution do you recommend?
   (It is a recommended, not a decision).
6. Why you recommend this?

Chapter 13

NABH, JCI: The Turning Point of Healthcare Quality System

"Hospitals do most of the right things, on most patients, most of the time. The checklist helps them to do all the right things, on all patients, all the time."

According to International Patient Safety Goal-4 (IPSG-4), the hospitals need to ensure the correct patient, correct site, correct procedure and correct surgery. WHO launched Safe Surgery Saves Lives program in 2009 to reduce the number of surgical deaths across the globe. In the complex setting of an operating room, any of the steps may be overlooked during the fast-paced preoperative, intraoperative, or postoperative preparations. So a customized checklist was introduced after sensitization and training of all operation theater (OT) users to reinforce accepted safety practices and foster better communication and team work between clinical disciplines. The aim of the checklist is to reduce the number of errors during surgery and to reduce postoperative complications. The use of the checklist reduced the rate of deaths and complications by more than one-third. The rate of major inpatient complications dropped from 11–7%, and the inpatient death rate following major operations fell from 1.5–0.8% after implementation of the checklist. Audit tool printed at the backside of the checklist is analyzed every month, to observe the shortcomings.

INTRODUCTION

Surgical care and its safe delivery affect the lives of millions of people. About 234 million major operations are performed worldwide every year and >1 million of these individuals die from complications. Surgical care has been an essential component of healthcare worldwide. There are three central problems in surgical safety—unrecognized as a public health issue, lack of data on surgery and outcomes and failure to use existing safety know-how. As the incidences of traumatic injuries, cancers and cardiovascular disease continue to rise, the impact of surgical intervention on public health systems will grow. There are between 1500 and 2500 wrong site surgery incidents every year in the US. In a survey of 1050 hand surgeons, 21% reported having performed wrong-site surgery at least once in their career.

To assist operating teams in reducing the number of these events, WHO Patient Safety—in consultation with surgeons, anesthetists, nurses, patient safety experts and patients around the world—has identified ten essential objectives for safe surgery. These are:

1. Operate on the correct patient at the correct site.
2. Use methods known to prevent harm from administration of anesthetics, while protecting the patient from pain.
3. Recognize and effectively prepare for life-threatening loss of airway or respiratory function.
4. Recognize and effectively prepare for risk of high blood loss.
5. Avoid inducing an allergic or adverse drug reaction for which the patient is known to be at significant risk.
6. Consistently use methods known to minimize the risk for surgical site infection.
7. Prevent inadvertent retention of instruments or sponges in surgical wounds.
8. Secure and accurately identify all surgical specimens.
9. Effectively communicate and exchange critical information for the safe conduct of the operation.
10. Hospitals and public health systems will establish routine surveillance of surgical capacity, volume and results.

MATERIALS AND METHODS

Execution of a customized version of WHO Safe Surgery checklist in all OTs was planned. Training programs for all the surgical staff was planned. A Steering Committee comprising of surgeons, anesthetists, technician, nurses, administration and quality department was formed which later transformed into implementation team. Role of implementation team was divided into three broad categories modification of current checklist, awareness and training, retrospective and prospective data collection. The surgical safety culture survey forms were circulated to all the OT personnel. Filled forms were collected, analyzed and discussed. It was decided that safe surgery checklist to be considered as a continuous quality improvement tool outside the medical record. Next an online survey was conducted for the staff that missed the first round of survey. Training of nurses, technicians, surgeons and anesthesiologists were conducted. Small group sessions with individual departments were planned. Also 'Incident Report Committee# was reconstituted. A list of possible postsurgical complications were prepared which included 30-day mortality, postoperative blood transfusion of 4 or more units within 72 hours, pulmonary embolism, stroke, infection of surgical site, cardiac arrest requiring CPR, myocardial infarction, major disruption of wound, unplanned return to OR, coma of >24 hours, unplanned intubation, sepsis/septic shock/SIRS, acute renal failure, ventilator use for 48 hours or more, VAP, vascular graft failure.

In order to implement the checklist during surgery, a single person must be made responsible for performing the safety checks on the list. It was decided that this designated checklist coordinator will often be a circulating nurse.

The checklist divides the operation into three phases, each corresponding to a specific time period in the normal flow of a procedure—the period before induction of anesthesia, the period after induction and before surgical incision, and the period during or immediately after wound closure but before removing the patient from the operating room. In each phase, the checklist coordinator must be permitted to confirm that the team has complete its tasks before it proceeds onward. As operating teams become familiar with the steps of the checklist, they integrate the checks into their familiar work patterns and verbalize their completion of each step without the explicit intervention of the checklist into its work with maximum efficiency and minimum disruption while aiming to accomplish the steps effectively.

All steps to be checked verbally with the appropriate team member to ensure that the key actions have been performed. Therefore, before induction of anesthesia, the person coordinating the checklist verbally review with the anesthetist and patient (when possible) that patient identity has been confirmed, that the procedure and site are correct and that consent for surgery has been given. The coordinator will visualize and verbally confirm that the operative site has been marked (if appropriate) and will review with the anesthetist the patient's risk of blood loss, airway difficulty and allergic safety check has been completed. Ideally, the surgeon be present during this phase as the surgeon may have a better idea of anticipated blood loss, allergies, or other complicating patient factors. However, the surgeon's presence is not essential for completing this part of the checklist.

Before skin incision, each team member introduces him or herself by name and role. If already partway through the operative day together, the team can simply confirm that everyone in the room is known to each other. The team confirms out loud that they are performing the correct operation on the correct patient and the correct site and then verbally review with one another, in turn, the critical elements of their plans for the operation, using the checklist for guidance.

They also confirm that prophylactic antibiotics have been administered within the previous 60 minutes and that essential imaging is displayed, as appropriate. Before leaving the operating room, the team reviews the operation that was performed, completion of sponge and instrument counts and the labeling of any surgical specimens obtained. It also reviews any equipment malfunctions or issues that need to be addressed. Finally, the team discusses key plans and concerns regarding postoperative management and recovery before moving the patient from the operating room.

Having a single person leading the checklist process is essential for its success. In the complex setting of an operating room, any of the steps may be overlooked during the fast-paced preoperative, intraoperative, or postoperative preparations. Designating a single person to confirm completion of each step of the checklist can ensure that safety steps are not omitted in the rush to move forward with the next phase of the operation. Until team members are familiar with the steps involved, the checklist process.

A possible disadvantage of having a single person lead the checklist is that an antagonistic relationship might be established with other operating team members. The checklist coordinator can and should prevent the team from progressing to the next phase of the operation until each step is satisfactorily addressed, but in doing so may alienate or irritate other team members. Therefore, hospitals must carefully consider which staff member is most suitable for this role and empower the designated staff.

RESULTS AND ANALYSIS

The goal of checklist is not role recitation or to frustrate workflow. The checklist is intended to give teams a simple, efficient set of priority checks for improving effective teamwork and communication and to encourage active consideration of the safety of patients in every operation performed. In a survey of 100 (30 doctors, 40 nurses, 30 technicians), 78.6% mentioned the checklist was easy to use. 79.2% says the checklist has improved operating room safety while 21% are not sure and 18.3% says communication has improved through use of the checklist. Finally 78.2% say, if I were to be operated, I would surely want the checklist to be used.

Wrong site draped in one surgery, radial pack gauze missing, graft size not prepared, blood not arranged for a surgery, allergy not mentioned in preoperative checklist and evaluation form, antibiotic prophylaxis not given before time out, before sign in, the need to secure central IV access not evaluated, are among the few errors prevented by the use of the checklist. Doing this has improved the chances of detection of possible errors and has helped the unit in implementing timely interventions to prevent serious outcomes. Hence, the checklist solves two purposes—ensuring consistency in patient safety and introducing (or maintaining) a culture that values achieving it.

Impact on Financials

Implementation of checklist leads to: (1) less SSI due to timely administered of antibiotics, 1 hour prior to surgery, (2) decreased ALOS, (3) decreased rate of return to OT, (4) elimination of error mitigates chances of litigation and compensation.

Impact on Patients

(1) Financial savings due to decrease ALOS on account of decrease complications, decrease duration of surgery, (2) Better outcome on account of (a) better planning, safer anesthesia, (b) timely administration of correct medication and elimination of errors, and (3) Patient safety.

Impact on Employees

(1) Team work and better communication, (2) Smoother and quicker processes, (3) Decreased turnaround time, (4) Skill enhancement, (5) Improved staff morale, and (6) Secure working environment.

To build a culture of safety in our healthcare organizations, healthcare leaders must ensure that, in their organizations, 'incidents,' such as surgical mishaps must be routinely reported without the fear of unjust retribution on the part of the unfortunate healthcare worker. When people are not afraid to report adverse incidents because of the existence of a 'just culture' where, when things go wrong, no one is immediately assigned blame (blame culture), only then will we be able to collect accurate and honest data about incidents, analyze them and learn important lessons from them and, in the process, improve our systems and processes so that the care that we provide will be safer.

DISCUSSION

The checklist should be modified to account for differences among facilities with respect to their processes, the culture of their operating rooms and the degree of familiarity each team member has with each other. However, removing safety steps because they cannot be accomplished in the existing environment or circumstances is strongly discouraged. The safety steps should inspire effective change that will bring an operating team to comply with each and every element of the checklist.

Modification of the checklist should be undertaken with a critical eye. Surgeons, anesthetists, and nurses should be involved in the modification process and the resulting checklist tried in simulated and real-life situations in order to ensure its functionality. Actively seeking inputs from nurses, anesthetists, surgeons and others are important not only in helping to make appropriate modification but also in creating the feeling of 'ownership' that is central to adoption and permanent practice change.

Monitoring and evaluation of outcomes is an essential component of surgical care. Many facilities and departments already engage in this process; additional data collection is neither recommended nor encouraged if such a system is already in place and proves useful to the clinicians and staff as a means of improving the quality of care. However, in hospitals where results of surgical care are not routinely tracked and postoperative complications are not recorded, or where surveillance mechanisms are not sufficient to identify poor practices, patient safety checklists become law in Nevada. Now government is picking up the baton.

CONCLUSION

The aim of this checklist is to reinforce accepted safety practices and foster better communication and teamwork between clinical disciplines. The checklist is intended as a tool for use by clinicians interested in improving the safety of their operations and reducing unnecessary surgical deaths and complications. Advantages of using a checklist are customizable to local setting and needs, Deployable in an incremental fashion, supported by scientific evidence and expert consensus, evaluated in diverse settings around the world, ensures adherence to established safety practices, minimal resources required to implement a far-reaching safety intervention.

The goal of the surgical safety checklist is to help insure that teams consistently follow critical safety steps and thereby minimize the most common and avoidable risk that endanger lives and safety of surgical patients. It evaluates the current state of safety practices and standards at our facility and identifies area for improvement.

Use of the surgical safety checklist has demonstrably improved compliance with basic standards of surgical care in diverse hospitals around the world. While the relationship between adherence to standards and decreases in complication rates is likely multifactorial, improving the safety and reliability of surgical care can save lives and promote confidence in the health system.

Leave aside the other advantages, if 2 minutes taken to read aloud one sheet of paper could prevent wrong surgeries (both on wrong patients and on wrong site), it would be more than worth its weight in gold. The moral, legal and financial cost of wrong surgery is unquantifiable.

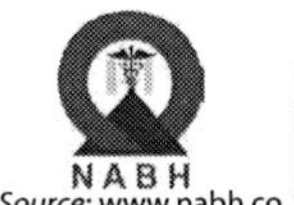

Source: www.nabh.co

NABH: THE TURNING POINT OF HEALTHCARE QUALITY SYSTEM

The healthcare sector in India has witnessed marked changes over the past few years. There is a growing demand for quality healthcare services. That has called for a closer look at the healthcare delivery systems and the necessity to introduce quality assurance mechanisms. The accreditation of hospitals assumes particular significance in this context. Accreditation relies on establishing technical competence of healthcare organizations in terms of certain standards in delivering services. With medical tourism/medical value travel to India gaining momentum, it was essential to cater to this select clientele. The obvious answer to this was accreditation conforming to global standards. A few Indian hospitals applied for and received accreditation by the Joint Commission International (JCI). There was a strongly felt need to establish a national accreditation structure, suitable to Indian conditions as well as credible internationally. A concrete step towards accreditation was finally taken with the launching of the hospital accreditation programme by the Quality Council of India (QCI) in 2006, with the setting up of the National Accreditation Board for Hospitals and Healthcare Providers (NABH) to establish and operate accreditation programmes for healthcare organizations.

The NABH standards provide a framework for quality assurance and quality improvement, while focusing on patient safety and quality of care. The standards are in consonance with the framework specified by ISQua (International Society for Quality in Healthcare Inc). Initial responses indicate that with accreditation in place, visible benefits have been noticed. These include a strong culture of safety that has been inculcated, a decrease in the incidence of adverse events, constant monitoring of quality within the system, etc. The best impact assessment criteria would be the success rates for various diagnostic and therapeutic procedures and the cure rates for various therapeutic applications. However, such comprehensive quantitative data is not available at present to measure parameters like infection control rates, mortality rates, surgical outcomes, etc. Apart from selecting outcome criteria, a patient satisfaction survey could also be carried out to capture the interpersonal aspects of care. NABH would need to start a process of impact assessment postaccreditation, on the basis of quantitative indicators. The possible parameters for assessment need to be determined and a standardized mechanism of measurement needs to be evolved to enable uniform assessment of hospitals, benchmarked against established national standards.

It is now well established that with the transformation taking place in the healthcare sector today, there is an obvious need for healthcare entities to focus on quality, and ultimately move towards accreditation. Accreditation of hospitals in India has so far been confined to metros and urban areas and has gained currency with corporate players and private healthcare providers. This has touched only a fringe of the healthcare delivery system in the country. While appreciating that the concept is as yet in its nascent stage, it is imperative that accreditation attains wider reach and gains greater acceptability, particularly in nonurban areas and eventually the rural hinterlands. It is essential to look at the possible steps required to carry the process forward.

To cater to its growing demand, NABH would soon roll out a slew of initiatives to strengthen its functioning.

Seeing the reams of files awaiting inspection at NABH's office in Delhi, who would believe that the quality and accreditation wave in healthcare started in India only a few years back! With 201 hospitals already NABH accredited and over 569 applications awaiting response, there's no denying that NABH accreditation has become a rage. The swelling demand for an accreditation that comes under the purview of the quasi-Government body? Quality Council of India? is quite an interesting phenomenon. And to think that most of the board members are veteran administrators from private and public sectors doing honorary work and the assessors also don't get major monetary benefit! But the most interesting development in recent times has been change of the old guard and constitution of a new board. The pre- and postimpact of accreditation can be seen in structures processes and outcomes of the HCOs as one proceeds towards the accreditation. However, the patient is the biggest beneficiary of quality drive.

As the awareness increased amongst the healthcare organizations about quality, and dialogue initiated between NABH and government, industry and organizations, scenario started changing. Department of AIDS Control, Ministry of Health and Family Welfare relied on NABH to start an accreditation program for opioid substitution therapy (OST) Centers after getting convinced that this will lead to better care and safety of patients visiting such centers. Central Government Health Scheme of Government of India and Ex-Servicemen Contributory Health Scheme of Ministry of Defense requires private hospitals to gain accreditation in order to be empanelled with them. It has helped boosting the concept of quality and patient safety across such hospitals. Recently, officials of Government Sponsored Health

Insurance Schemes (Rajiv Aarogyasri, Vajpayee Aarogyasri, Chief Minister's Comprehensive Health Insurance Scheme, Jeevandayi Aarogya Yojana, Rashtriya Swasthya Bima Yojana) have initiated discussion on improving quality of care in hospitals empanelled under these schemes. There are thousands of hospitals covered under these schemes and therefore, this move may bring drastic change in the care delivery. It is important to note that major discussion points were defining Standard Treatment Protocols, alignment of empanelment criteria with NABH accreditation standards and role of NABH in improving quality. There are number of workshops on Infection Control and Patient Safety being organized by hospitals and industry. In variably, NABH remains a partner/organizer in all such events. A very unique and innovative program 'Safe-I' has recently been started which focuses on infection control and prevention in hospitals. To strengthen patient care and safety, another innovative program on 'Nursing Excellence': is going to be launched soon. Strong need has already been felt about collecting data and analysis in order to gain insight on what is happening after implementing accreditation/quality improvement activities in relation to care and safety. NABH has recently started collecting quarterly data from accredited organizations on select indicators, however, a robust analysis and feedback mechanism is lacking. They are in the process of developing better tools to collect, analyze and disseminate data to the participating organizations. Need for a research/study in this area is to be emphasized.

In India, ISQua has played a vital role in the journey of healthcare quality and patient safety. NABH standards for hospital accreditation and entire organization follow ISQua International Principles and Standards. This has helped Indian accreditation program to convince people and stakeholders about the role and importance of quality and safety.

India's quality movement got its richly-deserved recognition when a constituent board of the Quality Council of India (QCI), the NABH, was invited by the Philippines healthcare sector to improve the quality of healthcare at their facilities. The move was part of the Philippines agenda of providing universal access to high-quality healthcare conforming to international benchmarks. The NABH-I's foray to the Philippines also means that the country's medical tourism products and programmes would be developed and brought up to be at par with the best in the world. This is an opportunity for the Philippines to benchmark with the best in the world. Accreditation with NABH-International will result in healthcare organizations that are globally competitive and attuned to the needs and requirements of international patients. While medical travel does generate drive for international accreditation, it ultimately benefits larger segment of society within the country, as it triggers quality improvement opportunity for health industry. Developed and successfully implemented in India, NABH standards have been accredited by ISQua—the international body that grants approval to healthcare accreditation programmes—as a seal of excellence under its International Accreditation Programme in 2008. With that NABH has acquired a unique status: it has become one of the few accrediting organizations in the world to achieve this recognition. "This is the first time that the NABH is taking its services outside India. We chose Philippine to be our first international venture because we believe that the Philippines faces similar healthcare challenges as India." In the first two years of NABH implementation, the quality of healthcare delivery in India improved a lot. "It helped us become one of the leading providers of healthcare in the world. We would like to carry out the same mission in the Philippines". Launched under the aegis of NABH-I's exclusive Philippines' representative HealthCORE. The globally-recognized accreditation programme has a wide vision: it seeks to improve the conditions, systems, processes and skills of healthcare facilities and professionals in the country through internationally recognized and accredited standards. NABH will help training of consultants and assessors for the hospitals, spas, clinics and other healthcare services providers in the Philippines. The Philippine general hospital along with two spas, a dental center, an ambulatory clinic and an eye center have been indentified under the pilot project for accreditation. The NABH accreditation was less costly than other similar groups like the Joint Commission International (JCI). All these bodies, including NABH, are accredited by the International Society for Quality in Healthcare (ISQua). "With NABH International's stringent accreditation process, we can ensure that our hospitals will provide safe and effective healthcare of the highest quality and best value. At its heart, NABH is all about improving the overall healthcare system for the benefit of patients."

According to NABH Engineering services of a hospital are the key to conversion of all the inputs into a successful output. Quality assurance is outcome oriented and process driven. It is outcome, i.e. the patient improvement and satisfaction, which is the most important. However, outcome depends on the effectiveness of the process of delivery of patient care which in turn depends on the efficiency of the engineering department. Although some components like electric supply, communication and information technology (IT) are of crucial significance (without which patient care will come to a standstill), all components are important in the sense that any problem with any component is going to affect the outcome of patient care and satisfaction. For effective and optimum level of functioning, therefore, it is essential that the infrastructure be of high quality. Every hospital must have a proper well staffed and equipped department of engineering services and must implement the maintenance program in a well planned and efficient manner. This is one department where one can say with certainty that a penny spent is worth a pound saved.

TOOLS USED FOR MAKING NABH POPULAR

- *Awareness of the concept*: The concept of accreditation can only spread with rising awareness and change in mindsets about the necessity to focus on quality, which may not be an immediate revenue earner, but will spell long-term benefits.
- *Role of the government*: A body of opinion suggests that the Ministry of Health and Family Welfare can act as a key enabler in popularizing the concept of accreditation through public awareness and sensitization programmes via the print and electronic media. The stakeholders—healthcare providers and patients alike—must be convinced of the long-term benefits of accreditation as against any immediate short-term gains/increase in revenue prospects. Government resources need to be allocated for the purpose.
- *CGHS empanelment*: Central Government Health Scheme (CGHS) empanelment could serve as a driver propelling smaller healthcare organizations/newly set-up hospitals to go in for accreditation. It could be made mandatory that accreditation would serve as a basic criterion for empanelment under the Central Government Health Scheme.
- *Costs of accreditation*: A potent factor weighing for/against accreditation may well be the costs of accreditation and the capabilities of smaller healthcare providers to raise resources for the purpose. An incentive to public hospitals may be considered in the form of the hospitals being allowed to levy user charges and thereafter utilizing the proceeds to better hospital services.
- *Role of industry*: Industry bodies could also play a key role in spreading awareness and sensitizing stakeholders.
- *Corporates driving accreditation*: It would be useful to understand that corporates can play a major role in driving the accreditation process. They could take a lead in ensuring that their medical care tie-ups are with accredited hospitals.
- *Insurance companies driving accreditation*: Globally, medical insurance is linked to accredited delivery centers. Once there are a sizeable number of accredited hospitals, a directive mandating medical reimbursement to be allowed only from accredited hospitals will be a welcome move, which is likely to induce hospitals to embrace accreditation.

- *Packaged preaccreditation programmes*: In addition to sensitization programmes aimed at inducing small healthcare providers to go in for accreditation, on a more practical level, it would be extremely useful to these providers if packaged programmes for accreditation could be offered to them in terms of the budget to be allotted for the purpose, and the provision of advisory/technical services through a panel of consultants. This would enable the healthcare providers to get a one-time preaccreditation packaged service. This will minimize efforts that would otherwise be necessary to seek out consultants for each individual technical/advisory service that will be required prior to accreditation.

INITIATIVE BY GOVERNMENT OF GUJARAT FOR NABH

In an effort to improve the quality of healthcare in the state, the Government of Gujarat has introduced total quality management (TQM) system in its key medical institutions. The system covers the state's Medical College Hospitals and District Hospitals, as per the NABH and NABL standards. A look at the state's successful journey towards quality in its healthcare systems. It's a success story par excellence. Less than 18 months after the state government signed a memorandum of understanding (MoU) with Quality Council of India (QCI), a quality revolution of sorts has taken place in Gujarat's healthcare systems. An essential component of this change is the growing recognition of the need for quality in health. programmes, which have, in the past, been beset with such problems as limited capacity, lack of programme standards and guidelines, and an obsession with quantified targets rather than client satisfaction. Worried by the lack of adequate standards; in public health services and the absence of written policies and procedures for healthcare delivery, the Government of Gujarat has identified quality health services and the efficiency of government-managed hospitals as key contributors for building trust and confidence for the hospitals in the hearts of the citizen of the state.

The new quality parameters introduced by the state government seek to address problems of poor sanitation and cleanliness in hospitals, staff shortage in every category, damaged and pathetic condition of the building and campus, poor signage system in hospitals, absence of patient satisfaction monitoring system, lack of a measurable parameter for patient safety and absence of legal compliances. The total quality management (TQM) system was introduced to tackle all these problems, as also the issues of lack of accountability and planning in delivery of care to patients, lack of blood bank/storage facility in some hospitals, and the absence of quality standards such as medical audit, management of medication, patient care, facility management and safety, information management system and infection control.

The idea behind the introduction of the TQM system was to provide quality healthcare by improving health infrastructure of the state and meeting the healthcare needs and expectations of the common man of Gujarat at all levels of the healthcare delivery system, as per the National Healthcare Quality Standards. The new system sought to develop a healthcare system based on Total Quality Management principles and application of information technology to achieve efficiency in operations, as well as faster and standard communication across the state, using the latest IT solutions. Simultaneously, it strived to develop a pool of healthcare professionals in the public health sector, trained in the implementation of healthcare quality standards and information technology, to bring productivity and effectiveness in the healthcare delivery system of the state. Under the system, a policy framework for NABH and NABL accreditation of public hospitals and laboratories, as approved by the state government, was launched, and empanelment of NABH and NABL consultants was undertaken in coordination with QCI.

Appointment of assistant hospital administrators (AHAs) for Government Hospitals/Medical Colleges in a phased manner, and training at various levels, were among the key mechanisms of the TQM system which also involved the development of quality steering committee for the state at all levels and nomination of district quality assurance officers. In the brief period of its implementation so far, the TQM system has led to major benefits for the state's healthcare system, as evidenced in the growing level of patient satisfaction and significant improvement in the various performance measures, as evaluated by medical, administrative, financial and infrastructural indicators.

Patients have benefited immensely in terms of the quality of care, access to quality focused organizations and to privileged medical staff, better safety conditions and pain management, safer transport and continuity of care. The benefits of TQM have not, however, been limited to the patients. The hospital staffs have also gained in terms of their professional development, increased professional satisfaction, leadership and ownership, and a good working environment. For the community at large, this has translated into a quality revolution, marked by access to comparative database and disaster preparedness (epidemic and physical). Needless to say, a commitment has been made.

A commitment to continued training of personnel to imbibe quality as a culture among its people. A commitment to strictly adhere to the quality manual in all its operations. A commitment to be abreast of the latest technology to become innovative. A commitment to be the best. And as it goes along, the state government plans to extend its TQM system to the medical colleges, district hospitals, blood banks and laboratories across the state accredited by NABH/ NABL. It also plans to work in close coordination with QCI to develop a sustainable and viable quality accreditation programme for CHCs and PHCs which can be replicated nationally, while managing work-load with assured quality.

INTRODUCTION TO NABH

National Accreditation Board for Hospitals and Healthcare Providers (NABH) is a constituent board of Quality Council of India, set-up to establish and operate accreditation programme for healthcare organizations. The board is structured to cater to much desired needs of the consumers and to set benchmarks for progress of health industry. The board while being supported by all stakeholders including industry, consumers, government, has full functional autonomy in its operation. NABH was established in 2006 with a vision to be apex national healthcare accreditation and quality improvement body, functioning at par with global benchmarks. NABH has its mission operate accreditation and allied programs in collaboration with stakeholders focusing on patient safety and quality of healthcare based upon national/international standards, through process of self and external evaluation. There are four main following core values on which NABH works:

1. *Credibility*: Provide credible and value addition services.
2. *Responsiveness*: Willingness to listen and continuously improving service.
3. *Transparency*: Openness in communication and freedom of information to its stakeholders.
4. *Innovation*: Incorporating change, creativity, continuous learning and new ideas to improve the services being provided.

NABH PROVIDES ACCREDITATION TO HEALTHCARE SETUPS

- Allopathic clinics
- AYUSH hospitals
- Blood banks
- Dental facilities
- Hospitals
- Medical imaging services
- Medical laboratory programme

- OST center
- PHC/CHC accreditation
- Small healthcare organizations
- Wellness center

NABH STRUCTURE (FLOW CHART 13.1)

Flow chart 13.1 NABH structure

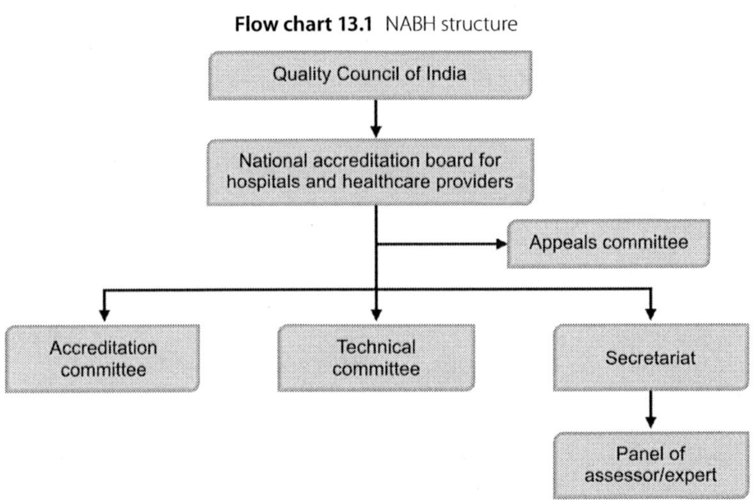

Accreditation Committee

The main functions of accreditation committee are as follows:

- Recommending to board about grant of accreditation or otherwise based on evaluation of assessment reports and other relevant information.
- Approval of the major changes in the scope of accreditation including enhancement and reduction, in respect of accredited hospitals.
- Recommending to the board on launching of new initiatives.

Technical Committee

The main functions of technical committee are as follows:

- Drafting of accreditation standards and guidance documents
- Periodic review of standards.

Appeals Committee

The appeal committee addresses appeals made by the hospitals against any adverse decision regarding accreditation taken by the NABH. The adverse decisions may relate to the following:

- Refusal to accept an application
- Refusal to proceed with an assessment
- Corrective action requests
- Changes in accreditation scope
- Decisions to deny, suspend or withdraw accreditation, and
- Any other action that impedes the attainment of accreditation.

NABH SECRETARIAT

The secretariat coordinates the entire activities related to NABH accreditation to hospitals and healthcare organizations.

ORGANIZATIONAL STRUCTURE

Panel of assessors and experts NABH has a panel of trained and qualified assessors for assessment of hospitals.

- *Principal assessor*: The principal assessor is overall responsible for conducting the preassessments and final assessments of the hospitals.
- *Assessors*: NABH has empanelled experts for assessment of hospitals. They are trained by NABH on hospital accreditation and various assessment techniques. The assessors are responsible for evaluating the hospital's compliance with NABH standards.

HOSPITAL ACCREDITATION

Hospital accreditation is a public recognition by a National Healthcare Accreditation Body, of the achievement of accreditation standards by a Healthcare Organization, demonstrated through an independent external peer assessment of that organization's level of performance in relation to the standards.

In India, heath system currently operates within an environment of rapid social, economical and technical changes. Such changes raise the concern for the quality of healthcare. Hospital is an integral part of healthcare system. Accreditation would be the single most important approach for improving the quality of hospitals. Accreditation is an incentive to improve capacity of national hospitals to provide quality of care. National accreditation system for hospitals ensure that hospitals, whether public or private, national or expatriate, play there expected roles in national heath system.

Confidence in accreditation is obtained by a transparent system of control over the accredited hospital and an assurance given by the accreditation body that the accredited hospital constantly fulfills the accreditation criteria.

NABH provides accreditation to hospitals in a nondiscriminatory manner regardless of their ownership, legal status, size and degree of independence. International society for quality in healthcare (ISQua) has accredited 'Standards for Hospitals,' 3rd edition, November 2011 developed by National Accreditation Board for Hospitals and Healthcare Providers (NABH, India) under its International Accreditation Programme for a cycle of 4 years (April 2012 to March 2016). The approval of ISQua authenticates that NABH standards are in consonance with the global benchmarks set by ISQua. The hospitals accredited by NABH have international recognition as ISQua is an international body which grants approval to accreditation bodies in the area of healthcare as mark of equivalence of accreditation program of member countries. NABH is a member of ISQua Accreditation Council. NABH is an institutional member as well as a member of the Accreditation Council of the International Society for Quality in HealthCare (ISQua). NABH is the founder member of proposed Asian Society for Quality in Healthcare (ASQua) being registered in Malaysia. NABH is a member of International Steering Committee of WHO Collaborating Center for Patient Safety as a nominee of ISQua Accreditation Council. Hence, it provides boost to medical tourism.

NABH standards for hospitals prepared by technical committee contains complete set of standards for evaluation of hospitals for grant of accreditation. The standards provide framework for quality of care for patients and quality improvement for hospitals. The standards help to build a quality culture at all level and across all the function of hospital. NABH first edition came in 2006 with 10 chapters, 100 standards and 503 objective elements. Second edition in 2009 where objective elements increases from 503 to 514 and now in 3rd edition NABH standards has ten chapters incorporating 102 standards and 636 objective elements.

NABH STANDARDS

Patient Centered Standards

- Access, assessment and continuity of care (AAC)
- Care of patient (COP)
- Management of medication (MOM)
- Patient right and education (PRE)
- Hospital infection control (HIC).

Organization Centered Standards

- Continuous quality improvement (CQI)

- Responsibility of management (ROM)
- Facility management and safety (FMS)
- Human resource management (HRM)
- Information management system (IMS).

ASSESSMENT CRITERIA

A hospital willing to be accredited by NABH must ensure the implementation of NABH standards in its organization. The assessment team will check the implementation of NABH standards in organization. The hospital shall be able to demonstrate to NABH assessment team that all NABH standards, as applicable, are followed.

PREPARING FOR NABH ACCREDITATION

Hospital management shall first decide about getting accreditation for its hospital from NABH. It is important for a hospital to make a definite plan of action for obtaining accreditation and nominate a responsible person to co-ordinate all activities related to seeking accreditation. An official nominated should be familiar with existing hospital quality assurance system.

Hospital shall procure a copy of standards from the NABH Secretariat against payment. Further clarification regarding standards can be got from NABH Secretariat in person, by post, by e-mail or on telephone.

The hospital looking for accreditation shall understand the NABH assessment procedure. The hospitals shall ensure that the standards are implemented in the organization.

The hospitals can download the application form for NABH accreditation from the web-site. The applicant hospital must have conducted self-assessment against NABH standards at least 3 months before submission of application and must ensure that it complies with NABH standards.

NABH ACCREDITATION PROCEDURE

Application for Accreditation

The hospital shall apply to NABH in the prescribed application form. The application shall be accompanied with the following:

- Prescribed application fee as detailed in the application form
- Signed copy of 'Terms and Conditions for Maintaining NABH Accreditation,' available free on the web-site
- Filled in self-assessment toolkit, available free on the web-site

- Quality/hospital manual (as per NABH standards) and other NABH relevant documents, i.e. different policies and procedures of the hospital.

Self-assessment toolkit is for self-assessing itself against NABH standards. The self-assessment shall be done by the hospital in a stringent manner and if at the time of preassessment it is found that there is a significant difference between the self-assessment and the preassessment report then the organization shall apply for final assessment not earlier than six months from the date of completion of preassessment. The applicant hospital must apply for all its facilities and services being rendered from the specific location. NABH accreditation is only considered for hospital's entire activities and not for a part of it.

Scrutiny of Application

NABH Secretariat receives the application form and after scrutiny of application for its completeness in all respect, acknowledgement letter for the application shall be issued to the hospital with a unique reference number. The hospital shall be required to quote this reference number in all future correspondence with NABH.

Preassessment

NABH appoints a Principal Assessor/Assessment Team who is responsible for preassessment of healthcare organization. NABH forwards the application form, documents, procedures, self-assessment toolkit to the Principal Assessor/Assessment Team.

Objective of Preassessment

- Check the preparedness of the hospital for final assessment
- Review the scope of accreditation and ascertain the requirement of the number of assessors and the duration of the accreditation
- Review of the documentation system of the hospital
- Explain the methodology to be adopted for assessment.

The principal assessor shall submit a preassessment report in the format specified in the document 'Preassessment Guidelines and Forms'. Copy of the report is handed over to the organization after the assessment and original sent to NABH Secretariat. The hospital shall be required to pay the requisite annual fee before the final assessment.

Final Assessment

The hospital is required to take necessary corrective action to the nonconformities pointed out during the preassessment. The final assessment involves comprehensive review of hospital functions and services. NABH shall appoint an assessment team. The team shall include principal assessor (already appointed) and the assessors. The total number of assessors appointed shall depend on the number of beds and services provided. The date of final assessment shall be agreed upon by the hospital management and assessors. Assessment shall be conducted on hospital's department and services.

Based on the assessment by the assessors, the assessment report is prepared by the principal assessor in a format prescribed by NABH.

The details of nonconformity(ies) observed during the assessment are handed over to the hospital by the principal assessor and detailed assessment report is sent to NABH.

Scrutiny of Assessment Report

NABH shall examine the assessment report. The report is taken to the accreditation committee. Depending on the score and compliance to standard would decided the award of accreditation or otherwise as per details given below:

- *Preaccreditation entry level*: Conditions for qualifying to this award are as below:
  - All the regulatory legal requirements should be fully met
  - No individual standard should have more than two zeros
  - The average score for individual standard must not be less than five
  - The average score for individual chapter must be more than five
  - The overall average score for all standards must exceed five.

  The validity period for preaccreditation entry level stage is from a minimum 6 months to a maximum of 18 months. It means that a hospital placed under this award cannot apply for assessment before six months.
- *Preaccreditation progressive level*: Conditions for qualifying to this award are as below:
  - All the regulatory legal requirements should be fully met
  - No individual standard should have more than two zeros
  - The average score for individual standard must not be less than five
  - The average score for individual chapter must be more than six
  - The overall average score for all standards must exceed six.

  The validity period for preaccreditation progressive level stage is from a minimum 3 months to a maximum of 12 months. It means that a hospital placed under this award cannot apply for assessment before 3 months.
- *Accredited*: Conditions for qualifying for accreditation are as below:
  - All the regulatory legal requirements should be fully met
  - No individual standard should have more than one zero to qualify

- The average score for individual standards must not be less than five
- The average score for individual chapter must not be less than seven
- The overall average score for all standards must exceed seven.

The validity period for accreditation is 3 years subject to terms and conditions.

Note: The awards are only valid till the next assessment or until that last date of validity, whichever is earlier. Awards cannot be renewed. Depending upon the progress, the organization is eligible to get either a preaccreditation entry level award, preaccreditation progressive level award or accredited. If the organization under the stage of preaccreditation entry level and preaccreditation progressive level does not show any improvement during the next assessment they shall be encouraged to apply afresh. Issue of accreditation certificate NABH shall issue an accreditation certificate to the hospital with a validity of three years. The certificate has a unique number and date of validity. The certificate is accompanied by scope of accreditation. The applicant hospital must make all payment due to NABH, before the issue of certificate. All decision taken by NABH regarding grant of accreditation shall be open to appeal by the hospitals, to chairman NABH.

Surveillance and reassessment accreditation to a hospital shall be valid for a period of three years. NABH conducts one surveillance of the accredited hospitals in one accreditation cycle of three years. The surveillance visit will be planned during the 2nd year, i.e. after 18 months of accreditation. The hospitals may apply for renewal of accreditation at least six months before the expiry of validity of accreditation for which reassessment shall be conducted. NABH may call for unannounced visit, based on any concern or any serious incident reported upon by an individual or organization or media.

BENEFITS OF ACCREDITATION

"A public recognition of the achievement of accreditation standards by a healthcare organization, demonstrated through an independent external peer assessment of that organization's level of performance in relation to the standards".

Accreditation benefits all stake holders. Patients are the biggest beneficiary. Accreditation results in high quality of care and patient safety. The patients get services by credential medical staff. Rights of patients are respected and protected. Patient satisfaction is regularly evaluated.

The staff in a accredited healthcare organization are satisfied lot as it provides for continuous learning, good working environment, leadership and above all ownership of clinical processes.

Accreditation to a healthcare organization stimulates continuous improvement. It enables the organization in demonstrating commitment to quality care. It raises community confidence in the services provided by the healthcare organization. It also provides opportunity to healthcare unit to benchmark with the best.

Finally, accreditation provides an objective system of empanelment by insurance and other third parties. Accreditation provides access to reliable and certified information on facilities, infrastructure and level of care.

Hospital accreditation is a public recognition by a National Healthcare Accreditation Body, of the achievement of accreditation standards by a Healthcare Organization, demonstrated through an independent external peer assessment of that organization's level of performance in relation to the standards.

In India, Heath System currently operates within an environment of rapid social, economical and technical changes. Such changes raise the concern for the quality of healthcare. Hospital is an integral part of healthcare system. Accreditation would be the single most important approach for improving the quality of hospitals. Accreditation is an incentive to improve capacity of national hospitals to provide quality of care. National accreditation system for hospitals ensure that hospitals, whether public or private, national or expatriate, play there expected roles in national heath system.

Confidence in accreditation is obtained by a transparent system of control over the accredited hospital and an assurance given by the accreditation body that the accredited hospital constantly fulfills the accreditation criteria.

Benefits for Hospitals

Accreditation to a hospital stimulates continuous improvement. It enables hospital in demonstrating commitment to quality care. It raises community confidence in the services provided by the hospital. It also provides opportunity to healthcare unit to benchmark with the best.

Benefits for Hospital Staff

The staff in an accredited hospital is satisfied lot as it provides for continuous learning, good working environment, leadership and above all ownership of clinical processes. It improves overall professional development of clinicians and para medical staff and provides leadership for quality improvement with medicine and nursing.

Benefits to Paying and Regulatory Bodies

Finally, accreditation provides an objective system of empanelment by insurance and other third parties. Accreditation provides access to reliable and certified information on facilities, infrastructure and level of care.

CONCLUSION

In our view we call it a great success because the success story delivered by leading states like Gujarat, Andhra Pradesh and Kerala where NABL and NABH accreditation program are implemented throughout the state. This will definitely encourage and motivate other states to follow their steps towards the delivery of quality of care and competence not only in Government hospital and laboratories but also in corporate healthcare divisions. A team from Government of Gujarat health and family welfare department was formed to represent the government institution for NABH and NABL accreditation program. Organizers and viewers appreciated this giant success.

During the last five years accreditation process focused on various aspects of patient safety and patient rights which the patients rightly deserve. Medical errors and negligence reporting, incident and sentinel event reporting and action taken reports, medical audits seem to have greatly improved leading to better quality care in accredited hospitals. Qualified and trained NABH auditors, during their pre and final audit do a meticulous and a fair evaluation which has won the appreciation of the hospital management professionals around the country.

Hospitals working towards NABH accreditation perceive that the inspection by NABH authorities is a learning and course correction exercise to improve quality of care instead of doubting it as fault finding mission. According to NABH sources there are 201 hospitals accredited for a three-year cycle and there are 569 hospitals waiting in the wings at different stages for approval. This is a clear sign that accreditation of hospitals is catching up faster than expected.

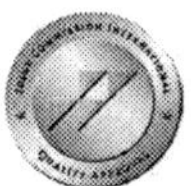

JOINT COMMISSION INTERNATIONAL (JCI) IN INDIAN HEALTHCARE

INTRODUCTION

India is one of the leading players in healthcare domain in the present world. Large number of well trained physicians and supporting staff, most modern medical technology and highly affordable cost structure make India one of the favorite healthcare destination. India is having a good number of JCI accredited hospitals in its major cities.

The low cost of healthcare is not the only driving force of medical tourism in India. The level of healthcare service in the leading hospitals and medical centers are on par to what is being offered in US and UK hospitals and superior to most Asian countries. Patients from Western nations who opt for top notch accredited facilities will receive the same type of medical services in a manner that they are accustomed to, as doctors, nurses and other health professionals are trained and certified to Western standards and practices. JCI Accreditation of Indian Hospitals is a recognition worldwide that Indian Healthcare is not behind others countries.

The new guidelines will help in increasing the market base for JCI in India as hospitals, which are into medical tourism in a big way, are mostly inclined towards JCI. With the patient being well informed, they expect quality and safety from hospitals. Another reason for healthcare organizations opting for JCI is that the medical professionals are keen on working with associations which are JCI-accredited.

"This step is a good marketing tool from JCI's side, as the guidelines will benefit the hospitals and thus more hospitals will be inclined towards JCI".

"In the US, almost 50% of the healthcare guidelines focus on patient safety. For India too, it should be a welcome change".

"The way things are moving in the Indian healthcare industry, patient safety is on the front seat. Hence, JCI guidelines will surely be welcomed."

Also, as JCI is the closest to The Joint Commission but a bit toned down where guidelines are concerned, JCI's market is on a rise in India.

INDIA FRIENDLY

JCI is planning to capture the Indian healthcare market.

India is a good healthcare investment destination, but currently we are not looking at any specific target number of hospitals that must be JCI accredited. But we are working at increasing our presence here. JCI recently established offices in Dubai and Singapore for easy access to Asian countries.

In India, more money is being pumped into healthcare, and health insurance is being introduced in a big way. Healthcare NGO's are more organized, and common people have access to health information, which makes India a preferable destination.

To increase its market presence, JCI is planning to collaborate with National Accreditation Board for Hospitals and Healthcare Providers (NABH). Meanwhile, JCI has started with awareness programmes too. End of last month saw educational workshops arranged by JCI at the national capital on the occasion of International Healthcare Quality Conclave conducted by Indian Healthcare Quality Forum in association with Quality Council of India (QCI) and JCI.

This collaboration is a good step for sharing ideas and working together towards common healthcare goals of quality in hospitals and patient safety. In addition, JCI is starting training for healthcare professionals from each region of each continent to become JCI consultants.

It will be sometime until the positive effects of new JCI guidelines actually start showing on the Indian healthcare industry as a whole. In the meantime, individual hospitals, which are JCI-accredited, will keep on reaping the benefits.

Joint Commission is not the only accreditation agency in the healthcare industry, but it is by far the largest and most prestigious. Receiving Joint Commission accreditation gives hospitals and other healthcare providers a leg up in the process of providing their consumers the highest level of service. Preparing for a Joint Commission survey can be a challenging process for any healthcare provider. At a minimum, a hospital must be completely familiar with the current standards, examine current processes, policies and procedures relative to the standards and prepare to improve any areas that are not currently in compliance. To obtain accreditation, healthcare organization staff members must be able to demonstrate proficiency across specific job competencies and receive performance evaluations based on specific job descriptions. The hospital must be in compliance with the standards for at least four months prior to the initial survey. Success factors easy-to-use healthcare industry solution, health practices, helps you simplify the Joint Commission survey process.

Top reasons for seeking Joint Commission accreditation in India are:

- Provides a competitive edge in the marketplace
- Educates staff regarding best practices and improves business operations, reducing risks
- Provides professional advice and boosts the quality of staff recruitment and development
- Improves quality, safety and overall healthcare experience for patients, families and staff
- Recognized by insurers and third parties and may fulfill regulatory requirements in select states.

From this list, you begin to gain insight into a few key benefits of Joint Commission accreditation. Administratively, it increases your ability to recruit and retain high-performing clinical and administrative staff that will provide patients the quality care they expect and deserve. Additionally, it is a valuable marketing tool for attracting consumers who seek only 'accredited' providers for their healthcare needs, thus keeping healthcare organizations in business. The objective of the Joint Commission's survey is not only to evaluate the hospital, but also to provide education and guidance that will help staff continue to improve the hospital's performance. Prospective patients who are looking for the highest-quality care possible will find research supporting the assumption that Joint Commission accredited hospitals have a marked improvement in quality of care when compared to nonaccredited hospitals. Additionally, a majority of state governments recognize Joint Commission accreditation as a condition of licensure and receiving medical insurance reimbursement. Some general and professional liability insurance companies strongly encourage external accreditations. Prior to billing Medical Insurance Companies, they will ask for accreditation, conditions of participation and/or a certificate of compliance. The survey process evaluates actual care processes by tracing patients through their care cycle, analyzing key operational systems that directly impact the quality and safety of patient care. All healthcare organizations, other than laboratories, are subject to a three-year accreditation cycle. The Joint Commission will provide the organization's accreditation decision, the date that accreditation was awarded, and any standards that were cited for improvement. Organizations deemed to be in compliance with all or most of the applicable standards are awarded the decision of accreditation. There are only so many hours in every day. By streamlining your preparation for the Joint Commission accreditation process you can spend more time focusing on what's really important—your core business objective to find high-performing employees to provide high-quality healthcare to all.

ABOUT JOINT COMMISSION INTERNATIONAL

Joint Commission International (JCI) is the international arm of The Joint Commission, the leading healthcare accreditor in the US Since 1994, JCI has been working with healthcare organizations, ministries of health, and global organizations in more than 90 countries. JCI has accredited and certified more than 410 public and private healthcare organizations over 45 countries since accrediting our first hospital in 1999. JCI is committed to making a difference in healthcare, and believes everything healthcare providers do must lead to a better experience for patients and must always acknowledge the human side of healthcare.

- JCI is dedicated to improving the quality, safety and efficiency of healthcare services around the globe. JCI offers accreditation programs and other assessment tools to provide objective evaluations of the quality and safety of healthcare organizations.

- JCI accreditation assists international healthcare organizations, clinical care programs, public health agencies, health ministries and others in evaluating, improving, and demonstrating the quality and safety of patient care in their nations.
- JCI is an affiliate of the most trusted name in accreditation—The Joint Commission. For more than 75 years, The Joint Commission and its predecessor organization, The American College of Surgeons, have been dedicated to improving the quality of healthcare organizations in the United States and around the world.
- JCI accreditation standards set uniform, achievable expectations for structures, processes and outcomes for hospitals, medical transport organizations, clinical laboratories, ambulatory care centers, primary care centers, and organizations providing care continuum services. The accreditation process is designed to accommodate specific legal, religious and cultural factors within a country. To ensure their international applicability, JCI standards were developed by a 16-member international task force, representing seven major world regions: Western Europe; the Middle East; Latin and Central America; Asia and the Pacific Rim; North America; Central and Eastern Europe; and Africa.
- As of October 2009, JCI's Disease or Condition-Specific Care Certification program has a new name: Clinical Care Program Certification (CCPC). Fifteen clinical care programs are eligible for certification under the CCPC program.
- JCI has extensive experience working with public and private healthcare organizations and local governments in more than 90 countries. In 2009, JCI celebrated the 10th anniversary of the first healthcare organization to be awarded accreditation under its globally developed international standards for hospitals. In 1999, Hospital Israelita Albert Einstein in Sao Paulo, Brazil, became the first organization accredited by JCI. There are more than 410 accredited organizations and certified programs in over 45 countries. Check JCI's website, www.jointcommissioninternational.org for the most up-to-date listing.
- In September 2007, JCI received accreditation by the International Society for Quality in Healthcare (ISQua). A nonprofit, independent organization with members in more than 70 countries, ISQua is known as the accreditor of accrediting bodies. Accreditation by ISQua provides assurance that the standards, training and processes used by JCI to survey the performance of healthcare organizations meet the highest international benchmarks for accreditation entities.

- In August 2005, the World Health Organization (WHO) designated JCI and The Joint Commission as the world's first and only WHO Collaborating Center dedicated solely to patient safety. By collaborating with ministries of health, national patient safety organizations and experts, healthcare professional organizations, and patient/consumer groups, the Collaborating Center focuses worldwide attention on patient safety solutions, patient safety practices and other issues related to reducing safety risks to patients.
- JCI offers international conferences and symposia on quality and patient safety issues, audio conferences, standards manuals and other quality improvement publications. In addition, individuals can subscribe to JCInsight, JCI's official bimonthly online newsletter and they automatically receive JCI Accreditation Exclusive, JCI's complimentary online quarterly bulletin for accredited organizations and certified programs. To receive your copy, visit http://www.jointcommissioninternational.org/Accredited-Organization-Resource-Center/

Mission of JCI: (Transforming patient care across the globe)

The mission of JCI is to continuously improve the safety and quality of care in the international community through the provision of education and advisory services and international accreditation and certification.

Vision of JCI: All people always experience the safest, highest quality, best-value healthcare across all settings.

HISTORY OF CONTINUAL IMPROVEMENT BY JOINT COMMISSION INTERNATIONAL

Founded in 1951, the Joint Commission evaluates and accredits more than 20,000 healthcare organizations and programs in the United States. An independent, not-for-profit organization, the Joint Commission is the nation's oldest and largest standards-setting and accrediting body in healthcare. To earn and maintain the Joint Commission's Gold Seal of Approval™, an organization must undergo an on-site survey by a Joint Commission survey team at least every three years (Laboratories must be surveyed every two years). The Joint Commission provides accreditation services for the following types of organizations:

- General, psychiatric, children's and rehabilitation hospitals
- Critical access hospitals
- Homecare organizations, including medical equipment services and hospice services
- Nursing homes and other long-term care facilities

- Behavioral healthcare organizations, addiction services
- Ambulatory care providers, including group practices and office-based surgery practices
- Independent or free-standing clinical laboratories.

The Joint Commission also awards Disease-Specific Care Certification to organizations that provide disease-specific care and chronic care services, and an advanced level of certification is offered for: chronic kidney disease, chronic obstructive pulmonary disease, heart failure, inpatient diabetes and primary stroke centers. The Joint Commission also has a Healthcare Staffing Services Certification program.

JCI'S RELATIONSHIP TO THE JOINT COMMISSION

JCI is the international arm of the Joint Commission (USA); JCI's mission is to improve the quality and safety of healthcare in the international community. For more than 75 years, the Joint Commission (USA) and its predecessor organization have been dedicated to improving the quality and safety of healthcare services. Today, the Joint Commission is the largest accreditor of healthcare organizations in the United States—it surveys nearly 16,000 healthcare programs through a voluntary accreditation process. The Joint Commission and JCI are both nongovernmental, not-for-profit United States corporations.

JCI accreditation is a variety of initiatives designed to respond to a growing demand around the world for standards-based evaluation in healthcare. The purpose is to offer the international community standards based, objective processes for evaluating healthcare organizations. The goal of the program is to stimulate demonstration of continuous, sustained improvement in healthcare organizations by applying international consensus standards, International Patient Safety Goals, and data measurement support.

BENEFITS TO INDIAN HOSPITALS ONCE THEY GET JCI ACCREDITATION

Improved Patient Safety and Quality

The most important reason to seek accreditation is to improve the quality of patient care. JCI Accreditation signifies your commitment to quality, safety and continuous improvement.

Accreditation by JCI meets a need for recognition of quality healthcare providers throughout the world.

Recognition for Your Organization

JCI Accreditation recognizes your organization's performance in complying with international healthcare quality standards. These standards are intended to help organizations:

- Achieve the highest level of performance possible
- Improve patient outcomes
- Create an environment for continuous improvement.

JCI standards represent a worldwide consensus on quality patient care that reflects state-of-the-art healthcare practices and healthcare delivery trends. Accreditation engages the organization's governing board, professional staff and administration in a cooperative effort to continuously improve patient care.

Increased Community Confidence

JCI accreditation makes a strong statement to your community about your desire to provide the highest quality healthcare services. For patients, businesses, health ministries and others, accreditation serves as an index that your organization meets international standards for quality.

Education on Best Practices

As part of the accreditation process, JCI survey team members offer your organization counsel on how to enhance organization performance. This is an added value of JCI accreditation.

Hospitals participating in the Joint Commission's accreditation process receive expert assistance and support from individual account executives and standards implementation and patient safety experts. Joint Commission certified surveyors provide a rigorous evaluation of the hospital's patient care processes and helpful expert advice on how to improve. Twenty (20) accreditation services are provided exclusively for Joint Commission accredited organizations. From a "Value" perspective, the average cost of Joint Commission hospital accreditation has historically been about 10% to 15% of the fees hospitals pay for their annual financial audit. Internal application of Lean and Six Sigma methods at the Joint Commission has led to improved customer service, reduced costs and no fee increase for 2009 and 2010. A 1% fee increase was instituted in 2011.

1. *Account executives*: The organizations are paired with an account executive dedicated to help each customer have a positive accreditation experience and address any accreditation process questions or concerns, they may have.

2. *Joint commission connect*: Each organization's specific extranet site provides authorized individual access to all important accreditation related information including the Accreditation Decision Report, e.app, Periodic Performance Review, historical files, ORYX data and the Evidence of Standards Compliance process.
3. *Expert analysis of sentinel events*: Feedback and assistance with the completion of Root Cause Analyzes.
4. *Targeted solutions tool™*: Customized solutions to serious quality and safety problems such as hand hygiene, hand-off communications and surgical site infection. Through the involvement of leading hospitals in the Joint Commission's Center for Transforming Healthcare, detailed information is being provided to Joint Commission-accredited hospitals about problem-specific root causes and identified solutions customized and targeted to the specific circumstances of individual hospitals.
5. *Expert and experienced surveyors*: The Joint Commission employs all of its field staff (surveyors), prohibits them from providing accreditation/certification-related consulting services and requires that they pass both a comprehensive written certification examination and a preceptorship training program. Many surveyors have conducted hundreds of surveys and average about 20 per year while simultaneously maintaining their clinical and professional experiences in the field.
6. *Comprehensive on-site survey and tracer methodology*: Certified and experienced surveyors with relevant knowledge of the healthcare settings, they survey, perform patient tracers and care systems tracers to determine, from the patient's viewpoint, the quality and safety of care being provided. These unannounced surveys result in a Report of Survey Findings and an official Accreditation Decision Report.
7. *Edition*: This electronic searchable standards manual provides online access to the most up-to-date content in a single location. Edition allows the organization to tailor the information, they need and that applies to their unique services and includes full text searching, history tracking and standards filtering.
8. *National patient safety goals*: Assessment of compliance with the safety goals and related requirements.
9. *Periodic performance review*: An electronic PPR tool is provided to each accredited organization as an efficient and effective method for assessing organizational compliance with national standards. Joint Commission expert staff provides telephone counseling and support to assist hospitals effectively complete their self-assessment of performance.
10. *Improvement assistance*: From clinical specialists in the Standards Interpretation Group. Inquiries from accredited organizations are given

a higher priority than non-accredited organizations and a call center priority routing system for customers has been implemented. Joint Commission accredited organizations receive expedited assistance by completing the Online Submission Form on their Joint Commission extranet site.

11. *Accreditation process guide*: A step-by-step review of how the hospital accreditation process works. The accreditation manual provides a comprehensive review of the accreditation process which includes a description of the survey agenda, patient tracers, accreditation decision process, the PPR process, and post-survey activity.
12. *Survey activity guide*: This comprehensive 65-page guide provides detailed information on what to expect during each segment of the on-site survey from the Surveyor Preliminary Planning Session to the Exit Conference.
13. *Online electronic payment option*: Customers can use Visa, MasterCard, American Express, Discover, or E-check to pay their deposit, annual fee and on-site fees online via the Joint Commission Connect extranet site.
14. *Strategic surveillance system (S3)*: Hospitals receive on their extranet site a comprehensive Performance Risk Assessment dashboard report that includes a risk assessment based on the Priority Focus Areas and comparative data depicting the hospital's performance in relation to leading and poor performing hospitals.
15. *Disease-specific care certification*: For an added fee, accredited organizations may seek special certification for the services, they provide to patients with chronic illnesses. Advanced programs are available for primary stroke centers, and chronic obstructive pulmonary disease (COPD), inpatient diabetes, chronic kidney disease and heart failure programs.
16. *Educational programs and publications*: A wide variety of programs and materials are made available through Joint Commission Resources (JCR). Topics include infection prevention and control, medication safety, environment of care and accreditation and certification requirements. Beginning in January 2010, Joint Commission-accredited and certified organizations will pay lower fees for educational programs and publications than other customers.
17. *Performance measurement analysis*: Each hospital is provided on a quarterly basis with both Control Charts and Comparison Charts as a set of *ORYX Performance Measurement Reports* for each and all reported measures. The reports include two years of data and also feed into the Strategic Surveillance System reports organizations receive as a management tool from the Joint Commission.

18. *Relief from state and federal agency inspections*: The Centers for Medicare and Medicaid Services (CMS) and 46 state agencies substantially rely on the Joint Commission's accreditation of hospitals in lieu of conducting their own inspections.
19. *The leading practice library*: It is a complimentary tool available to organizations that are currently accredited or certified by the Joint Commission. The documents in the Library are real life solutions that have been successfully implemented by healthcare organizations and reviewed by Joint Commission standards experts.
20. *Recognition of excellence*: Successful achievement of Joint Commission accreditation or certification earns the Joint Commission's Gold Seal of Approval™; the internationally-recognized symbol of healthcare quality.
21 *Standards boosterpaks™*: It provide all the information in a single source needed to understand and correctly interpret a standard.

Other Benefits of Joint Commission Accreditation in India

- *Helps organize and strengthen patient safety efforts*: Patient safety and quality of care issues are at the forefront of Joint Commission standards and initiatives.
- *Strengthens community confidence in the quality and safety of care, treatment and services*: Achieving accreditation makes a strong statement to the community about an organization's efforts to provide the highest quality services.
- *Provides a competitive edge in the marketplace*: Accreditation may provide a marketing advantage in a competitive healthcare environment and improve the ability to secure new business.
- *Improves risk management and risk reduction*: Joint Commission standards focus on state-of-the-art performance improvement strategies that help healthcare organizations continuously improve the safety and quality of care, which can reduce the risk of error or low quality care.
- *May reduce liability insurance costs*: By enhancing risk management efforts, accreditation may improve access to and reduce the cost of liability insurance coverage.
- *Provides education to improve business operations*: Joint Commission Resources, the Joint Commission's not-for-profit affiliate, provides continuing support and education to accredited organizations with services to help organizations in a variety of settings.
- *Provides professional advice and counsel, enhancing staff education*: Joint Commission surveyors are experienced healthcare professionals

trained to provide expert advice and education during the on-site survey.

- *Provides a customized, intensive review*: Joint Commission surveyors come from a variety of healthcare industries and are assigned to organizations that match their background. The standards are also specific to each accreditation program so each survey is relevant to your industry.
- *Enhances staff recruitment and development*: Joint Commission accreditation can attract qualified personnel who prefer to serve in an accredited organization. Accredited organizations also provide additional opportunities for staff to develop their skills and knowledge.
- *Provides deeming authority for medicare certification*: Some accredited healthcare organizations qualify for medicare and medicaid certification without undergoing a separate government quality inspection, which eases the burdens of duplicative federal and state regulatory agency surveys.
- *Recognized by insurers and other third parties*: In some markets, accreditation is becoming a prerequisite to eligibility for insurance reimbursement and for participation in managed care plans or contract bidding.
- *Provides a framework for organizational structure and management*: Accreditation involves not only preparing for a survey, but maintaining a high level of quality and compliance with the latest standards. Joint Commission accreditation provides guidance to an organization's quality improvement efforts.
- *May fulfill regulatory requirements in select states*: Laws may require certain healthcare providers to acquire accreditation for their organization. Those organizations already accredited by the Joint Commission may be compliant and need not undergo any additional surveys or inspections.
- *Provides practical tools to strengthen or maintain performance excellence*: The Leading Practice Library offers good practices submitted by accredited organizations. The Targeted Solutions Tool, an interactive web-based tool from the Joint Commission Center for Transforming Healthcare, allows accredited organizations to measure their organization's performance and help them find customized solutions for challenging healthcare problems.
- *Aligns healthcare organizations with one of the most respected names in healthcare*: Being accredited by the Joint Commission helps organizations position for the future of integrated care.

Recent Studies Support the Value of Joint Commission Accreditation

- Longo study showed that accreditation is a significant factor in whether facilities engaged in actions widely recognized to improve patient safety; advocates accreditation as a means for improving healthcare.
- *Health affairs* report indicated that Joint Commission accreditation requirements influenced hospitals' efforts toward implementing patient safety initiatives.
- *Study in hospital* topics found accreditation to be effective in driving efforts to reduce errors.

The process of Joint Commission International accreditation has set many of the fundamental principles that guide healthcare organizations today. Many of these principles are routine in healthcare today but were revolutionary in their time.

Some examples:

Medical records

- First required in 1917, many considered the medical record unnecessary
- Today the medical record is inarguably the central point of information gathering for treatment decisions, research, patient monitoring, outcomes measurement, and even billing.

Infection control programs

- In the mid-1950s, patients, especially surgery patients and newborns, acquired infections in epidemic proportions
- In the 1950s, hospitals were required to appoint infection control committees to direct activities aimed at curbing epidemics of infections
- Infection control programs were created that reduced the spread of devastating infectious agents.

Fire safety

Nonsmoking standards for hospitals were developed due to the adverse effects of passive nonsmokers and significant fire hazards.

Advance directives

- Protects patients from a life or death they would not have wished
- Requires organizations to establish Do-Not-Resuscitate (DNR) standards and request an advance directive from each patient so the individual's wishes can be documented in the patient chart
- In the 1980s only 20% of hospitals addressed this issue; since the implementation of the standard, nearly 100% of accredited organizations are in compliance with the standard.

ACCREDITATION: THE VALUE EQUATION

- Joint Commission International has conducted descriptive research with a sample of accredited hospitals to determine the value of accreditation
- Accredited hospitals in India report significant improvements:
  - Leadership
  - Medical records management
  - Infection control
  - Reduction in medication errors
  - Staff training and professional credentialing
  - Improved quality monitoring.

WORLD-CLASS VIA ACCREDITATIONS

Medical tourism has played a catalytic role in making the Indian hospital strive for world-class quality standards.

The fact that medical tourism in India is happening, is no longer news. But prediction of its huge growth potential certainly is. Abacus International, a UK-based healthcare consultancy believes that the lure of low-cost, high quality healthcare in Asia will attract more than 1.3 million tourists a year to the key locations—Thailand, Singapore, India, South Korea and Malaysia. The medical tourism market is expected to be worth US$ 4 billion by 2012.

Rising healthcare costs in the US have forced the uninsured and under-insured patients to look at cheaper healthcare alternatives outside the US. But while high costs have been an important driver, the factor that has actually pushed the patients to undertake the long journey is that the hospitals in Asia have made an effort to match the quality standards that exist in the US and other western countries. They did so by striving to achieve the global accreditations like Joint Commission International (JCI). "An accreditation is a way to distinguish a hospital," says Anne Rooney, Executive Director of International Services at JCI. That's why Indian Hospitals are striving for JCI accreditation.

However, the importance of international accreditations to Indian hospitals goes far beyond just attracting foreign tourists. Better quality of healthcare and higher standards of patient safety help the hospitals to give the best treatment to a patient—irrespective of nationality—in the least possible time and with minimal wastage and lesser medical errors. While for the patients this means better treatment, for hospitals it is reduced wastage and lower costs in the long run. With accreditations, quality no longer remains the job of a few but it gets woven into the fabric of function involving all processes and people to pursue the same goal.

ACCREDITATIONS: RESHAPING INDIAN HEALTHCARE

Healthcare in Asia has emerged as a major focus area, with many nations recovering from the Asian Crisis as also the increasing prosperity China and India have begun to experience as a result of their policy reforms. There is a greater need to revamp the healthcare systems for better quality of healthcare. Attempts are on to benchmark with the best globally. India established the National Accreditation Board for Hospitals and Healthcare Providers (NABH) for accreditation of hospitals in the country recently. Absence of such standards always put the patients at risk. A survey by the World Health Organization (WHO) found the incidence of hospital—acquired infections to be highest in the Southeast Asian region at 10%, only marginally behind the Eastern Mediterranean region at 11.8%, which topped the list.

But there has been a gradual increase in the awareness regarding the importance of quality, thanks mainly to the increasing role of private players in the sector, especially in countries like India and China, where private sector hospitals have aggressively pursued accreditation. Medical tourism has played a catalytic role in making the Indian hospitals strive for world-class quality standards following JCI standards. Despite accreditations being a voluntary process, the competition to attract foreign tourists has been driving hospitals towards them. This of course is good news for domestic patients as well since they will be able to access the best healthcare without having to travel a lot.

Among the various international accreditations available, the one awarded by JCI, the international arm of the US-based accreditation body Joint Commission on Accreditation for Healthcare Organizations (JCAHO), has become very popular. High standards, wide scope and rigorous process of evaluation have made JCI accreditation a 'gold standard' in hospital accreditation. Already, as many as 22 Indian hospitals have got themselves accredited. And this number is going up with a few others preparing for it.

The other option that could soon be available for hospitals is the NIAHO—ISO certification developed by the TUVHS America. This program combines two independent sets of standards—ISO 9001 Quality Management standards and Hospital Conditions and Participation standards set by the Medicare program in the US. This new system has a wider scope than ISO 9001:2000 certification, which focuses largely on the administrative processes. However, it is yet to receive the final approval from the Centers for Medicare and Medicaid Services (CMS) of the US. Only then it will be able to accredit hospitals internationally.

THE ACCREDITATION PROCESS

The accreditation process for any hospital, the accreditation process represents bringing about a significant change in the way it functions. A comprehensive accreditation, such as that of JCI, needs to be implemented organization-wide, with the involvement of all the employees who take part in the patient's journey from admission to discharge. In JCI, there are 565 standards divided into 197 core standards that must be met to achieve accreditation and 368 other standards that lead organizations to best practice levels. These standards are further divided into 1033 measurable parameters, which focus on aspects such as patient safety, patient rights, facilities, and physicians' credentials besides policies and procedures of the organization. To get accredited a hospital will have to fully meet most of these parameters and the remaining ones at least partially. Singapore's National Health Center (NHC), which got accredited in November 2005, met 1013 of the 1033 parameters successfully. The JCI accreditation is valid for 3 years and has to be renewed on a regular basis.

CHAPTERS IN JOINT COMMISSION INTERNATIONAL ACCREDITATION

- Access to and continuity of care
- Patient and family rights
- Assessment of patient
- Care of patient
- Patient and family education
- Prevention and control of infection
- Staff qualification and education
- Governance, leadership and direction
- Facility management and safety
- Management of information
- Quality improvement and patient safety.

Implementation Requirements

- Standardize processes
- Clearly communicate new policies to the employees
- Improve documentation
- Improve facilities to increase patient safety
- Expand the scope of the Quality Management Committee
- Plan and document Continuous Medical Education (CME) for all staff

- Implement new and stricter credentialing and privileging criteria for medical staff
- Streamline the monitoring of clinical outcomes
- Change the maintenance records of medical equipment according to the standards
- Improve communication with the patient
- Practice strict control over patient information

The accreditation process typically lasts for about 2 years and involves two surveys by a team of consultants from JCI who also educate the hospital staff about various standards and their implementation. Here, the role of the top management becomes very crucial since it is their commitment that in turn influences the commitment of the whole organization. "It takes strong commitment from the top management" says Rooney and adds that the point-of-care staff, nursing staff, physicians and other employees of the hospitals too play a crucial role, as they have to adapt to a whole new way of functioning (Fig. 13.1).

The benefits are multi-fold. Both the healthcare provider and customer stand to gain if an organization complies with the standards. The benefits that ensure accreditations include better care for the patients, a customer-centric approach, improved branding as a result of increased confidence

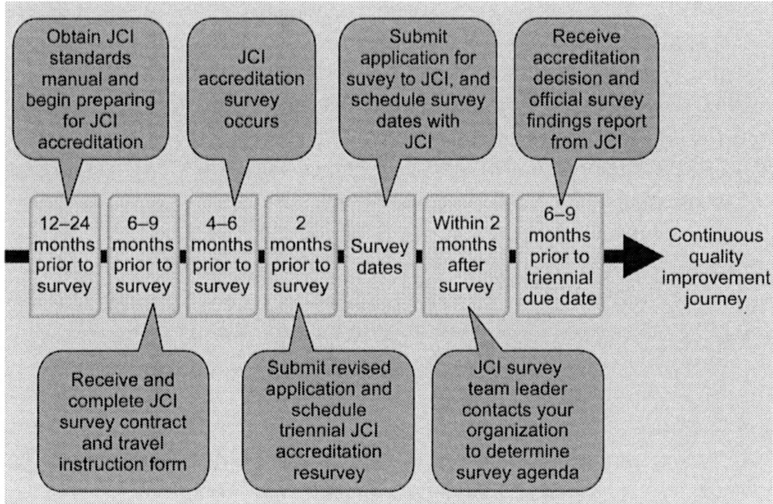

Fig. 13.1 Accreditation timeline process
Source: Joint Commission International

within the community, high employee morale and continuous monitoring of standards. Over a period of time the hospital would experience cost reductions as efficiency go up and more is achieved through less effort. Medical errors that cost hospitals thousands of dollars every year could be reduced as well. The final beneficiaries would be the patients since the new processes would be designed to meet their requirements and they have access to the best treatment. Says Rooney, "It's interesting to note that some organizations have reduced medication errors by almost 75% to 80%. That obviously translates into a better patient experience." Further, as processes get streamlined and designed around the patient needs, there is also a better chance for the hospital to provide evidence-based medicine to their patients.

Implementing the exacting standards of accreditation is usually a tough task to begin with. With so many standards to deal with, there is a need for meticulous planning and thorough implementation, which involves active participation of all the employees. As the process aims to influence the functioning of the organization itself, change management—the process of generating a buyin by all, attains utmost importance prior to implementation. "Organizations that do this well really get to see a huge difference in the way they manage their hospitals", claims Rooney.

AFFORDABILITY

While the benefits of international accreditation are quite attractive, the fact is that accreditations such as JCI's could be very expensive for a majority of medium-to-smaller hospitals in the region. A JCI accreditation would cost a hospital approximately US$ 100,000 and this does not include the expenses incurred for upgrading its facilities. The Apollo Indraprastha Hospital in New Delhi, India—first hospital in India to get the JCI accreditation—spent close to ₹ 30 crore (US$ 600,000 approximately) to upgrade its facilities. Medium-sized hospitals may not have such financial muscle!

While this being the limitation, accreditations also give rise to another possibility—national level accreditations with standards designed on the lines of international accreditations and customized to the needs of the local hospitals. In this scenario, the cost tends to come down significantly. The NABH could perform this very function helping smaller hospitals improve quality of healthcare and patient safety without having to spend huge amounts of money. While this may or may not result in them being able to attract international patients, it would certainly help in improving the quality of care in the hospitals.

THE FUTURE

With an opportunity worth US$ 4 billion around, competition for medical tourists is bound to heat up and more hospitals are likely to queue up for international accreditations.

Accreditation organizations would have to work closely with the governments of various Asian countries to make this happen lest the world-class healthcare facilities would be confined only to a small portion of the population. As more hospitals start acquiring accreditations, domestic patients too would prefer to opt the accredited hospitals for treatment. This scenario will eventually push a general move towards improvement in quality of care. The peer pressure is two-fold—those who can afford accreditations start drawing blueprint for the same whereas those who cannot start learning about how to improve the status quo. This sort of a trend is already evident. "A recently held five-day practicum at Singapore was fully booked about six weeks in advance! This shows that there is a very strong interest in education about quality standards in Asia," points Rooney.

To be successful, the hospitals that are gearing up to acquire accreditations, would do well to remember what Phillip Crosby, initiator of the Zero Defect concept said, "It (quality) has to be the fabric of the organization, not part of the fabric."

BIBLIOGRAPHY

1. Bratzler. The surgical infection prevention and surgical care improvement projects: national initiatives to improve outcomes for patients having surgery. Am J Surg. CID 2006;43:328.
2. Classen DC, Evans RS, Pestotnik SL, Horn SD, Menlove RL, Burke JP. The timing of prophylactic administration of antibiotics and the risk of surgical-wound infection. New England J Med. 1992a;326(5):281-6.
3. Gawande AA, Thomas EJ, et al. The incidence and nature of surgical adverse events in Colorado and Utah in 1992. Surgery. 1999;126:66-75.
4. Haynes AB, Weiser TG, et al. A surgical safety checklist to reduce morbidity and mortality in global population. N Eng J Med. 2009;360:491-9.
5. Joint Commission, Sentinel Event Statistics, 2006.
6. Safe surgeries save life initiative. Implementation Guidelines. Quality in Medical Care Section, Medical Development Division, Ministry of Health Malaysia, November 2009 guidelines.
7. Seiden, Archives of Surgery, 2006.
8. Weiser TG, Regenbogen SE, Thompson KD, et al. An estimation of the global volume of surgery: a modeling strategy based on available data. Lancet. 2008;372:139-44.
9. World Alliance for Patient Safety. WHO guidelines for safe surgery. Geneva: World Health Organization, 2009.

Chapter 14

Six Sigma Concept in Healthcare

INTRODUCTION

Six Sigma is an approach originally developed by Motorola in 1980s to systematically improve processes by eliminating defects(G) which will result to reduction of process variation.

At Motorola, they think Six Sigma as a metric, a methodology and a management system at the same time.

The term "Six Sigma" refers to the ability of highly capable processes to produce output at defect levels below 3.4 defects per (one) million opportunities (DPMO).

Objective of the Course

Six Sigma's goal is to improve processes by reducing levels of output defects at levels below 3.4 defects per (one) million opportunities (DPMO).

Field of Application

To improve production processes, service delivery processes, administration processes, etc.

Related Tools

FMEA, QFD, Paretto Diagram, Fishbone Diagram, Control Chart, Process Maps, Histograms, Check Sheets, Gannt Chart.

Description

At Motorola, Six Sigma has been and still is defined as a quality improvement program with a goal of reducing the number of defects to as low as 3.4 parts per million opportunities. In fact, there is a difference in the true value of Six Sigma and Motorola's value of Six Sigma. The explanation of this difference is beyond the scope of this tool.

Six Sigma Evolution

Motorola is the creator of the formal Six Sigma methodology. The first proponents of Six Sigma after Motorola were GE Aircraft Engines, Texas Instruments, Allied Signal, Eastman Kodak, Borg-Warner Automotive, GenCorp, Navistar International.

Although Six Sigma has been developed in industry, in recent years started to apply in the service sector, and in healthcare more specific, although the big challenge in services is the identification of the appropriate metrics, and gathering and exploitation of credible data which are not produced from a manufacturing process which is in statistical control, rather than responses produced from human behavior.

On the other hand, the basic Six Sigma objective for eliminating errors is more than appropriate as a target especially in the very sensitive for human life healthcare sector.

The first healthcare organization that implemented fully Six Sigma was Commonwealth Health Corp (CHC) with partnership with General Electric.

Six Sigma Explanation

Six Sigma is, basically, a process quality goal, where sigma is a statistical measure of variability in a process.

One puzzling aspect of the 'official' Six Sigma literature is that it states that a process operating at Six Sigma will produce 3.4 parts-per-million (PPM) nonconformances. However, if a special normal distribution table is consulted, one finds that the expected nonconformances are 0.002 PPM (2 parts-per-billion, or PPB). The difference occurs because Motorola presumes that the process mean can drift 1.5 sigma in either direction. The area of a normal distribution beyond 4.5 sigma from the mean is indeed 3.4 PPM. Since control charts will easily detect any process shift of this magnitude in a single sample, the 3.4 PPM represents a very conservative upper bound on the nonconformance rate.

In contrast to Six Sigma quality, the old three sigma quality standard of 99.73% translates to 2,700 PPM failures, even if we assume zero drift.

Six Sigma Methodology

The basic approach is to measure performance on an existing process, compare it with a statistically valid ideal and figure out how to eliminate any variation.

It starts with a detailed analysis to quantify and measure factors that are critical to our customers' success, and to find ways to remove obstacles (defects) to that success.

Customer requirements, both external and internal, are paramount in choosing which Six Sigma projects to undertake.

When Six Sigma was first launched at GE Aircraft Engines, a four-step methodology (DMAIC) was followed. Recently, the Define phase has been added to recognize the importance of having a well-scoped project and to be in line with the current practices across GE. The DMAIC model is consisted of the following descrete phases:

Phase 1: Define (D)

Who are the customers and what are their priorities?

A Six Sigma project team identifies a project suitable for Six Sigma efforts based on business objectives as well as customer needs and feedback. As part of the definition phase, the team identifies those attributes, called CTQs (critical to quality characteristics), that the customer considers to have the most impact on quality.

Phase 2: Measure (M)

How is the process measured and how is it performing?

The team identifies the key internal processes that influence CTQs and measures the defects currently generated relative to those processes.

Phase 3: Analyze (A)

What are the most important causes of defects?

The team discovers why defects are generated by identifying the key variables that are most likely to create process variation.

Phase 4: Improve (I)

How do we remove the causes of the defects?

The team confirms the key variables and quantifies their effects on the CTQs. It also identifies the maximum acceptable ranges of the key variables and validates a system for measuring deviations[(G)] of the variables. The team modifies the process to stay within the acceptable range.

Phase 5: Control (C)

How can we maintain the improvements?

Tools are put in place to ensure that under the modified process the key variables remain within the maximum acceptable ranges over time.

In some cases, the 5 steps mentioned above, should be supplemented by the 'recognize' of the problem prior to 'define', and 'standardize' and 'integrate' as final steps of the process helping to incorporate the solution into the organization permanently.

Organizational Infrastructure

The implementation of Six Sigma is a very intensive, long-lasting, and resource demanding job, and needs many people to get trained and involved. Experience of big organizations that implemented Six Sigma, have shown that the appropriate organizational infrastructure is required in terms of roles and responsibilities of personnel.

A successful model of organisational structure in deploying Six Sigma is to implement various levels of expertise as described in Table 14.1:

- *Champions* are fully trained business leaders who promote and lead the deployment of Six Sigma in a significant area of the business;
- *Master black belts* are fully-trained quality leaders responsible for Six Sigma strategy, training, mentoring, deployment, and results;
- *Black belts* are fully-trained Six Sigma experts who lead improvement teams, who work projects across the business and mentor green belts;
- *Green belts* are full-time teachers with quantitative skills as well as teaching and leadership ability; they are fully-trained quality leaders;
- Responsible for Six Sigma strategy, training, mentoring, deployment, and results; and
- *Team members* are individuals who support specific projects in their area.

Table 14.1 Six Sigma responsibility matrix

Phase	Responsibility
Recognize	Champions
Define	Champions/master black belts
Measure	Black belts
Analyze	Black belts
Improve	Black belts
Control	Black belts
Standardize	Champions
Integrate	Champions

Other Six Sigma Related Models

The basic model for Six Sigma implementation is the DMAIC already described. However, the success of the model lead to variations or improvements of the initial approach, or even complementary models aim to enhance DMAIC.

Design for Six Sigma (DFSS) is a systematic methodology utilizing tools, training and measurements to design products and processes that meet customer expectations at Six Sigma quality levels. DFSS is deployed via a framework known as DMADV. Six Sigma DMADV process (define, measure, analyze, design, verify) is an improvement system used to develop new processes or products at Six Sigma quality levels.

WHAT IS SIX SIGMA?

Six Sigma at many organizations simply means a measure of quality that strives for near perfection. It is a disciplined, data-driven approach and methodology for eliminating defects (driving towards six standard deviations between the mean and the nearest specification limit) in any process—from manufacturing to transactional and from product to service.

The statistical representation of Six Sigma describes quantitatively how a process is performing. To achieve Six Sigma, a process must not produce more than 3.4 defects per million opportunities. A Six Sigma defect is defined as anything outside of customer specifications. A Six Sigma opportunity is then the total quantity of chances for a defect.

Six Sigma was originally developed as a set of practices designed to improve manufacturing processes and eliminate defects, but its application was subsequently extended to other types of business processes as well. In Six Sigma, a defect is defined as anything that could lead to customer dissatisfaction.

Six Sigma asserts that:

- Continuous efforts to achieve stable and predictable process results (i.e. reduce process variation) are of vital importance to business success.
- Manufacturing and business processes have characteristics that can be measured, analyzed, improved and controlled.
- Achieving sustained quality improvement requires commitment from the entire organization, particularly from top-level management.

Features that set Six Sigma apart from previous quality improvement initiatives include:

- A clear focus on achieving measurable and quantifiable financial returns from any Six Sigma project.
- An increased emphasis on strong and passionate management leadership and support.

- A special infrastructure of 'Champions', 'Master Black Belts', 'Black Belts', etc. to lead and implement the Six Sigma approach.
- A clear commitment to making decisions on the basis of verifiable data, rather than assumptions and guesswork.

The term 'Six Sigma' is derived from a field of statistics known as process capability studies. Originally, it referred to the ability of manufacturing processes to produce a very high proportion of output within specification. Processes that operate with 'Six Sigma quality' over the short-term are assumed to produce long-term defect levels below 3.4 defects per million opportunities (DPMO). Six Sigma's implicit goal is to improve all processes to that level of quality or better.

METHODS

Six Sigma projects follow two project methodologies inspired by Deming's Plan-Do-Check-Act Cycle. These methodologies comprise five phases each and are known by the acronyms DMAIC and DMADV.

- DMAIC (Define, Measure, Analyze, Improve and Control) is used for projects aimed at improving an existing business process.
- DMADV (Define, Measure, Analyze, Design and Verify) is used for projects aimed at creating new product or process designs.

DMAIC

The five phases in the DMAIC project methodology are:

- ***Define*** high-level project goals and the current process.
- ***Measure*** key aspects of the current process and collect relevant data.
- ***Analyze*** the data to verify cause-and-effect relationships. Determine what the relationships are, and attempt to ensure that all factors have been considered.
- ***Improve*** or optimize the process based upon data analysis using techniques like Design of experiments.
- ***Control*** to ensure that any deviations from target are corrected before they result in defects. Set-up pilot runs to establish process capability, move on to production, set-up control mechanisms and continuously monitor the process.

DMADV

The five phases in the DMADV project methodology are:

- ***Define*** design goals that are consistent with customer demands and the enterprise strategy.

- *Measure* and identify CTQs (characteristics that are **C**ritical **T**o **Q**uality), product capabilities, production process capability, and risks.
- *Analyze* to develop and design alternatives, create a high-level design and evaluate design capability to select the best design.
- *Design* details, optimize the design, and plan for design verification. This phase may require simulations.
- *Verify* the design, set-up pilot runs, implement the production process and hand it over to the process owners.

DMADV is also known as DFSS, an abbreviation of "**D**esign **F**or **S**ix **S**igma".

Quality Management Tools and Methods used in Six Sigma

Within the individual phases of a DMAIC or DMADV project, Six Sigma utilizes many established quality management tools that are also used outside of Six Sigma. An overview of the main methods used are following:

- 5 Whys
- Analysis of variance
- ANOVA Gauge repeatability and reproducibility
- Axiomatic design
- Business process mapping
- Catapult exercise on variability
- Cause and effects diagram (also known as fishbone or Ishikawa diagram)
- Chi-square test of independence and fits
- Control chart
- Correlation
- Cost-benefit analysis
- CTQ tree
- Quantitative marketing research through use of enterprise feedback management (EFM) systems
- Design of experiments
- Failure mode and effects analysis
- General linear model
- Histograms
- Homoscedasticity
- Quality function deployment (QFD)
- Pareto chart
- Pick chart
- Process capability
- Regression analysis
- Root cause analysis
- Run charts

- SIPOC analysis (**S**uppliers, **I**nputs, **P**rocess, **O**utputs, **C**ustomers)
- Stratification
- Taguchi methods
- Taguchi loss function
- Thought process map
- TRIZ (Theory of Inventive Problem Solving).

The term 'Six Sigma process' comes from the notion that if one has six standard deviations between the process mean and the nearest specification limit, as shown in the graphic, there will be practically no items that fail to meet specifications.

Concepts of Six Sigma resource as initiated by Motorola in 1985.

In order to understand Six Sigma, you must understand how Cpk compares to PPM.

Lets get real here. Is it truly necessary to go for zero defects? Why is not 99.9% defect-free good enough? Here are some examples of what life would be like if 99.9% were 'good enough':

- 1 hour of unsafe drinking water every month.
- 2 long or short landings at every American airports each day.
- 400 letters per hour which never arrive at their destination.
- 500 incorrect surgical operations each week.
- 3,000 newborns accidentally falling from the hands of nurses or doctors each year.
- 4,000 incorrect drug prescriptions per year.
- 22,000 checks deducted from the wrong bank account each hour.
- 32,000 missed heartbeats per person per year.

Here are some examples of what life would be like at Six Sigma

- 13 wrong drug prescriptions per year.
- 10 newborns accidentally falling from the hands of nurses or doctors each year.
- 1 lost article of mail per hour.

Suddenly, the quest for Six Sigma is not so bad.

SIX STEPS TO SIX SIGMA

- Step #1: Identify the product you create or the service you provide
  In other words. What do you do?
- Step #2: Identify the customer(s) for your product or service, and determine what they consider important, i.e. customer requirements
  In other words. Who uses your product and services?
- Step #3: Identify your needs (to provide product/service so that it satisfies the customer)

In other words. What do you need to do your work?

- Step #4: Define the process for doing your work
  In other words. How do you do your work?
- Step #5: Mistake-proof the process and eliminate wasted efforts using
  In other words. How can you do your work better?
- Step #6: Ensure continuous improvement by measuring, analyzing and controlling the improved process using DMAIC (Define, Measure, Analyze, Improve and Control)
  In other words, How perfectly are you doing your customer-focused work?
- Step 6: Ensure continuous improvement by measuring, analyzing and controlling the improved process from Step #5.

SIX SIGMA

According to many business development and quality improvement experts, Six Sigma is now the most popular management methodology in history. Six Sigma is certainly a very big industry in its own right, and Six Sigma is now an enormous 'brand' in the world of corporate development. Six Sigma began in 1986 as a statistically-based method to reduce variation in electronic manufacturing processes in Motorola Inc in the USA. Today, twenty-something years on, Six Sigma is used as an all-encompassing business performance methodology, all over the world, in organizations as diverse as local government departments, prisons, hospitals, the armed forces, banks, and multinationals corporations. Six Sigma, it might seem, is taking over the world.

Interestingly while Six Sigma has become a very widely used 'generic' term, the name Six Sigma is actually a registered trademark of Motorola Inc., in the USA, who first pioneered Six Sigma methods in the 1980s. The original and technically correct spelling seems to be Six Sigma, rather than 6 Sigma, although in recent years Motorola and GE have each since developed their own sexy Six Sigma logos using the number six and the Greek sigma characters.

Six Sigma is now a global brand and something of a revolution. But what is Six Sigma?...

The answer is that Six Sigma is lots of things.

First, Six Sigma is arguably a very clever way of branding and packaging many aspects of Total Quality Management that exist in their own right, regardless of the development of Six Sigma.

Six Sigma is lots of different things because it had different meanings over time, and also because it is now interpreted in increasingly different ways. And Six Sigma is still evolving.

The *UK Department for Trade and Industry says Six Sigma is*:

"A data-driven method for achieving near perfect quality. Six Sigma analysis can focus on any element of production or service, and has a strong emphasis on statistical analysis in design, manufacturing and customer-oriented activities."

Six Sigma is a business improvement methodology that focuses an organization on:

- Understanding and managing customer requirements.
- Aligning key business processes to achieve those requirements.
- Utilizing rigorous data analysis to minimize variation in those processes.
- Driving rapid and sustainable improvement to business processes.

As a management system, Six Sigma is a high performance system for executing business strategy. Six Sigma is a top-down solution to help organizations:

- Align their business strategy to critical improvement efforts.
- Mobilize teams to attack high impact projects.
- Accelerate improved business results.
- Govern efforts to ensure improvements are sustained.

"...The Six Sigma Management System drives clarity around the business strategy and the metrics that most reflect success with that strategy. It provides the framework to prioritize resources for projects that will improve the metrics, and it leverages leaders who will manage the efforts for rapid, sustainable, and improved business results."

These Days A Lot Is Being Heard About Six Sigma Belts.

What Does Six Sigma Mean?

Six sigma is a process, which identifies the defects and fault within the working system and the processes of the company. It tries to reduce them to the minimum. It initiates toward goal defining, fault finding, performance measuring, process controlling, etc. in a company.

What is the Aim of Six Sigma?

Six Sigma's prime motive is to make the company excel in the products and services. The concept lies on the foundation of customer satisfaction. It quantifies the qualitative aspects of the system. It aims toward the best quality as far as products and services are concerned. Now, here an important thing comes and that is not every process in an industry or a company is measurable. For example, how can you measure the customer satisfaction or how can you measure the client loyalty or employee's efficiency. Well, in this case, the sales of the company and demand for the products along with revenue generation speak for itself. So, in that case you can definitely find out the positive results of Six Sigma process.

About Six Sigma Belts

Now, since you know what is Six Sigma it will be easier to understand about the Six Sigma belts. There are four levels in Six Sigma training. And each belt defines the expertise in that particular level. These levels in the respective order are yellow belt, green belt, black belt and master black belt. Now let us understand each level in detail.

- *Yellow belt:* This is the lowest level in Six Sigma. The person trained at this level holds the responsibility of smaller process improvement but is not in charge of a team under him. He has the basic knowledge about Six Sigma processes.
- *Green belt:* Green belt is the next level of expertise in Six Sigma processes. Usually, the person trained or certified with this level gets an opportunity to head and lead the project. Usually, the projects allotted to him are quite challenging and require him to be much responsible.
- *Black belt:* At this level, the person in charge needs to be responsible in Six Sigma implementation at all levels. He has many teams under him and he guides them and trains them to achieve the goals successfully. He also has to play the role of a mentor or teacher and teach his subordinates about Six Sigma programs. He leads the team and provides training to green belts and yellow belts.
- *Master black belt:* This is the highest level and the expert is the mentor of black belts. He is the trainer, the teacher and the person who is responsible for implementation of Six Sigma processes at all levels. He is the head and leads many projects at a time. A master black belt is responsible for company's strategies and training the black belts in Six Sigma methods.

The concept of Six Sigma methods started in the early eighties but has now become quite popular. When it started, the main aim was to give company a result oriented environment. But now, Six Sigma methods and programs are being used even at the stage of product development and service designing. The motive initially was to save Dollars but now it is to achieve the goals and discarding all the possible defects from the company's system. The demand for Six Sigma professionals and consultants have risen unbelievably and more and more companies want their project leaders to get trained in Six Sigma programs to the level of black belt.

SIX SIGMA AND HEALTHCARE

Six Sigma is gaining momentum in the US hospitals. Many hospitals are joining the ranks of leading healthcare institutions such as Stanford in the West to Yale-New Haven in the East. Six Sigma is a process to improve the quality and customer satisfaction while reducing the cost of delivery and enhancing the revenue. The Healthcare industry embraced Six Sigma only after it was fully developed, tested, and tried by many in the manufacturing sector. Companies such as Motorola, Allied Signal, Xerox, and General Electric used it to generate significant bottom line results coupled with increased customer satisfaction, and reduced product development time to market with higher quality products.

The Six Sigma approach optimizes the average (represented by Greek letter Mu) and reduces the variance (process represented by Greek letter Sigma or standard deviation) of a desired process. The desired outcome can be a reduction of the patient registration time in Emergency Department, lost charges for billing in Patient Financial Services, delinquent medical records, diagnostic results turn around times, accounts receivables days, patients' length of stay, or medication errors. The outcome can also be increased physician satisfaction, market share, and patient flow. To put Six Sigma in perspective, for instance, 200,000 wrong prescriptions per year amounts to 3.8 Sigma and 68 per year amounts to 6 Sigma.

More on Six Sigma?

Sigma has several meanings depending on the context. It could be:

- Greek alphabet
- Mathematical symbol for summation
- Statistical term for standard deviation
- Quality level indicator
- Management philosophy.

Sigma in this context refers to level of quality and a management philosophy. Six Sigma is six times sigma quality level as measured by defects or instances over the customer specified acceptable limit. This corresponds to only 3.4 defects per million opportunities (DPMO) or 99.9997% close to perfection. Most businesses are at three sigma quality level with 66,800 DPMO or 93.32%. The DPMO for various sigma levels are: One Sigma 691,500, two Sigma 308,500, three Sigma 66,800, four Sigma 6,200, five Sigma 230, and six Sigma 3.4.

There are businesses that operate at levels equal to Six Sigma and above. For instance, the airline industry.

How is Six Sigma Different from Previous TQM, CQI Type of Efforts?

Both TQM (Total Quality Management) and CQI (Continuous Quality Improvement) of the last two decades are also improvement programs. The key differences are:

- Customer centricity is the main theme of Six Sigma. It starts with the customer needs as captured via Voice of the Customer (VOC).
- Return on the investment is a key component of Six Sigma.

Which Hospitals have used Six Sigma?

There are many hospital systems or hospitals that use Six Sigma. Some use it system or hospital wide, some in selected areas or departments whereas others use it to solve specific issues. To name a few of the hospitals that use Six Sigma:

- Long Island Jewish, New York, USA
- Stanford Medical Center, California, USA; Northwestern Memorial, Illinois, USA
- MD Anderson, Texas, USA
- Virtua Health System, New Jersey, USA
- Charleston Area Medical Center, West Verginia, USA
- Boston Medical Center, Massachusetts, USA
- Yale New Haven Medical Center, Connecticut, USA
- Verdugo Hills Hospital, California, USA
- Johns Hopkins Hospital, Maryland, USA
- Good Samaritan Hospital, Dhio, USA
- Sir Gangaram Hospital, New Delhi, India.

How to Implement Six Sigma Program in a Hospital?

Here are some steps the hospital can follow to implement Six Sigma.

- Have a sponsor from the C-level, i.e. executive management.
- Develop a project team consisting of people with content and statistics knowledge.
- Have a Green Belt (GB), Black Belt (BB) or Master Black Belt (MBB) designated to mentor the project. If the hospital does not have trained/ certified people in Six Sigma, consider sending their resources will be allocated and the recommendations are likely to be taken seriously for implementation.
- Develop a realistic project plan and get the needed resources.

- Recognize that the effectiveness of the implementation is due to both the quality of the solution and acceptance of the change with a structured change management process.
- Establish a project review mechanism for the stakeholders to review the project status at designated milestones to ensure the project is on schedule.
- Provide necessary support to make sure the people provide data and participate in brainstorming sessions.
- Confirm that the anticipated improvements are achieved both intangible and tangible in the form of return on the investment (ROI).
- Make sure the plan to sustain the results from the pilot is defined.

SIX SIGMA IN HEALTHCARE

Six Sigma principles and the healthcare sector are very well matched because of the healthcare nature of very low or zero tolerance to mistakes and potentials for reducing medical errors.

In 1998, the Institute of Medicine released an assessment stating that 98,000 people die each year as a result of medical errors, highlighting the necessity for quality improvements. Additionally an estimated £400 million is being paid in clinical negligence claims and adverse incidents resulted in approximately £2 billion per annum. Those are some examples that can easily point out the vital importance of quality in healthcare services, and the significant need for implementation of quality management principles and techniques to improve performance, quality levels, and customer satisfaction.

Six Sigma projects in healthcare industry have focused on direct care delivery, administrative support and financial administration. From emergency room to boardroom, Six Sigma can reduce variability and waste by translating to fewer errors, better processes, improved patient care, greater patient satisfaction rates, and happier, more productive employees. To achieve these goals, the DMAIC must be implemented.

However, applying Six Sigma in healthcare is not always the easiest thing to do. Some of challenges someone has to face, as stated by Mehmet Tolga Taner and Bulent Sezen and Jiju Antony are the initial investment in Six Sigma Belt System training, the absence or difficulty to obtain the baseline data on process performance, the identification of processes which can be measured in terms of defects or errors per million opportunities, the psychology of the workforce, the extensive use of statistical language.

Benefits

Some of the benefits of implementing Six Sigma are:

- Improve responsiveness to and focus on the customer.
- Improve product and service performance.
- Improve financial performance and profitability by reducing quality costs and defects.
- Achieve and maintain measurable quality standards.

A longer list of improvements could be achieved through Six Sigma projects in healthcare are listed in the "An overview of Six Sigma applications in healthcare industry" article.

SUCCESS STORIES OF SIX SIGMA

Some Six Sigma success stories and results are presented here to point out benefits measured in numbers that have been accomplish by implementing Six Sigma.

- Motorola has reported over US$17 billion in savings from Six Sigma as of 2006.
- In 1997 alone GE invested US$380 million in Six Sigma ± mostly for training. However, there was payback in the same year ± GE received about US$700 million in documented benefits from increased productivity.
- GE Medical Systems alone saved US$40 million in 1997 (Conlin, 1998).
- Product development cycles have also improved at GE Harris Energy Control System, LLC. In the past it typically took 12–18 months to develop their Energy Management Systems. After implementing Six Sigma processes, they were able to develop and introduce two new Internet.
- Based management information products in just 3 months. The products were identified during a Six Sigma review of critical customer needs.
- Allied Signal, has shown an incredible upturn since it introduced Six Sigma. In 1992, annual sales were about US$13 billion from a workforce of 102,00. Sales (in February 1998) were estimated around US$14 billion with a workforce of 77,000. Productivity in 2Q1998 rose above the long-term target of 6% a year.

PREREQUISITES OF SIX SIGMA

- Strong and insisting management commitment and involvement.
- Strong 'quality culture.'

- Excessive intensive training (GE has implemented a full 13 days of training for every employee).
- Advanced knowledge of statistical techniques, extremely rigorous data collection and statistical analysis.
- Organizational infrastructure, meaning support systems, specific roles and responsibilities, team working culture.
- IT infrastructure and data gathering systems.

THE RED CROSS HOSPITAL CASE STUDY

Red Cross Hospital in Beverwijk, the Netherlands, is a 384-bed, medium-sized general hospital, with a staff of 930 and a budget of $70 million. In addition to being a general healthcare provider, Red Cross Hospital is the base for a 25-bed national burn care center that provides services to all of the Netherlands. In 2002, it admitted 11,632 patients, performed 8,269 outpatient treatments and received 190,218 visits to its outpatient units. During the past 4 years, Red Cross Hospital's management and employees invested significant resources in building and quality assurance system, and at the end of 2000, the hospital was awarded an ISO 9002 certification. After that, management began undertaking quality improvement projects on a regular basis, but it was doing so without the benefit of Six Sigma's project management system.

At the end of 2001, they started the implementation of Six Sigma with one-day training course for the management team. The quality manager and 16 employees continued with an in-company Belt training. More groups have followed up to 2004. Projects were implemented in several areas of interest from patient logistics to medication and the length of stay in the hospital, and all show that Six Sigma, despite its origin from industry, can work equally well in healthcare.

Sample Project: Shortening the Length of Stay of Gynecology Patients

Due to the fact that in Netherlands, hospitals receive, as part of their budgets, a fixed amount of money for every admission, reducing the length of stay of patients has a direct impact on the financial results of the hospital because more patients can be admitted.

Define Phase

The objective of this project was to shorten the stay of gynecology patients who had to undergo an abdominal uterus extirpation (AUE) or a vaginal uterus extirpation (VUE). The financial benefits of this project were estimated to be €57,800. An additional benefit was the possible reduction in the waiting lists for these types of gynecological procedures. The duration of the project was estimated to be 6 months. The project was carried out by two Green Belts in training. Both Green Belts had one day per week available to spend on the project.

Measure Phase

The so-called critical to quality (CTQ) characteristic is the length of stay of patients with AUE or VUE. This CTQ was defined as the length of the stay measured in days. The requirement on the CTQ was to shorten the length of stay as much as possible with no additional discomfort to the patients. The measurement of the length of stay by an information system has been validated.

Analyze Phase

Data for the year 2002 were used. There appeared to be a few outliers, which were analyzed and excluded from the data by performing a capability analysis. The average stay in the hospital of patients with VUE or AUE was 7 days, and the standard deviation was 2 days. Based on the current performance, the Green Belts decided that the objective of this project was to reduce the length of stay for AUE or VUE patients to 4.5 days with a standard deviation of 0.6 days. This objective should result in a financial benefit of €63,520.

Factors influencing the length of stay were listed by using a cause and effect diagram and a failure mode and effect analysis (FMEA).

Improve Phase

The most relevant factors influencing the length of the stay were found to be:

- Treatment protocols of patients with AUE or VUE; and situation at home, i.e. whether there are relatives who can take care of the patients after discharge.

Changes in the protocols of AUE or VUE patients, such as skipping the presurgery day, directly reduced the length of stay of the patient. The other most fruitful improvements are listed further.

- An outpatient clinic to prepare the patient for the operation (this action reduces the length of stay of patients by one day)
- Improved protocols
- Check on the situation at home and offer home care if needed; and
- Information about the length of the stay given to the patient in advance.

Control Phase

All of the above-mentioned improvements were implemented in March 2004. At that time, the average length of stay is 5.2 days and the standard deviation is 0.9 days (based on 15 patients). Further reduction in the length of stay is expected after this initial phase.

Quality Approaches and Models

DFSS—(Design for Six Sigma) is a systematic methodology utilizing tools, training and measurements to enable us to design products and processes that meet customer expectations and can be produced at Six Sigma quality levels.

DMAIC—(Define, Measure, Analyze, Improve and Control) is a process for continued improvement. It is systematic, scientific and fact based. This closed-loop process eliminates unproductive steps, often focuses on new measurements, and applies technology for improvement.

Six Sigma—A vision of quality which equates with only 3.4 defects per million opportunities for each product or service transaction. Strives for perfection.

QUALITY TOOLS

Associates are exposed to various tools and terms related to quality. Below are just a few of them:

- *Control chart*: Monitors variance in a process over time and alerts the business to unexpected variance which may cause defects.
- *Defect measurement*: Accounting for the number or frequency of defects that cause lapses in product or service quality.
- *Pareto diagram*: Focuses on efforts or the problems that have the greatest potential for improvement by showing relative frequency and/or size in a descending bar graph. Based on the proven Pareto principle: 20% of the sources cause 80% of any problems.
- *Process mapping*: Illustrated description of how things get done, which enables participants to visualize an entire process and identify areas of strength and weaknesses. It helps reduce cycle time and defects while recognizing the value of individual contributions.
- *Root cause analysis*: Study of original reason for nonconformance with a process. When the root cause is removed or corrected, the nonconformance will be eliminated.
- *Statistical process control*: The application of statistical methods to analyze data, study and monitor process capability and performance.

- *Tree diagram*: Graphically shows any broad goal broken into different levels of detailed actions. It encourages team members to expand their thinking when creating solutions.

QUALITY TERMS

- *Black belt*: Leaders of team responsible for measuring, analyzing, improving and controlling key processes that influence customer satisfaction and/or productivity growth. Black Belts are full-time positions.
- *Control*: The state of stability, normal variation and predictability. Process of regulating and guiding operations and processes using quantitative data.
- *CTQ*: Critical to quality (Critical "Y")—Element of a process or practice which has a direct impact on its perceived quality.
- *Customer needs, expectations*: Needs, as defined by customers, which meet their basic requirements and standards.
- *Defects*: Sources of customer irritation. Defects are costly to both customers and to manufacturers or service providers. Eliminating defects provides cost benefits.
- *Green belt*: Similar to Black Belt but not a full-time position.
- *Master black belt*: First and foremost teachers. They also review and mentor Black Belts. Selection criteria for Master Black Belts are quantitative skills and the ability to teach and mentor. Master Black Belts are full-time postions.
- *Variance*: A change in a process or business practice that may alter its expected outcome.

Lean Six Sigma

A business improvement framework that integrates the Six Sigma methodology with the cost reduction benefits of the Lean production approach. Lean production techniques are included as part of the Motorola University Black Belt program.

MINITAB

A software package used to implement Six Sigma and other quality initiatives. It provides data analysis and graphical data presentations and offers many statistical procedures, ranging from simple to advanced.

Sigma Level

A metric that counts defects per million opportunities (or DPMO). A metric of Six Sigma equates to 3.4 DPMO.

Six Sigma Black Belt

A Six Sigma expert highly skilled in the application of rigorous statistical tools and methodologies to drive business process improvement.

Six Sigma Certification

A confirmation of a person's capabilities with respect to successfully leading and supporting Six Sigma project teams. It entails learning the appropriate skills, passing a written proficiency test, and displaying competency in a real-world environment. Achieving Six Sigma certification is a way to demonstrate your energy and intent to be a leader within the quality profession.

Six Sigma Champion

The Champions typically have day-to-day responsibility for the business process being improved and their role is to ensure the Six Sigma project team has the resources required to successfully execute the project.

Six Sigma Consultant

A company or individual with experience and expertise in Six Sigma business improvement implementations who is hired for a limited time to advise and facilitate Six Sigma implementation.

Six Sigma Consulting

A service provided to organizations to help improve business processes, services, and/or products using the Six Sigma methodology. Guidance may be provided on specific topics or on strategic planning for Six Sigma implementations.

Six Sigma Green Belt

A Six Sigma practitioner trained in the methodology and tools to be need to work effectively on a process improvement team. Green Belts may act as team members under the direction of a Black Belt or may lead their own less complex, high impact projects.

Six Sigma Leadership Principles

A set of guiding principles required to help leadership identify the best way to drive results and support teams. The four principles are Align, Mobilize, Accelerate, and Govern.

Six Sigma Master Black Belt

A Black Belt achieves 'Master' status after demonstrating experience and impact over some period of time. Master Black Belts address the most complex process improvement projects and provide coaching and training to Black Belts and Green Belts.

Six Sigma Quality

A level of quality that represents only 3.4 defects per million opportunities.

Six Sigma Software

A computer program that provides data analysis, project management, resource management and reporting functionality for Six Sigma projects and overall implementations.

Six Sigma Sponsor

A member of the leadership team that is responsible for selecting Six Sigma projects and is ultimately accountable for a project's results.

X's

Often referred to as Big X's, these are the factors or variables that will have the greatest impact on the Big Y's.

Y's

Often referred to a "Big Y's", these are the business results that matter. Big Y's represent measures directly linked to critical customer requirements.

BASIC CONCEPT AND MOST FREQUENTLY USED FORMULA'S IN SIX SIGMA

Histograms

- Each vertical bar represents an interval of data or a category of data
- The X-axis is showing the measurements

- The Y-axis is showing the frequency
- All bars are adjacent and will not overlap since they represent a certain interval (group) of measurements at a specified frequency.

The histogram, when made up of normally distributed data, will form a 'bell' curve when a smooth probability density function is produced using kernel smoothing techniques. This line that generalizes the histogram appears to look like a bell.

Often the more data being analyzed and with more resolution will create more bars since more intervals or categories of data are available to plot. The more measurements and at various frequencies will create more bars and fill up more of the area under the probability density function.

To assess the data there should be at least 5 bars or intervals and at least 30 data points.

There are a variety of histograms (Fig. 14.1), for most practical purposes understanding these basic components will be sufficient.

Left-Skewed Distribution (Negatively Skewed)

These histograms have the curve on the right side or the most common values on the right side of the distribution. The data extends much farther out to the left side. These distributions are common where there is an upper specification limit or it is not possible to exceed an upper value, also known as boundary limit. This may occur if a customer has requested the process run at towards the upper specification limit as opposed to targeting the mean.

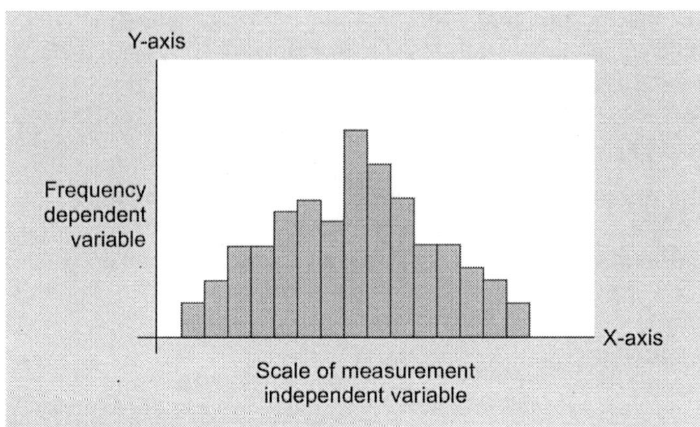

Fig. 14.1 Variety of histograms

The measure of central location is the median.

Mean < Median < Mode

Right Skewed Distribution (Positively Skewed)

The distribution of the data reaches far out to the right side. This may be caused by a process having a lower boundary. Cost or time plots commonly exhibit this behavior.

The measure of central location is the median.

Mode < Median < Mean

If most common value is 10, the middle most value is 15, and the average of the data set is 20, then the distribution is right skewed.

Mode = 10

Median = 15

Mean = 20

Bimodal Distribution

These histograms appear to have two or more (polymodal) behaviors occurring in one process and appear to have two points of central location. This can be caused by two sets of data being analyzed as one that are from different populations such as plotting the heights of females and males as one distribution.

Uniform Distribution

The distribution is flat or not exhibiting much of a bell shape and has no appearance of a central location. This may occur when all values between a lower specification limit (LSL) and upper specification limit (USL) are weighted equally acceptable. In other words, values very close to the limits are as good as a value in the middle.

Normal Distribution

Points are evenly distributed among a central value or location.

The mean is used to describe the central location of distribution. The median, mode, and mean are all close to the same value and the coefficient of skewness is close to zero.

Coefficient of Skewness (Fig. 14.2)

Karl Pearson is credited with developing the formula below to measure the coefficient of skewness. The formula compares the median with the standard deviation of the same distribution.

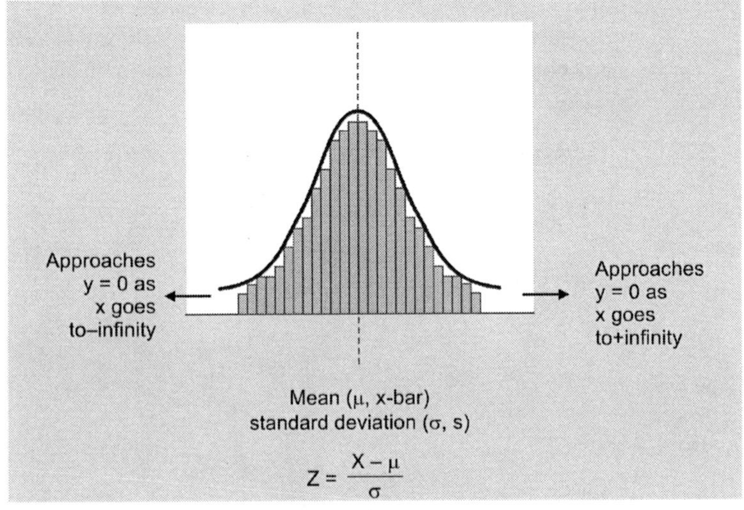

Fig. 14.2 Coefficient of skewness

$$S_k = \frac{3(\mu - \text{median})}{\sigma}$$

If:

$S_k > 0$ then skewed right distribution

$S_k = 0$ then normal distribution

$S_k < 0$ then skewed left distribution

DEFECTS PER UNIT (DPU)

The average number of defects per unit. The ratio of defects to unit is the universal measure of quality.

Given:

D: Number of defects

U: Number of units

Formula:

$$DPU = \frac{\textit{Total number of defects}}{\textit{Total units}} = \frac{D}{U}$$

DPU may be estimated if the Throughput Yield (also called First Pass Yield) is known:

$$DPU = -\ln TPY$$

Table 14.2 exemplified defect per unit. Let us say that ten nails were produced at a manufacturing facility and each nail has five ways (opportunities) it can be defective. If any one of the five characteristics fails, then the entire nail is considered defective.

Table 14.2 Six Sigma responsibility matrix

Nail	Length	Diameter	Pisting	Hardness	Material	Defective	No. of defects per nail
Nail#1		×			×	Yes	2
Nail#2	×					Yes	1
Nail#3						No	0
Nail#4		×	×	×		Yes	3
Nail#5				×	×	Yes	2
Nail#6	×	×			×	Yes	3
Nail#7	×	×	×	×		Yes	4
Nail#8			×	×		Yes	2
Nail#9						No	0
Nail#10				×	×	Yes	2

There is a possibility of 50 total defects if each nail had all five characteristics (opportunities) fail. The total number of defects (D) is 2 + 1 + 3 + 2 + 3 + 4 + 2 + 2 = 19.

The number of defectives is 8.

8 out of 10 nails contained one or more defects qualifying them as *defective*.

From the table:

D = 19 total defects were found

U = 10 units (nails).

Defect Per Unit (DPU) = 1.9 defects per nail

If all these defects could come from a SINGLE process (not in reality for this case, these types of defects occur from different operations), rearranging the formula above the TPY is:

$$\text{TPY} = e^{-\text{DPU}} = 2.71828^{-1.9} = 0.1496 = 14.96\%$$

DEFECTS PER MILLION OPPORTUNITIES (DPMO)

Defects per million opportunities factors in the total opportunities for defect occurrence existing in a process. DPMO is considered long-term measurement of a process and this can be directly converted into a long-term Z-statistic (sigma value). Given:

D: No. of defects

O: No. of opportunities for a defect

U: No. of units

TOP: Total number of opportunities = U × O

Formula: DPMO = DPO × 1,000,000

Note:

DPMO is NOT the same as PPM since it is possible that each unit (part) being appraised may be found to have multiple defects of the same type or may have multiple types of defects. A part is defective if it has one or more defects. The number of defectives can never exceed the number of defects.

If each part only has one characteristic that can be a defect, then DPMO and PPM will be the same.

DPMO will always exceed or equal PPM for a given yield or sigma level of performance.

Example

Table 14.3 shows example of defect per million opportunities (DPMO). Nail #1 it has two types of defects. Therefore, it is ONE defective nail that contains TWO defects.

Table 14.3 Example of DPMO

Nail	Length	Diameter	Pisting	Hardness	Material	Defective	No. of defects per nail
Nail#1		×			×	Yes	2
Nail#2	×					Yes	1
Nail#3						No	0
Nail#4		×	×	×		Yes	3
Nail#5			×	×	×	Yes	2
Nail#6	×	×			×	Yes	3
Nail#7	×	×	×	×		Yes	4
Nail#8			×	×		Yes	2
Nail#9						No	0
Nail#10				×	×	Yes	2

Summary of Table

D = 19 total defects
O = 5 opportunities (categories of defect types)
U = 10 nails
TOP = U × O = 50 total opportunities
DPU = D/U = 19/10 = 1.9 defects per unit
DPO = D/TOP = 19/50 = 0.38
DPMO = 380,000
Out of a million opportunities, the long-term performance of the process would create 380,000 defects.

Using Excel to Calculate Sigma and DPMO

There are a couple of processes which commonly used Microsoft Excel functions that converts Defects per Million Opportunities (DPMO) to a process sigma (Z-score) and vice versa.
To convert from DPMO to process sigma:
Process Sigma = NORMSINV × (1 – (DPMO/1,000,000)) + 1.5

To convert from process sigma to DPMO:
DPMO = 1,000,000 × (1 – (NORMSDIST * (process sigma – 1.5))

Note:
A Six Sigma quality process refers to the process short-term performance or how it is performing currently when there are 3.4 DPMO. Over the long-term, this Six Sigma process is estimated to shift –1.5 sigma (lower) and will perform at a 4.5 sigma level, which produces 1,350 DPMO.

Get the DPMO Calculator (Table 14.4)

Enter your values in the white cells and everything else is calculated. Notes are in the actual template that offer more guidance and information on each row.

Table 14.4 DPMO calculator

Units	1,221
Opportunities/Unit	12
Actual no. of defective units	219
No. of units with zero defects	1,002
TOP	14,652

Contd...

Contd...

Actual no. of total defects	726
DPU	0.5945946
DPO	0.0495495
DPMO	49,550
Percent defective	17.94%
Percent defects	4.95%
Final yield	82.06388%
Process yield	95.04505%
Shift	0.00
Process sigma	1.649

BINOMIAL DISTRIBUTION

The binomial distribution is a discrete distribution displaying data that has only *two outcomes* and each trial includes *replacement.*
Such as:

- Pass/Fail
- Go/No-Go
- Success/Failure
- In/Out
- Hot/Cold
- Male/Female
- Defective/Not defective
- Right-Handed/Left-Handed
- High/Low
- Heads/Tails.

Assumptions

- Each trial has only two outcomes
- The experiment has unidentical trials
- Each trial is independent of the other trials
- The probability of getting one outcome (success) p is held constant and the probability of getting the other outcome (failure) is also held constant (1 – p)
- Includes replacement for each trial can be used to approximate without replacement trials but it is suggested to use hypergeometric distribution formulas.

Lets evaluate the assumptions.

A coin flip is an example of two outcomes and each flip has the same chance for both outcomes (meaning independent). Flipping the coin n amount of times means there are n identical trials. Nothing changes from one flip to another and the odds are the same for each flip.

$$\text{Mean} = \mu = E(x) = np$$
$$\text{Variance} = \sigma^2 = np(1\text{-}p)$$
$$\text{Standard Deviation} = \sigma = \sqrt{np(1-p)}$$

where

n = number of trials

p = probability of success

$1\text{-}p$ = probability of other outcome (failure)

The following formula is used to compute the number of *experimental outcomes* resulting from x successes in n trials.

$$\frac{n}{x} = \frac{n!}{x!(n-x)!}$$

For example: 4! (4 factorial) = $4 \times 3 \times 2 \times 1 = 24$

The *Binomial Distribution Probability Function* is shown below:

$$P(x) = \frac{n!}{x!(n-x)!} p^x q^{n-x}$$

and x is the number of successes desired.

Example One

A manufacturing process creates 3.4% defective parts. A sample of 10 parts from the production process is selected. What is the probability that the sample contains exactly 3 defective parts?

Solution

There are two outcomes: Defective/not defective, therefore the binomial distribution equation is applied.

$p = 0.034$

$n = 10$

then $q = 1 - p = 1 - 0.034 = 0.966$ (96.6%)

Need the probability that $x = 3$.

Substitute the values into the Binomial Probability Function and solve:

$$P(x) = \frac{10!}{3!(10-3)!}(0.034^3)(0.966^7)$$
$$P(x) = 120(0.034^3)(0.966^7)$$
$$P(x) = 003702 = 0.372\%$$

Example Two

Forty-five percent of all registered voters in a national election are female. A random sample of 8 voters is selected. The probability that the sample contains 2 males is:

Solution

55% are male and there are two outcomes: Male/Female

$n = 8$

$p = 0.55$ (55%)

$q = 1 - p = 0.45$

Need the probability that $x = 2$

$$P(x) = \frac{8!}{2!(8-2)!}(0.55^2)(0.45^6)$$

$$P(x) = 28(0.55^2)(0.45^6)$$

$$P(x) = 0.07033$$

$$= 7.03\%$$

Example Three

Seventy nine percent of the students of a large class passed the final examination. A random sample of 4 students are selected to be analyzed by the school. What is the probability that the sample contains *fewer* than 2 students that passed the examination?

There are two outcomes: Pass/Fail

$p = 0.79$

$n = 4$

Need the probability that $x < 2$.

Note that we need to compute $p\,(x < 2)$. So, it is necessary to add the $P\,(x = 0)$ to the $P\,(x = 1)$.

Each $P\,(x = 0)$ and $P\,(x = 1)$ must be calculated separately and added.

$p\,(x < 2) = p\,(x = 0) + p\,(x = 1)$

Substitute the following values into the Binomial equation to find $p\,(x = 0)$:

$n = 4$

$p = 0.79$

$q = 1 - p = 1 - 0.79 = 0.21$

$x = 0$

Plus

$n = 4$

$p = 0.79$

$q = 1 - p = 1 - 0.79 = 0.21$

$x = 1$

$$P(x)=\frac{n!}{x!(n-x)!}p^x q^{n-x}$$

$$P(0)=\frac{4!}{0!(4-0)!}(0.79^0)(0.21^4)$$

(0! = 1 and any number to the power of zero = 1)

$$P(0)=(1)(1)(0.21^4)=0.194\%$$

$$P(1)=\frac{4!}{1!(4-1)!}(0.79^1)(0.21^3)$$

$$P(1)=4(0.79)(0.009261)=2.926\%$$

Adding

$$P(0) + P(1) = 0.194\% + 2.926\% = 3.12\%$$

There is 3.12% chance of selecting fewer than 2 students that passed the examination when randomly selecting 4 students when 79% of them passed.

There are also Binomial tables that can be used when the input variables are known (and found within the table).

POISSON DISTRIBUTION

The Poisson distribution is a discrete distribution named after French mathematician Simeon-Denis Poisson.

Unlike the Binomial Distribution that has only two possible outcomes as a success or fail, this distribution focuses on the number of discrete occurrences over a defined interval.

The Poisson formula describes rare events and is also referred to as the law of improbable events. The formula is shown below to calculate the probability of occurrences over an interval.

$$P(x)=\frac{\lambda^x e^{-\lambda}}{x!}$$

where

$x = 0, 1, 2, 3, 4,....$

$e = 2.71828$

λ = long run average

The Poisson distribution exhibits the following:

- Discrete distribution
- Occurrences are independent of each other
- Occurrences range from 0 to infinity in an interval
- Describes rare events
- Describes discrete occurrences of defined interval

- Expected number of occurrences must be constant in a Poisson experiment, this is the value of *lambda* which must be a positive real number.

The Poisson distribution may apply when studying the:
- Number of customers per minute in a bookstore
- Number of transactions per hour at a bank
- Number of long distance telephone calls per day
- Number of cracks in a windshield after installation
- Number of cars passing through an intersection per day
- Number of late shipments per 1,000 shipments
- Number of pieces scrapped per 1,000,000 pieces produced
- Number of planes arriving per hour at airport
- Number of vacant houses per county in a state.

Example One

A new website has an average random hit rate of 2.9 unique visitors every 4 minutes.
What is the probability of getting exactly 50 unique visitors every hour?
Given information
x = exactly 50 unique visitor/1 hour
$e = 2.71828$
λ = lambda = 2.0 unique visitor/4 minutes
First step is to get the units of time to match:
x = exactly 50 unique visitors/1 hour
λ = 43.5 unique visitors/1 hour
(multiplied both numerator and denominator by 15)
Substitute into the Poisson probability equation:

$$P(x) = \frac{(43.5)^{50} e^{-43.5}}{50!} = 0.035$$

Note:
Never adjust the x value, this remains constant for each interval or experiment.

T-DISTRIBUTION

The various t-test are commonly applied during the *analyze* phase for Six Sigma project managers. You should be familiar with these tests and able to explain the results.

William Sealy Gosset is credited with first publishing the data of the test statistic and became known as the Student's t-distribution. It is generally used for sample sizes less than 30 ($n < 30$).

The *t*-distribution bell curve gets flatter as the Degrees of Freedom (DF) decrease.

Looking at it from the other perspective, as the DF increases, that means the number of samples (n) must be increasing thus the sample is becoming more representative of the population and then the sample statistics approach the population parameters. So as the these values come closer to one another the 'z' calculation and 't' calculation get closer and closer to same value.

Six Sigma used in t-distribution of various test as shown in Table 14.5.

Table 14.5 Various test of Six Sigma used in t-distribution

Comparison of means	Degrees of freedom	Application	Assumptions	Test statistics
One sample *Z*-test	Not applicable	Testing the difference of a sample mean, x-bar, with a known population mean, μ (fixed mean, historical mean, or targeted mean)	Normal distribution known population σ	$Z = \frac{\bar{X} - \mu}{\frac{\sigma}{\sqrt{n}}}$
One sample *t*-test	$n - 1$	Testing the difference of one sample mean, *x*-bar, with a known population mean, μ (fixed mean, historical mean, or targeted mean)	Normal distribution Popular standard deviation, σ is unknown	$t = \frac{\bar{X} - \mu}{\frac{\sigma}{\sqrt{n}}}$
Two sample *t*-test	$n_1 + n_2 - 2$	Testing difference of two sample means when population variances unknown but considered equal	Normal distribution Requires standard pooled deviation calculation, s_p	$t = \frac{\bar{X}_1 - \bar{X}_2}{S_p \sqrt{\frac{1}{n_1} + \frac{1}{n}}}$
Paired *t*-test	$n - 1$	Testing two sample means when their respective population standard deviations are unknown but considered equal. Data recorded in pairs and each pair has a difference, d	Normal distribution Two dependent samples. Always two-trailed test S_d = standard deviations of the differences of all samples	$t = \frac{\bar{d}\sqrt{n}}{S_d}$
One-way ANOVA	$n_2 - 1$ and $n_2 - 1$	Testing the difference of three or more population means	Normal distribution s_1^2 and s_2^2 represent sample variances	$F = \frac{(S_1)^2}{(S_2)^2}$

HYPOTHESIS TESTING

Before running test, try to visualize your data to get a better understanding of the projected outcome of expected result. Using tools such as Box Plot can provide a wealth of information.

Also, if the confidence interval contains the value of zero then insufficient evidence exist to suggest there is a statistical difference between the null and alternative hypothesis and accept the null.

Two Sample T-test

This test is used when comparing the means of:

- Two random independent samples are drawn, n_1 and n_2.
- Each population exhibit normal distribution.
- Equal standard deviations assumed for each population (Table 14.6).

The degrees of freedom (DF) = $n_1 + n_2 - 2$

Example:

The overall length of a sample of a part running of two different machines is being evaluated. The hypothesis test is to determine if there is a difference between the overall lengths of the parts made of the two machines using 95% level of confidence.

Machine 1:

Sample size: 22 parts

Mean: 28.4 mm

Sample standard deviation: 3.4 mm

Machine 2:

Sample size: 20 parts

Mean: 27.6 mm

Sample standard deviation: 2.2 mm

DF = $n_1 + n_2 - 2 = 22 + 20 - 2 = 40$ Alpha-risk = 1 – CI = 1 – 0.95 = 0.05

Establish the hypothesis test:

Null: Mean A equals the Mean B

Alternative: Mean A does not equal Mean B

This is two-tailed example since the direction (shorter or longer) is not relevant. All that is relevant is if there is a statistical difference or not.

Now, determine the range for which t-statistic and any values outside these ranges will result in rejecting the null and inferring the Alternative hypothesis.

Using the *t*-table below notice that:

-t(0.975) to t(0.975) with 40 DF equals a range of -2.021 to 2.021.

If the calculated *t*-value from our example falls within this range then accept the Null hypothesis.

Note: Keep in mind Table 14.6 which is a one-tailed table so use the column 0.025 that corresponds to 40 DF and include both the positive and negative value.

Paired T-test

Use this test when analyzing the samples of a *before* and *after* situation and the number of samples must be the same.

$$DF = n - 1$$

The 'SD' is the standard deviation of the difference in all of the samples. The data is recorded in pairs and each pair of data has a difference, *d*.

Table 14.6 T-distribution table

df \ α	0.25	0.1	0.05	0.025	0.01	0.005	0.0025	0.001	0.0005
1	1.000	3.078	6.314	12.706	31.821	63.656	127.321	318.289	636.578
2	0.816	1.886	2.920	4.303	6.965	9.925	14.089	22.328	31.600
3	0.765	1.638	2.353	3.182	4.541	5.841	7.453	10.214	12.924
4	0.741	1.533	2.132	2.776	3.747	4.604	5.598	7.173	8.160
5	0.727	1.476	2.015	2.571	3.365	4.032	4.773	5.894	6.869
6	0.718	1.440	1.943	2.447	3.143	3.707	4.317	5.208	5.959
7	0.711	1.415	1.895	2.365	2.998	3.499	4.029	4.785	5.408
8	0.706	1.397	1.860	2.306	2.896	3.355	3.833	4.501	5.041
9	0.703	1.383	1.833	2.262	2.821	3.250	3.690	4.297	4.781
10	0.700	1.372	1.812	2.228	2.764	3.169	3.581	4.144	4.587
11	0.697	1.363	1.796	2.201	2.718	3.106	3.497	4.025	4.437
12	0.695	1.356	1.782	2.179	2.681	3.055	3.428	3.930	4.318
13	0.694	1.350	1.771	2.160	2.650	3.012	3.372	3.852	4.221
14	0.692	1.345	1.761	2.145	2.624	2.977	3.326	3.787	4.140
15	0.691	1.341	1.753	2.131	2.602	2.947	3.286	3.733	4.073
16	0.690	1.337	1.746	2.120	2.583	2.921	3.252	3.686	4.015
17	0.689	1.333	1.740	2.110	2.567	2.898	3.222	3.646	3.965
18	0.688	1.330	1.734	2.101	2.552	2.878	3.197	3.610	3.922
19	0.688	1.328	1.729	2.093	2.539	2.861	3.174	3.579	3.883
20	0.687	1.325	1.725	2.086	2.528	2.845	3.153	3.552	3.850
21	0.686	1.323	1.721	2.080	2.518	2.831	3.135	3.527	3.819
22	0.686	1.321	1.717	2.074	2.508	2.819	3.119	3.505	3.792

Contd...

Contd...

23	0.685	1.319	1.714	2.069	2.500	2.807	3.104	3.485	3.768
24	0.685	1.318	1.711	2.064	2.492	2.797	3.091	3.467	3.745
25	0.684	1.316	1.708	2.060	2.485	2.787	3.078	3.450	3.725
26	0.684	1.315	1.706	2.056	2.479	2.779	3.067	3.435	3.707
27	0.684	1.314	1.703	2.052	2.473	2.771	3.057	3.421	3.689
28	0.683	1.313	1.701	2.048	2.467	2.763	3.047	3.408	3.674
29	0.683	1.311	1.699	2.045	2.462	2.756	3.038	3.396	3.660
30	0.683	1.310	1.697	2.042	2.457	2.750	3.030	3.385	3.646
40	0.681	1.303	1.684	2.021	2.423	2.704	2.971	3.307	3.551
60	0.679	1.296	1.671	2.000	2.390	2.660	2.915	3.232	3.460
120	0.677	1.289	1.658	1.980	2.358	2.617	2.860	3.160	3.373

Confidence Interval Formula

$$\mu = \overline{x} \pm t_{a/2,n-1}\frac{S}{\sqrt{n}}$$

CHI-SQUARE DISTRIBUTION

The Chi-square distribution is most often for hypothesis tests and in determining confidence intervals.

- Chi-square test for independence in an 'Row × Column' contingency table.
- Chi-square test to determine if the standard deviation of a population is equal to a specified value.

Unlike the normal distribution, the Chi-square distribution is not symmetric. Separate tables exist for the upper and lower tails of the distribution.

This statistical test can be used to examine the hypothesis of independence between two attribute variables and determine if the attribute variables are related.

Assumptions

- Chi-square is the underlying distribution for these tests.
- Attribute data (X data and Y data are attribute).
- Observations must be independent.

Ideally used when comparing more than two samples, otherwise use the 2-Proportions Test (with two samples) or 1-Proportion Test (with one sample).

Formula

The sum of the expected frequencies is always equal to the sum of the observed frequencies.

The Chi-squared statistic can be used to:

- Test how well the distribution fits the population.
- Test association of two attribute variables.

$$\chi^2 = \sum_{j=1}^{g} \frac{(f_0 - f_e)^2}{f_e}$$

f_0 = observed frequencies
f_e = expected frequencies

Possible Applications

- Test to see if a particular region of the country is an important factor in the number wins for a baseball team.
- Determine if the number of injuries among a few facilities is statistically different.
- Determine if a coin or a set of dice is biased or fair.

Goodness of Fit (GOF) Hypothesis Test

The GOF test compares the frequency of occurrence from an observed sample to the expected frequency from the hypothesized distribution.

As in all hypothesis test, craft a statement without numbers and use simple terms for the team's understanding and then create the numerical or statistical version of the problem statement.

- State the practical problem.
- State the statistical problem.
- Develop null and alternative hypotheses.
- Create table of observed and expected frequencies.
- Calculate the test statistic.

The Degrees of Freedom = (No. of rows – 1) × (No. of columns – 1)

Two methods can be applied to test the hypotheses. The decision to reject the null (and infer the alternative hypothesis) if:

1. Calculate the critical value the Chi-squared test statistic and reject the null hypothesis if the calculated value is *greater than* the critical value
   OR
2. Reject the null hypothesis if the *p*-value is *less than* the alpha-risk. Your team determines the alpha-risk. For a Confidence Level of 95% the alpha-risk = 5% or 0.05.
   Using EXCEL to determine the *p*-value is done by:
   P-value = CHIDIST (Chi-square calculated, degrees of freedom)
   OR
   P-value = CHITEST (Observed range, expected range).

Critical Values of the Chi-Square Distribution (Tables 14.7 and 14.8)

Table 14.7 Upper-tail critical values of Chi-square distribution with v degrees of freedom

Probability less than the critical value					
v	*0.90*	*0.95*	*0.975*	*0.99*	*0.999*
1.	2.706	3.841	5.024	6.635	10.828
2.	4.605	5.991	7.378	9.210	13.816
3.	6.251	7.815	9.348	11.345	16.266
4.	7.779	9.488	11.143	13.277	18.467
5.	9.236	11.070	12.833	15.086	20.515
6.	10.645	12.592	14.449	16.812	22.458
7.	12.017	14.067	16.013	18.475	24.322
8.	13.362	15.507	17.535	20.090	26.125
9.	14.684	16.919	19.023	21.666	27.877
10.	15.987	18.307	20.483	23.209	29.588
11.	17.275	19.675	21.920	24.725	31.264
12.	18.549	21.026	23.337	26.217	32.910
13.	19.812	22.362	24.736	27.688	34.528
14.	21.064	23.685	26.119	29.141	36.123
15.	22.307	24.996	27.488	30.578	37.697
16.	23.542	26.296	28.845	32.000	39.252
17.	24.769	27.587	30.191	33.409	40.790
18.	25.989	28.869	31.526	34.805	42.312
19.	27.204	30.144	32.852	36.191	43.820

Contd...

Contd...

20.	28.412	31.410	34.170	37.566	45.315
21.	29.615	32.671	35.479	38.932	46.797
22.	30.813	33.924	36.781	40.289	48.268
23.	32.007	35.172	38.076	41.638	49.728
24.	33.196	36.415	39.364	42.980	51.179
25.	34.382	37.652	40.646	44.314	52.620
26.	35.563	38.885	41.923	45.642	54.052
27.	36.741	40.113	43.195	46.963	55.476
28.	37.916	41.337	44.461	48.278	56.892
29.	39.087	42.557	45.722	49.588	58.301
30.	40.256	43.773	46.979	50.892	59.703
31.	41.422	44.985	48.232	52.191	61.098
32.	42.585	46.194	49.480	53.486	62.487
33.	43.745	47.400	50.725	54.776	63.870
34.	44.903	48.602	51.966	56.061	65.247
35.	46.059	49.802	53.203	57.342	66.619
36.	47.212	50.998	54.437	58.619	67.985
37.	48.363	52.192	55.668	59.893	69.347
38.	49.513	53.384	56.896	61.162	70.703
39.	50.660	54.572	58.120	62.428	72.055
40.	51.805	55.758	59.342	63.691	73.402
41.	52.949	56.942	60.561	64.950	74.745
42.	54.090	58.124	61.777	66.206	76.084
43.	55.230	59.304	62.990	67.459	77.419
44.	56.369	60.481	64.201	68.710	78.750
45.	57.505	61.656	65.410	69.957	80.077
46.	58.641	62.830	66.617	71.201	81.400
47.	59.774	64.001	67.821	72.443	82.720
48.	60.907	65.171	69.023	73.683	84.037
49.	62.038	66.339	70.222	74.919	85.351
50.	63.167	67.505	71.420	76.154	86.661
51.	64.295	68.669	72.616	77.386	87.968
52.	65.422	69.832	73.810	78.616	89.272

Contd...

Contd...

53.	66.548	70.993	75.002	79.843	90.573
54.	67.673	72.153	76.192	81.069	91.872
55.	68.796	73.311	77.380	82.292	93.168
56.	69.919	74.468	78.567	83.513	94.461
57.	71.040	75.624	79.752	84.733	95.751
58.	72.160	76.778	80.936	85.950	97.039
59.	73.279	77.931	82.117	87.166	98.324
60.	74.397	79.082	83.298	88.379	99.607
61.	75.514	80.232	84.476	89.591	100.888
62.	76.630	81.381	85.654	90.802	102.166
63.	77.745	82.529	86.830	92.010	103.442
64.	78.860	83.675	88.004	93.217	104.716
65.	79.973	84.821	89.177	94.422	105.988
66.	81.085	85.965	90.349	95.626	107.258
67.	82.197	87.108	91.519	96.828	108.526
68.	83.308	88.250	92.689	98.028	109.791
69.	84.418	89.391	93.856	99.228	111.055
70.	85.527	90.531	95.023	100.425	112.317
71.	86.635	91.670	96.189	101.621	113.577
72.	87.743	92.808	97.353	102.816	114.835
73.	88.850	93.945	98.516	104.010	116.092
74.	89.956	95.081	99.678	105.202	117.346
75.	91.061	96.217	100.839	106.393	118.599
76.	92.166	97.351	101.999	107.583	119.850
77.	93.270	98.484	103.158	108.771	121.100
78.	94.374	99.617	104.316	109.958	122.348
79.	95.476	100.749	105.473	111.144	123.594
80.	96.578	101.879	106.629	112.329	124.839
81.	97.680	103.010	107.783	113.512	126.083
82.	98.780	104.139	108.937	114.695	127.324
83.	99.880	105.267	110.090	115.876	128.565
84.	100.980	106.395	111.242	117.057	129.804
85.	102.079	107.522	112.393	118.236	131.041
86.	103.177	108.648	113.544	119.414	132.277

Contd...

Contd...

87.	104.275	109.773	114.693	120.591	133.512
88.	105.372	110.898	115.841	121.767	134.746
89.	106.469	112.022	116.989	122.942	135.978
90.	107.565	113.145	118.136	124.116	137.208
91.	108.661	114.268	119.282	125.289	138.438
92.	109.756	115.390	120.427	126.462	139.666
93.	110.850	116.511	121.571	127.633	140.893
94.	111.944	117.632	122.715	128.803	142.119
95.	113.038	118.752	123.858	129.973	143.344
96.	114.131	119.871	125.000	131.141	144.567
97.	115.223	120.990	126.141	132.309	145.789
98.	116.315	122.108	127.282	133.476	147.010
99.	117.407	123.225	128.422	134.642	148.230
100.	118.498	124.342	129.561	135.807	149.449

Table 14.8 Lower-tail critical values of Chi-square distribution with v degrees of freedom

Probability less than the critical value					
v	*0.10*	*0.05*	*0.025*	*0.01*	*0.001*
1.	0.016	0.004	0.001	0.000	0.000
2.	0.211	0.103	0.051	0.020	0.002
3.	0.584	0.352	0.216	0.115	0.024
4.	1.064	0.711	0.484	0.297	0.091
5.	1.610	1.145	0.831	0.554	0.210
6.	2.204	1.635	1.237	0.872	0.381
7.	2.833	2.167	1.690	1.239	0.598
8.	3.490	2.733	2.180	1.646	0.857
9.	4.168	3.325	2.700	2.088	1.152
10.	4.865	3.940	3.247	2.558	1.479
11.	5.578	4.575	3.816	3.053	1.834
12.	6.304	5.226	4.404	3.571	2.214
13.	7.042	5.892	5.009	4.107	2.617
14.	7.790	6.571	5.629	4.660	3.041
15.	8.547	7.261	6.262	5.229	3.483
16.	9.312	7.962	6.908	5.812	3.942

Contd...

Contd...

17.	10.085	8.672	7.564	6.408	4.416
18.	10.865	9.390	8.231	7.015	4.905
19.	11.651	10.117	8.907	7.633	5.407
20.	12.443	10.851	9.591	8.260	5.921
21.	13.240	11.591	10.283	8.897	6.447
22.	14.041	12.338	10.982	9.542	6.983
23.	14.848	13.091	11.689	10.196	7.529
24.	15.659	13.848	12.401	10.856	8.085
25.	16.473	14.611	13.120	11.524	8.649
26.	17.292	15.379	13.844	12.198	9.222
27.	18.114	16.151	14.573	12.879	9.803
28.	18.939	16.928	15.308	13.565	10.391
29.	19.768	17.708	16.047	14.256	10.986
30.	20.599	18.493	16.791	14.953	11.588
31.	21.434	19.281	17.539	15.655	12.196
32.	22.271	20.072	18.291	16.362	12.811
33.	23.110	20.867	19.047	17.074	13.431
34.	23.952	21.664	19.806	17.789	14.057
35.	24.797	22.465	20.569	18.509	14.688
36.	25.643	23.269	21.336	19.233	15.324
37.	26.492	24.075	22.106	19.960	15.965
38.	27.343	24.884	22.878	20.691	16.611
39.	28.196	25.695	23.654	21.426	17.262
40.	29.051	26.509	24.433	22.164	17.916
41.	29.907	27.326	25.215	22.906	18.575
42.	30.765	28.144	25.999	23.650	19.239
43.	31.625	28.965	26.785	24.398	19.906
44.	32.487	29.787	27.575	25.148	20.576
45.	33.350	30.612	28.366	25.901	21.251
46.	34.215	31.439	29.160	26.657	21.929
47.	35.081	32.268	29.956	27.416	22.610
48.	35.949	33.098	30.755	28.177	23.295
49.	36.818	33.930	31.555	28.941	23.983
50.	37.689	34.764	32.357	29.707	24.674

Contd...

Contd...

51.	38.560	35.600	33.162	30.475	25.368
52.	39.433	36.437	33.968	31.246	26.065
53.	40.308	37.276	34.776	32.018	26.765
54.	41.183	38.116	35.586	32.793	27.468
55.	42.060	38.958	36.398	33.570	28.173
56.	42.937	39.801	37.212	34.350	28.881
57.	43.816	40.646	38.027	35.131	29.592
58.	44.696	41.492	38.844	35.913	30.305
59.	45.577	42.339	39.662	36.698	31.020
60.	46.459	43.188	40.482	37.485	31.738
61.	47.342	44.038	41.303	38.273	32.459
62.	48.226	44.889	42.126	39.063	33.181
63.	49.111	45.741	42.950	39.855	33.906
64.	49.996	46.595	43.776	40.649	34.633
65.	50.883	47.450	44.603	41.444	35.362
66.	51.770	48.305	45.431	42.240	36.093
67.	52.659	49.162	46.261	43.038	36.826
68.	53.548	50.020	47.092	43.838	37.561
69.	54.438	50.879	47.924	44.639	38.298
70.	55.329	51.739	48.758	45.442	39.036
71.	56.221	52.600	49.592	46.246	39.777
72.	57.113	53.462	50.428	47.051	40.519
73.	58.006	54.325	51.265	47.858	41.264
74.	58.900	55.189	52.103	48.666	42.010
75.	59.795	56.054	52.942	49.475	42.757
76.	60.690	56.920	53.782	50.286	43.507
77.	61.586	57.786	54.623	51.097	44.258
78.	62.483	58.654	55.466	51.910	45.010
79.	63.380	59.522	56.309	52.725	45.764
80.	64.278	60.391	57.153	53.540	46.520
81.	65.176	61.261	57.998	54.357	47.277
82.	66.076	62.132	58.845	55.174	48.036
83.	66.976	63.004	59.692	55.993	48.796
84.	67.876	63.876	60.540	56.813	49.557
85.	68.777	64.749	61.389	57.634	50.320

Contd...

Contd...

86.	69.679	65.623	62.239	58.456	51.085
87.	70.581	66.498	63.089	59.279	51.850
88.	71.484	67.373	63.941	60.103	52.617
89.	72.387	68.249	64.793	60.928	53.386
90.	73.291	69.126	65.647	61.754	54.155
91.	74.196	70.003	66.501	62.581	54.926
92.	75.100	70.882	67.356	63.409	55.698
93.	76.006	71.760	68.211	64.238	56.472
94.	76.912	72.640	69.068	65.068	57.246
95.	77.818	73.520	69.925	65.898	58.022
96.	78.725	74.401	70.783	66.730	58.799
97.	79.633	75.282	71.642	67.562	59.577
98.	80.541	76.164	72.501	68.396	60.356
99.	81.449	77.046	73.361	69.230	61.137
100.	82.358	77.929	74.222	70.065	61.918

How to Use This Table

This table contains the critical values of the Chi-square distribution. Because of the lack of symmetry of the Chi-square distribution, separate tables are provided for the upper and lower tails of the distribution.

A test statistic with v degrees of freedom is computed from the data. For upper-tail one-sided tests, the test statistic is compared with a value from the table of upper-tail critical values. For two-sided tests, the test statistic is compared with values from both the table for the upper-tail critical values and the table for the lower-tail critical values.

F-TABLE

The *F Distribution* is a continuous probability distribution based on the ratio of two random variances. It is formed from the ratios of two Chi-squared variables with the following formula:

$$F = \frac{X_1/\upsilon_1}{X_2/\upsilon_2}$$

X_1 and X_2 represent independent Chi-square variables
υ represents the degrees of freedom for each variable

Rarely is the probability density function calculated mathematically. Thankfully that work has been done and *F-tables* with the most common levels of significance and degrees of freedom exist for reference.

Be careful when using tables. Some tables are for one-tailed test and others cover two-tailed test.

For a one-tailed test, the null hypothesis is rejected when the test statistic is greater than the value given in the F-table.

DESIGN FOR SIX SIGMA (DFSS)

Design for Six Sigma is used to perfect product and processes before use or release. When a new product design or new process design is needed and expected to perform at a Six Sigma level from the start or level considered to be 'perfect' for the company or industry.

DMADV is another acronym sometimes used in place of DFSS, consisting of the following five steps:

Define: Design goals that satisfy customer demands, company and end-user.
Measure: Identify characteristics that are critical to quality, product capabilities, production process capability, and risks.
Analyze: Efficient product, process, or system design. Design alternatives, evaluate designs capability, reliability, and manufacturability, to select the best design.
Design: Using tools such as Axiomatic Design, refine and optimize the software, hardware, and system design.
Verify: Validate and quantify the design performance. Implement the production process. SIx Sigma GB or BB to hold final gate review and close the project, hand-off to the process owner.

The tools used in traditional DMAIC Six Sigma projects require a process or service that already exist with past performance. DFSS focuses on gathering the customer requirements and desires and designing them into a new product, process, or service. There is not always a baseline to compare past, current, and future results.

It is often the most expensive up-front and requires the highest level of effort but should deliver the most satisfying product, process, or service upon initiation. It will include most of the mistake proofing and will have attempted to reduce or eliminate all known risks before initiation.

Ultimately, the time, effort, and money devoted up-front will be more than offset with the long-term implementation of the new product, process, or service. There will be fewer failures, more satisfied customers, higher loyalty levels, and less reaction due to the proactivity of the DFSS team.

Some of the tools are also used in the DMAIC process. Some are unique to DFSS since they assist in new development instead of continual improvement.

HYPOTHESIS TESTING AND PARAMETRIC

Selecting the appropriate comparison test can be challenging especially in the learning stages. There are more than listed here. A Six Sigma project manager should understand the formulas and computations within the commonly applied tests.

Statistical software has simplified the work to the point where comprehension of these tests is convenient to overlook.

Parametric tests are used when:

- Normally distributed data
- Non-normal distribution but transformable
- Sample size is large enough to satisfy the Central Limit Theorem
- Require that the data be interval or ratio data.

Nonparametric tests are used when:

- The above criteria are not met or if distribution is unknown
- These tests are used when analyzing nominal or ordinal data
- Nonparametric test can also analyze interval or ratio data.

Comparison of Variances

Use the *F*-test or ANOVA for >2 variances. The *F*-test assumes the data is normal.

Levene's test is an option to compare variances of non-normal data.

Hypothesis Testing Steps

1. Define the problem.
2. State the objectives.
3. Establish the hypothesis.
4. State the null hypothesis (Ho).
5. State the alternative hypothesis (Ha).
6. Select the appropriate statistical test.
7. State the alpha risk level.
8. State the beta risk level.
9. Establish the effect size.
10. Create sampling plan, determine sample size.

Now, the physical part of the test:

11. Gather samples.
12. Collect and record data.
13. Calculate the test statistic.

14. Determine the *p*-value.

If *p*-value is less than alpha-risk, reject Ho and accept Ha.

If *p*-value is more than alpha-risk, fail to reject the null, Ho.

Try to re-run the test (if practical) to further confirm results. The next step is to take the statistical results and translate it to a practical solution.

It is also possible to determine the critical value of the test and use to calculated test statistic to determine the results. Either way, using the *p*-value approach or critical value should provide the same result.

Create a Visual Aid of the Test

To make the learning process easier, it is recommended that the problem be broken into *four* smaller steps.

Create a table similar to the one below and begin by completing the top two boxes. The bottom-left is the results from the test and then coverting those numbers into meaning is the practical result that belongs in the bottom-right box.

State the practical problem	**Write the statistical problem**
In simple words, write the statement and comparison being tested	Develop the null and alternate hypothesis. Determine level of confidence and power Determine degree of freedom
Find the statistical solution Document the test used and the final numerical statistics Calculate test statistic and/or *p*-value Compare test statistic to tabulated value and/or *p*-value to alpha risk	**State the practical solution** Interpret the numerical results into meaningful statement about the conclusions that can be drawn

The null hypothesis is refered to as 'Ho.'

The alternate hypothesis is referred to as 'Ha.'

This is the hypothesis being tested or the claim being tested. The null hypothesis is either 'rejected' or 'failed to reject.' Rejecting the null hypothesis means accepting the alternative hypothesis.

The null hypothesis is valid until it is proven wrong. This is done by collecting data and using statistics with a specified amount of certainty. The more samples of data usually equates as more evidence and reduces the risk of an improper decision.

The null hypothesis is never accepted, it can be 'failed to reject' due to lack of evidence, just as a defendant is not proven guilty due to lack of evidence. The defendant is not necessarily innocent but is determined 'not guilty.'

There is simply not enough evidence and the decision is made that no change exists so the defendant started the trial as not guilty and leaves the trial not guilty.

Selecting the Hypothesis Test

If you have One X and One Y variable and...

If 'Y' data is:

if 'X' data is :		Continuous or variable	Attribute or discrete
	Attribute or discrete	One-sample *t* One-way ANOVA Wilcoxon signed-rank (also Wilcoxon *T* test)	Proportions tests Chi-square for independence
	Continuous or variable	Simple regression	Simple logistic regression

If you have more than one X and One Y variable and...

If 'Y' data is:

if 'X' data is :		Continuous or variable	Attribute or discrete
	Attribute or discrete	2-sample t ANOVA Kruskal-Wallis Mann-Whitney Mood's median	Advanced logistic regression
	Continuous or variable	Multiple regression	

Chapter 15

Power of Six Sigma in HR Management

IMPROVE YOUR HR EXCELLENCE WITH SIX SIGMA

Applying Six Sigma in HR Excellence

Managing healthcare employees is critical to every organization's success. Rising costs are making healthcare unaffordable for millions, and 100,000 people die every year due to medical error. Healthcare must change—dramatically. The human resource department has been practically untouched by Six Sigma. Now many leading healthcare organizations are discovering a powerful toolset Six Sigma. HR should be considered as human capital. HR must ensure that there is good return on investment in human capital. HR functions include recruitment, innovation, change management, employee's management, compensation, skills development and training.

Did you know there is an important role for Human Resources (HR) in Six Sigma? HR professionals with the right skills can contribute to a Six Sigma initiative at both strategic and tactical levels in healthcare. This chapter describes the areas in which HR should play a role in Six Sigma and discusses how HR professionals can increase their chances of being included in Six Sigma decision-making and implementation. How does HR implement Six Sigma? and "What can HR do to help Six Sigma initiatives in an organization"? If you want to become a more effective leader and make a real impact in your organization's bottom line, then the Six Sigma is just the ticket.

To appreciate the important role HR has in Six Sigma, it is important to begin this discussion by having an understanding of what Six Sigma is, all the roles played by others in a Six Sigma implementation, and the factors critical to a successful implementation.

ROLE OF SIX SIGMA IN HUMAN RESOURCE MANAGEMENT

Many factors contribute to the success of Six Sigma in HR. Some of these factors will fall within HR's area of responsibility, such as:

- Understandable, objective and measurable position requirements and performance standards

- Hiring and candidate selection processes driven by the position requirements
- Identifying leaders for management positions
- Effective, objective and accurate performance appraisals
- Focusing training and development programs on specific position requirements and individual performance
- Integrating individual performance with overall performance and quality management system
- Eliminating waste and inefficiencies
- Tracking and measuring continuous improvement in your HR processes.

SIX SIGMA PROCESS

Flow chart 15.1 shows the steps of six sigma process.

Flow chart 15.1: Six sigma process

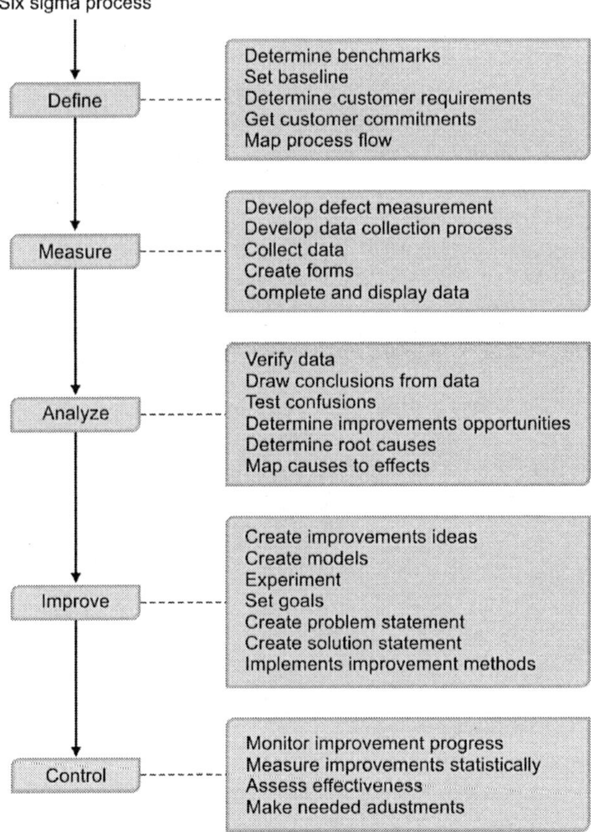

HOW IS SIX SIGMA DIFFERENT?

Six Sigma is really different from other approaches.
Six Sigma gives:

- A top-down approach, linked to strategy, sponsored by leaders
- Applicable to all business processes such as administrative, HR, marketing, R&D, etc.
- Fact based, data driven
- Results-oriented, hands-on way to develop critical managerial skills
- Projects based on top and bottom-line impact
- Exponential improvement targets.

When done correctly, Six Sigma becomes a way toward organization and cultural development. It is more than a set of tools!

DEFINITION OF SIX SIGMA

The term Six Sigma means standard deviation. Six Sigma is a goal for process improvement that forces us to put our vision of quality in numerical terms *(i.e. 3.4 defect parts per million)*. It is an organizational philosophy in establishing the belief of 'doing things right, first time and every time'.
More practical definition—"Data driven problem solving".

STEPS TO IMPLEMENT SIX SIGMA IN HR

- Establish a clear cut and significant role of HR for institutionalizing Six Sigma
- Establish Six Sigma objectives and role in HR
- Seek employee feedback and identify opportunities for improvement
- Establish Six Sigma goals for HR functions
- Formulate, prioritize projects and form teams
- Provide Six Sigma green belt/black belt training
- Implement DMAIC for breakthrough solution.

STEPS IN SIX SIGMA METHODOLOGY (DMAIC)

Define: Define the problem and improvement activity.

Measure: Measure the target metric and confirm that the measurement system is accurate. Measure the existing system. Establish valid and reliable metrics to help monitor progress towards the goals defined at the previous step. Begin by determining the current baseline. Use exploratory and descriptive data analysis to help you understand the data.

Analyze: Analyze the system to identify ways to eliminate the gaps between the current performance of the system or process and desired goal. Use statistics to find the root cause of the problem and generate a prioritized listing of them.

Improve: Enhance the healthcare delivery system. Be creative in finding new ways to do things better, cheaper, or faster. Use project management and other operations, planning and management tools to implement new approach. Use facts and statistical methods to validate improvement.

Control: Monitor the new system. Institutionalize the improved system by modifying.

Key players in Six Sigma initiatives are:
- Champions and sponsors
- Master black belt (MBB)
- Black belt (BB) and
- Green belt (GB).

Champion and sponsors: Six Sigma champions are high-level individuals who understand Six Sigma and are committed to its success. Sponsors are the owners of processes and systems who help initiate and co-ordinate Six Sigma improvement activities in their areas of responsibilities.

Master black belts (MBB): He/she plays a vital role as a leader, project selector, coach, mentor, manager and strategic business planner. An MBB in healthcare needs a variety of skills and information in order to function effectively. An MBB teaches other sigma students and helps them achieve green belt and black belt status.

Black belt: He/she is a person that is part of the leadership structure for process improvement team called 'black belts'. They are highly-regarded personnel who have an ability to lead teams as well as to advise the management.

Green belt: He/she is person trained in Six Sigma methodology and is a team member of a Six Sigma process improvement action team.

CRITICAL SUCCESS FACTORS FOR THE SIX SIGMA

- Top management leadership and commitment
- A well-implemented customer management system
- Continuous education and training system
- Design well-organized information and analysis system
- Identify well-implemented process management system
- A well-developed strategic planning system
- A well-developed human resource management system

- A well-developed competitive benchmarking system
- Black belt selection and retention.

Having the right people in the black belt role is critical to the success of a Six Sigma initiative. The training investment is substantial for this pivotal role. Further, black belts are the visible "face" of Six Sigma. They help shape the organization's impression of Six Sigma, and, consequently, the willingness of many to embrace the initiative. Therefore, you want to pick black belts very carefully (some organizations only select black belts from among those who have already been identified as "high potentials.").

HR professionals can help the Six Sigma leader find the right people for black belt roles and ensure they remain in those positions for the typical two-year rotation. Potential HR contributions in this area include:

- Building a competency model that will help identify candidates with the right mix of technical, team, and leadership skills and abilities.
- Creating job descriptions that help candidates fully understand the position and expectations prior to signing on.
- Developing a retention strategy that will help ensure black belts complete their rotation and the organization recoups its investment in training and development.

REWARDS AND RECOGNITION IN SIX SIGMA

Rewarding and recognizing black belts and Six Sigma teams is more complex than it may appear. Black belts join the Six Sigma initiative from various places in the organization where they are likely to have been at different job levels with differing compensation arrangements. Determining whether and how to make appropriate adjustments in level and compensation now that all these individuals are in the same role is both tricky and critical.

Similar complexities are involved at the project team level. Six Sigma projects led by black belts typically result in savings in the hundreds of thousands of dollars. Deciding how the team should be rewarded and recognized and who should get credit for what is not easy. Yet ignoring these issues can result in resentment, reluctance to work on Six Sigma projects, and the potential failure of the overall initiative.

HR professionals can help the Six Sigma leader tackle the challenge of establishing the right rewards/recognition. Potential HR contributions in this area include:

- Analyzing existing compensation arrangements to identify the extent to which those arrangements will support the Six Sigma initiative
- Creating a strategic compensation plan that will better support Six Sigma
- Developing a nonmonetary reward program for Six Sigma teams.

HOW TO CREATE A SIX SIGMA CULTURE

Many sponsors, champions, and leaders look to Six Sigma as a way to change an organization's culture to one that is more data-driven, proactive, decisive, and customer-oriented. But they often have little idea about how to achieve successful culture change.

HR professionals can help executives approach culture change in a way that addresses the underlying business goals without creating organizational resistance. Potential HR contributions in this area include:

- Working with Six Sigma sponsors, leaders, and champions to identify elements of the culture that might hinder the achievement of Six Sigma goals
- Advising on change plans that will target those specific cultural elements
- Identifying how Six Sigma can be rolled out in a way that works with, rather than against, the current culture.

CHANGE MANAGEMENT AND COMMUNICATIONS

Introducing Six Sigma into an organization is a major change that will have a profound effect on a broad group of stakeholders. Managers and employees at many levels of the organization will be asked to engage in new behaviors. In many cases, those leading other initiatives will see Six Sigma as a source of competition for resources, executive attention, and organizational power. Others may see it as an indictment of their past performance. Many will be confused about how Six Sigma fits with the large number of other ongoing organizational initiatives.

HR professionals can help reduce the uncertainty and anxiety surrounding Six Sigma and increase the levels of acceptance and cooperation in the organization. Potential HR contributions in this area include:

- Drafting a change management/communications plan that addresses the people side of the Six Sigma rollout.
- Helping create a "case for change" that describes:
  - The reasons for and benefits of Six Sigma
  - How the organization will help employees succeed in new ways of working
  - How Six Sigma fits with other ongoing initiatives
- Counseling Six Sigma leaders and champions on how their behavior can help or hinder Six Sigma's acceptance throughout the organization.

Being Included in Six Sigma

Just because HR professionals can play a role in the success of Six Sigma, it does not automatically follow that they will be asked to participate.

Unless you are in an organization that views HR as a partner in all business initiatives, you may have to push to be included in Six Sigma.

HR can greatly increase its chances of being included in the Six Sigma initiative by:

- Ensuring HR professionals have the right skills and knowledge
- Marketing its potential contribution early in the initiative.

Gaining the Right Skills and Knowledge

In addition to HR/organizational development-related areas, HR professionals need a familiarity with Six Sigma itself. Without a basic knowledge of the DMAIC method, supporting tools, roles, jargon, and even simple statistical methods, HR will not have the credibility it needs to be considered a potential contributor to the initiative.

The time to get this knowledge is now. Even if your organization is not rolling out—or even considering—Six Sigma today, there are two reasons why it is worth a HR professional's time to become familiar with the concepts now. If the organization does decide to implement Six Sigma, there will not be enough time to catch-up. HR has to be involved at the very beginning of the initiative. In addition, there are many applications of Six Sigma to HR's processes themselves, e.g. the payroll process, benefits administration, selection, and recruiting. HR might even consider setting an example for the rest of the organization by adopting Six Sigma techniques to enhance its own processes.

Marketing HR's Potential Contribution

The marketing challenge is two-fold. First, senior executives may not believe that the people issues are just as critical to Six Sigma's success as are its many technical components. In that case, HR will need to sell the importance of the people side. Second, executives must perceive HR as being able to make a significant contribution on the people side of Six Sigma. Besides ensuring that it has both the required skills and knowledge described above, HR can also meet these challenges by:

- Gathering data that supports the need for attention to the people side of Six Sigma. Potential sources include Six Sigma publications, case studies, conference sessions, and executives in companies that have already implemented Six Sigma
- Deriving lessons from previous organizational initiatives in which people issues and/or HR actions played an acknowledged role in success or failure

- Meeting with senior executives to discuss their business/Six Sigma goals and then identifying areas where HR could provide very specific and measurable help
- Speaking to Six Sigma Leaders and champions in the language of Six Sigma, not the language of HR. These executives are typically interested in improving efficiency (i.e. internal cost) and effectiveness (i.e., what the customer sees as "defects"). HR needs to understand what the executives care about and pitch HR's services in relevant terms
- Taking the lead and applying Six Sigma successfully within the HR function.

HR has a substantial role to play in the success of a Six Sigma initiative. But it will have the opportunity to contribute only if its professionals have the right skills and knowledge and are able to show Six Sigma executives the value they can add. Gain those skills now and make sure senior leadership knows how HR can help support the success of the initiative. Only then will they realize they just cannot do it without you!

Advantages of HR having Six Sigma

- Reduction in overtime
- Reduction in time and cost to hire employees
- Reduction in employee's retention or turnover
- Reduction in safety violations
- Reduction in cost of employee separation
- Fairness in internal inquires, payroll, performance appraisal and promotions
- Improvement and innovation of HR functions
- Achievement of corporate growth and profitability
- Innovative solutions and employees innovations.

If you make Six Sigma a strategy in your HR department, the end result will get reflected in sustainable bottom line improvement of hospital. The average time taken to develop a plan and improve a process takes 3–12 months, depending on the scope and goals of the organization.

Six Sigma Training Institutes

Following are the Six Sigma training institutes.

Indian Statistical Institute, Delhi Center

7, Shaheed Jeet Singh Marg, New Delhi - 110016

Phone: 011-41493968 (Direct), 41493981

Web: www.isid.ac.in

Six Sigma Accreditation Board
Six Sigma House, 10A
Sai Baba Enclave, Tehsil Road
Najafgarh, New Delhi
Phone: 011-25324000, 25324001
E-mail: sixsigmahealthcare@gmail.com
Web: www.sixsigmahealth.org

Indian Institute of Management Bangalore
Bannerghatta Road, Bengaluru 560 076
Karnataka, India
Phone: 080-26993742/3264/3475
Fax: 080-26584004/26584050
E-mail: edp@iimb.ernet.in
Website: http://www.iimb.ernet.in

Quality Council of India
Institution of Engineers Building, IInd Floor
2-Bahadur Shah Zafar Marg, New Delhi-110002, India
Tel: 91-11-2337 9321, 2337 9260, 2337 0567, 2337 8057
Fax: 91-11-2337 9621.
E-mail: sg@qcin.org, nrbpt@qcin.org, nabcb@qcin.org

BSI-Bangalore
BSI Management Systems India Pvt Ltd.
34/1, BHCS-BTM Layout
Phase 1, 2nd Stage
Bengaluru 560 076
India
Telephone: +91 (0)80 4113 4654
E-mail: bsibangalore@bsigroup.com
Fax: +91 (0)80 4113 4655

EdistaLearning
1013-14A, Ansal Tower
38, Nehru Place
New Delhi-110 019
E-mail: edistaindia@edistalearning.com

Online Six Sigma Learning Institutes

- Professional Training and Development Centre (PTADC) Web: www.ptadc.com.
- Six Sigma Training and Certification, Web: www.6sigma.us.
- More Steam University, Web: www.moresteam.com.

Chapter 16

High Altitude Medical Services

DEFINITIONS

Altitude

Altitude is a distance measurement, usually in the vertical or 'up' direction, between a reference datum and a point or object. The reference datum also often varies according to the context. Although the term altitude is commonly used to mean the height above sea level of a location, in geography, the term elevation is often preferred for this usage.

High Altitude

1,500–3,500 m (4,900–11,500 ft): The onset of physiological effects of diminished inspiratory oxygen pressure (PiO_2) includes decreased exercise performance and increased ventilation (lower arterial PCO_2). Minor impairment exists in arterial oxygen transport (arterial oxygen saturation (SaO_2) at least 90%), but arterial PO_2 is significantly diminished. Because of the large number of people who ascend rapidly to altitudes between 2,400 and 4,000 m, high-altitude illness is common in this range.

Very High Altitude

3,500–5,500 m (11,500–18,000 ft): Maximum SaO_2 falls below 90% as the arterial PO_2 falls below 60 mm Hg. Extreme hypoxemia may occur during exercise, during sleep, and in the presence of high altitude pulmonary edema or other acute lung conditions. Severe altitude illness occurs most commonly in this range.

Extreme Altitude

Above 5,500 m (18,000 ft): Marked hypoxemia, hypocapnia, and alkalosis are characteristic of extreme altitudes. Progressive deterioration of physiologic function eventually outstrips acclimatization. As a result, no permanent human habitation occurs above 6,000 m. A period of acclimatization is necessary when ascending to extreme altitude; abrupt ascent without supplemental oxygen for other than brief exposures invites severe altitude sickness.

EFFECTS OF HIGH ALTITUDE ON HUMAN BEINGS

The *effects of high altitude on humans* are considerable. The percentage saturation of hemoglobin with oxygen determines the content of oxygen in our blood. After the human body reaches around 2,100 m (7,000 f) above sea level, the saturation of oxidized hemoglobin begins to plummet. However, the human body has both short-term and long-term adaptations to altitude that allow it to partially compensate for the lack of oxygen. Athletes use these adaptations to help their performance. There is a limit to the level of adaptation; mountaineers refer to the altitudes above 8,000 m (26,000 ft) as the 'death zone', where no human body can acclimatize.

The human body can perform best at sea level, where the atmospheric pressure is 101,325 Pa or 1013.25 millibars (or 1 atm, by definition). The concentration of oxygen (O_2) in sea-level air is 20.9%, so the partial pressure of O_2 (PO_2) is 21.136 kPa. In healthy individuals, this saturates hemoglobin, the oxygen-binding red pigment in red blood cells.

Atmospheric pressure decreases exponentially with altitude while the O_2 fraction remains constant to about 100 km, so PO_2 decreases exponentially with altitude as well. It is about half of its sea-level value at 5,000 m (16,000 ft), the altitude of the Everest Base Camp, and only a third at 8,848 m (29,029 ft), the summit of Mount Everest. When PO_2 drops, the body responds with altitude acclimatization.

Mountain medicine recognizes three altitude regions that reflect the lowered amount of oxygen in the atmosphere:

- High altitude = 1,500–3,500 m (4,900–11,500 ft)
- Very high altitude = 3,500–5,500 m (11,500–18,000 ft)
- Extreme altitude = above 5,500 m (18,000 ft).

Travel to each of these altitude regions can lead to medical problems, from the mild symptoms of acute mountain sickness to the potentially fatal high altitude pulmonary edema (HAPE) and high altitude cerebral edema (HACE). The higher the altitude, the greater the risk. Research also indicates elevated risk of permanent brain damage in people climbing to extreme altitudes. Expedition doctors commonly stock a supply of dexamethazone, or 'dex,' to treat these conditions on site.

Humans have survived for two years at 5,950 m (19,520 ft) (475 millibars of atmospheric pressure), which is the highest recorded permanently tolerable highest altitude; the highest permanent settlement known,

La Rinconada, is at 5,100 m (16,700 ft). At extreme altitudes, above 7,500 m (24,600 ft) (383 millibars of atmospheric pressure), sleeping becomes very difficult, digesting food is near-impossible, and the risk of HAPE or HACE increases greatly.

Long-term Effects

One hundred and forty million people live at altitudes above 2,500 m (8,200 ft). Studies have found that these populations, especially people living in the Andes and in the Himalayas, have ways of compensating for the lower oxygen levels that are different from people living at sea level. Compared with acclimatized newcomers, native Andean and Himalayan populations have better oxygenation at birth, enlarged lung volumes throughout life, and a higher capacity for exercise. Tibetans demonstrate a sustained increase in cerebral blood flow, lower hemoglobin concentration, and less susceptibility to chronic mountain sickness (CMS) than other high altitude populations. These adaptations may reflect their longer history of high altitude habitation.

There is a significantly lower mortality rate for permanent residents at higher altitudes. Similarly, there is a dose response relationship between increasing elevation and decreasing obesity prevalence in the United States. This is not explained by migration alone. On the other hand, people living at higher elevations also have a higher rate of suicide in the United States. Similar findings were observed for both firearm-related suicides (59% of suicides) and nonfirearm-related suicides. The correlation between elevation and suicide risk was present even when the researchers control for known suicide risk factors, including age, gender, race and income. Research also indicates that oxygen levels are unlikely to be a factor, considering that there is no indication of increased mood disturbances at high altitude in those with sleep apnea or in heavy smokers at high altitude. The cause for the increased suicide risk is unknown so far.

Acclimatization to Altitude

The human body can adapt to high altitude through immediate and long-term acclimatization. At high altitude, in the short-term, the lack of oxygen is sensed by the carotid bodies, which causes an increase in the breathing rate (hyperventilation). However, hyperventilation also causes the adverse effect of respiratory alkalosis, inhibiting the respiratory center from enhancing the respiratory rate as much as would be required. Inability to increase the breathing rate can be caused by inadequate carotid body response or pulmonary or renal disease.

In addition, at high altitude, the heart beats faster; the stroke volume is slightly decreased; and nonessential bodily functions are suppressed, resulting in a decline in food digestion efficiency (as the body suppresses the digestive system in favor of increasing its cardiopulmonary reserves).

Full acclimatization, however, requires days or even weeks. Gradually, the body compensates for the respiratory alkalosis by renal excretion of bicarbonate, allowing adequate respiration to provide oxygen without risking alkalosis. It takes about four days at any given altitude and can be enhanced by drugs such as acetazolamide. Eventually, the body has lower lactate production (because reduced glucose breakdown decreases the amount of lactate formed), decreased plasma volume, increased hematocrit (polycythemia), increased RBC mass, a higher concentration of capillaries in skeletal muscle tissue, increased myoglobin, increased mitochondria, increased aerobic enzyme concentration, increase in 2,3-BPG, hypoxic pulmonary vasoconstriction, and right ventricular hypertrophy. Pulmonary artery pressure increases in an effort to oxygenate more blood.

Full hematological adaptation to high altitude is achieved when the increase of red blood cells reaches a plateau and stops. The length of full hematological adaptation can be approximated by multiplying the altitude in kilometers by 11.4 days. For example, to adapt to 4,000 m (13,000 ft) of altitude would require 45.6 days. The upper altitude limit of this linear relationship has not been fully established.

Altitude and Athletic Performance

For athletes, high altitude produces two contradictory effects on performance. For explosive events (sprints up to 400 m, long jump, triple jump) the reduction in atmospheric pressure means there is less resistance from the atmosphere and the athlete's performance will generally be better at high altitude. For endurance events (races of 800 m or more), the predominant effect is the reduction in oxygen, which generally reduces the athlete's performance at high altitude. Sports organizations acknowledge the effects of altitude on performance: the International Association of Athletics Federations (IAAF), for example, have ruled that performances achieved at an altitude greater than 1,000 m will be approved for record purposes, but carry the notation of 'A' to denote they were set at altitude. The 1968 Summer Olympics were held at altitude in Mexico City. With the best athletes in the world competing for the most prestigious title, most short sprint and jump records were set there at altitude. Other records were also set at altitude in anticipation of those Olympics. Bob Beamon's record in the long jump held for almost 23 years and has only been beaten once without altitude or wind assistance. Many of the other records set at Mexico City were later surpassed by marks set at altitude.

Athletes can also take advantage of altitude acclimatization to increase their performance. The same changes that help the body cope with high altitude increase performance back at sea level. However, this may not always be the case. Any positive acclimatization effects may be negated by a detraining effect as the athletes are usually not able to exercise with as much intensity at high altitudes compared to sea level.

This conundrum led to the development of the altitude training modality known as 'Live-High, Train-Low', whereby the athlete spends many hours a day resting and sleeping at one (high) altitude, but performs a significant portion of their training, possibly all of it, at another (lower) altitude. A series of studies conducted in Utah in the late 1990s by researchers Ben Levine, Jim Stray-Gundersen, and others, showed significant performance gains in athletes who followed such a protocol for several weeks. Other studies have shown performance gains from merely performing some exercising sessions at high altitude, yet living at sea level.

The performance-enhancing effect of altitude training could be due to increased red blood cell count, more efficient training, or changes in muscle physiology.

ALTITUDE SICKNESS

Altitude sickness—also known as *acute mountain sickness (AMS), altitude illness, hypobaropathy, 'the altitude bends'*, or *soroche*—is a pathological effect of high altitude on humans, caused by acute exposure to low partial pressure of oxygen at high altitude. It commonly occurs above 2,400 m (8,000 ft). It presents as a collection of nonspecific symptoms, acquired at high altitude or in low air pressure, resembling a case of "flu, carbon monoxide poisoning, or a hangover". It is hard to determine who will be affected by altitude sickness, as there are no specific factors that correlate with a susceptibility to altitude sickness. However, most people can ascend to 2,400 m (8,000 ft) without difficulty.

Acute mountain sickness can progress to high altitude pulmonary edema (HAPE) or high altitude cerebral edema (HACE), which are potentially fatal.

Chronic mountain sickness, also known as *Monge's disease*, is a different condition that only occurs after very prolonged exposure to high altitude.

Causes

The available amount of oxygen to sustain mental and physical alertness decreases with altitude. Available oxygen drops as the air density itself, the number of molecules (of both oxygen and nitrogen) per given volume, drops as altitude increases.

However, the percentage of oxygen in air, at 21%, remains almost unchanged up to 21,000 m (69,000 ft). The RMS velocities of diatomic nitrogen and oxygen are very similar and thus no change occurs in the ratio of oxygen to nitrogen.

Dehydration due to the higher rate of water vapor lost from the lungs at higher altitudes may contribute to the symptoms of altitude sickness.

The rate of ascent, altitude attained, amount of physical activity at high altitude, as well as individual susceptibility, are contributing factors to the onset and severity of high-altitude illness.

Altitude sickness usually occurs following a rapid ascent and can usually be prevented by ascending slowly. In most of these cases, the symptoms are temporary and usually abate as altitude acclimatization occurs. However, in extreme cases, altitude sickness can be fatal.

Signs and Symptoms

People have different susceptibilities to altitude sickness; for some otherwise healthy people, acute altitude sickness can begin to appear at around 2000 m (6,500 ft) above sea level, such as at many mountain ski resorts, equivalent to a pressure of 80 kPa. This is the most frequent type of altitude sickness encountered. Symptoms often manifest themselves 6–10 hours after ascent and generally subside in 1–2 days, but they occasionally develop into the more serious conditions. Symptoms include headache, fatigue, stomach illness, dizziness, and sleep disturbance. Exertion aggravates the symptoms.

The Lake Louise assessment system of AMS is based on a self-report questionnaire as well as a quick clinical assessment.

Those individuals with the lowest initial partial pressure of end-tidal PCO_2 (the lowest concentration of carbon dioxide at the end of the respiratory cycle, a measure of a higher alveolar ventilation) and corresponding high oxygen saturation levels tend to have a lower incidence of acute mountain sickness than those with high end-tidal PCO_2 and low oxygen saturation levels.

Primary Symptoms

Headaches are the primary symptom used to diagnose altitude sickness, although a headache is also a symptom of dehydration. A headache occurring at an altitude above 2,400 m (8,000 ft = 76 kPa), combined with anyone or more of the following symptoms, may indicate altitude sickness:

- Lack of appetite, nausea, or vomiting
- Fatigue or weakness
- Dizziness or lightheadedness
- Insomnia
- Pins and needles
- Shortness of breath upon exertion
- Nosebleed
- Persistent rapid pulse
- Drowsiness
- Excessive flatulation
- General malaise
- Peripheral edema (swelling of hands, feet, and face).

Severe Symptoms

Symptoms that may indicate life-threatening altitude sickness include:

- Pulmonary edema (fluid in the lungs)
  - Symptoms similar to bronchitis
  - Persistent dry cough
  - Fever
  - Shortness of breath even when resting
- Cerebral edema (swelling of the brain)
  - Headache that does not respond to analgesics
  - Unsteady gait
  - Gradual loss of consciousness
  - Increased nausea
  - Retinal hemorrhage.

The most serious symptoms of altitude sickness arise from edema (fluid accumulation in the tissues of the body). At very high altitude, humans can get either high altitude pulmonary edema (HAPE), or high altitude cerebral edema (HACE). The physiological cause of altitude-induced edema is not conclusively established. It is currently believed, however, that HACE is caused by local vasodilation of cerebral blood vessels in response to hypoxia, resulting in greater blood flow and, consequently, greater capillary pressures. On the other hand, HAPE may be due to general vasoconstriction in the pulmonary circulation (normally a response to regional ventilation-perfusion mismatches) which, with constant or increased cardiac output, also leads to increases in capillary pressures. For those suffering HACE, dexamethasone may provide temporary relief from symptoms in order to keep descending under their own power.

The HAPE can progress rapidly and is often fatal. Symptoms include fatigue, severe dyspnea at rest, and cough that is initially dry but may progress to produce pink, frothy sputum. Descent to lower altitudes alleviates the symptoms of HAPE.

The HACE is a life-threatening condition that can lead to coma or death. Symptoms include headache, fatigue, visual impairment, bladder dysfunction, bowel dysfunction, loss of coordination, paralysis on one side of the body, and confusion. Descent to lower altitudes may save those afflicted with HACE.

Physiology

The physiology of altitude sickness is based on the following equation:

$$V_{gas} = A/TD_k(P_1 - P_2)$$

where V_{gas} is the diffusion rate, A is the area of the lung, T is the thickness of the lung membranes, P_1 and P_2 are the differences in partial pressure of any gas-but most importantly CO_2 and O_2-where in high altitudes the partial pressure differences for O_2 are low and the differences in partial pressures for CO_2 are high. Thus, CO_2 will have a high diffusion out and O_2 will have a low diffusion though the alveolar membranes and into the blood.

The body's response to high altitude includes the following:

- ↑Erythropoietin → ↑hematocrit and hemoglobin
- ↑2,3-DPG (allows ↑ release of O_2 and a right shift on the Hb-O_2 disassociation curve)
- ↑renal excretion of bicarbonate (use of acetazolamide can augment for treatment)
- Chronic hypoxic pulmonary vasoconstriction (can cause Right Ventricular Hypertrophy).

DEATH ZONE

- The death zone, in mountaineering, refers to altitudes above a certain point, where the amount of oxygen is insufficient to sustain human life. This point is generally tagged as 8,000 m (26,000 ft) (less than 356 millibars of atmospheric pressure). The concept of the *death zone* (originally the *lethal zone*) was first conceived by Edouard Wyss-Dunant, a Swiss doctor, in an article about acclimatization published in the journal of the Swiss Foundation for Alpine Research.
- Many deaths in high-altitude mountaineering have been caused by the effects of the death zone, either directly (loss of vital functions) or

indirectly (wrong decisions made under stress, physical weakening leading to accidents). In the death zone, the human body cannot acclimatize. An extended stay in the zone without supplementary oxygen will result in deterioration of bodily functions, loss of consciousness and, ultimately, death.

- Scientists at the High Altitude Pathology Institute in Bolivia dispute the existence of a death zone, based on observation of extreme tolerance to hypoxia in patients with chronic mountain sickness and normal fetuses *in utero*, both of which present PaO_2 levels similar to those at the summit of Mount Everest.

PREVENTION

Ascending slowly is the best way to avoid altitude sickness. Avoiding strenuous activity such as skiing, hiking, etc. in the first 24 hours at high altitude reduces the symptoms of acute mountain sickness (AMS). Alcohol and sleeping pills are respiratory depressants, and thus slow down the acclimatization process and should be avoided. Alcohol also tends to cause dehydration and exacerbates AMS. Thus, avoiding alcohol consumption in the first 24–48 hours at a higher altitude is optimal.

Pre-acclimatization

Pre-acclimatization is when the body develops tolerance to low oxygen concentrations before ascending to an altitude. It significantly reduces risk because less time has to be spent at altitude to acclimatize in the traditional way. Additionally, because less time has to be spent on the mountain, less food and supplies have to be taken up. Several commercial systems exist that use altitude tents, so called because they mimic altitude by reducing the percentage of oxygen in the air while keeping air pressure constant to the surroundings.

Altitude Acclimatization

Altitude acclimatization is the process of adjusting to decreasing oxygen levels at higher elevations, in order to avoid altitude sickness. Once above approximately 3,000 m (10,000 ft = 70 kPa), most climbers and high-altitude trekkers take the ‘climb-high, sleep-low’ approach. For high-altitude climbers, a typical acclimatization regimen might be to stay a few days at a base camp, climb-up to a higher camp (slowly), and then return to base camp. A subsequent climb to the higher camp then includes an overnight stay. This process is then repeated a few times, each time extending the time spent at higher altitudes to let the body adjust to the oxygen level there, a process that involves the production of additional red blood cells. Once the climber has acclimatized to a given altitude, the process is repeated with camps placed at progressively higher elevations. The general rule of thumb is to ascend no more than 300 m (1,000 ft) per day to sleep. That is, one can climb from 3,000 (10,000 ft = 70 kPa) to 4,500 m (15,000 ft = 58 kPa) in one day, but one should then descend back to 3,300 m (11,000 ft = 67.5 kPa) to sleep. This process cannot safely be rushed, and this is why climbers need to spend days (or even weeks at times) acclimatizing before attempting to climb a high peak. Simulated altitude equipment that produces hypoxic (reduced oxygen) air can be used to acclimate to high altitude, reducing the total time required on the mountain itself.

Altitude acclimatization is necessary for some people who move rapidly from lower altitudes to intermediate altitudes (e.g. by aircraft and ground transportation over a few hours), such as from sea level to 8,000 ft (2,400 m) as in many Colorado, USA mountain resorts. Stopping at an intermediate altitude overnight can alleviate or eliminate occurrences of AMS.

MEDICAL TREATMENT

The drug acetazolamide (trade name Diamox) may help some people making a rapid ascent to sleeping altitude above 2,700 m (9,000 ft), and it may also be effective if started early in the course of AMS. Acetazolamide can be taken before symptoms appear as a preventive measure at a dose of 125 mg twice daily. The Everest Base Camp Medical Center cautions against its routine use as a substitute for a reasonable ascent schedule, except where rapid ascent is forced by flying into high altitude locations or due to terrain considerations. The Center suggests a dosage of 125 mg twice daily for prophylaxis, starting from 24 hours before ascending until a few days at the highest altitude or on descending; with 250 mg twice daily recommended for treatment of AMS. The Centers for Disease Control and Prevention (CDC) suggest the same dose for prevention of 125 mg acetazolamide every 12 hours. Acetazolamide, a mild diuretic, works by stimulating the kidneys to secrete more bicarbonate in the urine, thereby acidifying the blood. This change in pH stimulates the respiratory center to increase the depth and frequency of respiration, thus speeding the natural acclimatization process. An undesirable side-effect of acetazolamide is a reduction in aerobic endurance performance. Other minor side-effects include a tingle-sensation in hands and feet, and it can make carbonated drinks taste 'flat'. Although a sulfonamide, acetazolamide is a nonantibiotic and has not been shown to cause life-threatening allergic cross-reactivity in those with a self-reported sulfa allergy. Dosage of 1000 mg/day will produce a 25% decrease in performance, on top of the reduction due to high-altitude exposure. The CDC advises that Dexamethasone be reserved for treatment of severe AMS and HACE during descents, and notes that Nifedipine may prevent HAPE.

A single randomized controlled trial found that sumatriptan may help prevent altitude sickness. Despite their popularity, antioxidant treatments have not been found to be effective medications for prevention of AMS. Interest in phosphodiesterase inhibitors such as sildenafil has been limited by the possibility that these drugs might worsen the headache of mountain sickness. A promising possible preventive for altitude sickness is myo-inositol trispyrophosphate (ITPP), which increases the amount of oxygen released by hemoglobin.

Prior to the onset of altitude sickness, ibuprofen is a suggested non-steroidal anti-inflammatory and painkiller that can help alleviate both the headache and nausea associated with AMS. It has not been studied for the prevention of cerebral edema (swelling of the brain) associated with extreme symptoms of AMS.

For centuries, indigenous peoples of the Americas such as the Aymaras of the Altiplano, have chewed coca leaves to try to alleviate the symptoms of mild altitude sickness. In Chinese and Tibetan traditional medicine, an extract of the root tissue of *Radix rhodiola* is often taken in order to prevent the same symptoms, though neither of these therapies has been proven effective in clinical study.

Oxygen Enrichment

In high-altitude conditions, oxygen enrichment can counteract the hypoxia related effects of altitude sickness. A small amount of supplemental oxygen reduces the equivalent altitude in climate-controlled rooms. At 3,400 m (11,155 ft = 67 kPa), raising the oxygen concentration level by 5% via an oxygen concentrator and an existing ventilation system provides an effective altitude of 3,000 m (10,000 ft = 70 kPa), which is more tolerable for surface-dwellers.

Other Methods

Increased water intake may also help in acclimatization to replace the fluids lost through heavier breathing in the thin, dry air found at altitude, although consuming excessive quantities ('over-hydration') has no benefits and may cause dangerous hyponatremia. It is a good idea to limit alcohol intake the first day or so at higher elevation as well.

Oxygen from gas bottles or liquid containers can be applied directly via a nasal cannula or mask. Oxygen concentrators based upon pressure swing adsorption (PSA), VSA, or vacuum-pressure swing adsorption (VPSA) can be used to generate the oxygen if electricity is available. Stationary oxygen concentrators typically use PSA technology, which has performance degradations at the lower barometric pressures at high altitudes. One way to compensate for the performance degradation is to utilize a concentrator with more flow capacity. There are also portable oxygen concentrators that can be used on vehicular DC power or on internal batteries, and at least one system commercially available measures and compensates for the altitude effect on its performance up to 4,000 m (13,000 ft). The application of high-purity oxygen from one of these methods increases the partial pressure of oxygen by raising the FiO_2 (fraction of inspired oxygen).

Treatment

The only reliable treatment and in many cases the only option available is to descend. Attempts to treat or stabilize the patient *in situ* at altitude are dangerous unless highly controlled and with good medical facilities. However, the following treatments have been used when the patient's location and circumstances permit:

- Oxygen may be used for mild to moderate AMS below 3,700 m (12,000 ft) and is commonly provided by physicians at mountain resorts. Symptoms abate in 12–36 hours without the need to descend.
- For more serious cases of AMS, or where rapid descent is impractical, a Gamow bag, a portable plastic hyperbaric chamber inflated with a foot pump, can be used to reduce the effective altitude by as much as 1,500 m (5,000 ft). A Gamow bag is generally used only as an aid to evacuate severe AMS patients, not to treat them at altitude.
- Acetazolamide 250 mg twice daily dosing assists in AMS treatment by quickening altitude acclimatization. A study by the Denali Medical Research Project concluded: "In established cases of acute mountain sickness, treatment with acetazolamide relieves symptoms, improves arterial oxygenation, and prevents further impairment of pulmonary gas exchange."
- The folk remedy for altitude sickness in Ecuador, Peru and Bolivia is a tea made from the coca plant. See mate de coca.
- Steroids can be used to treat the symptoms of pulmonary or cerebral edema, but do not treat the underlying AMS.

- Two studies in 2012 showed that Ibuprofen 600 milligrams three times daily was effective at decreasing the severity and incidence of AMS. But it was not clear if this affected HAPE or HACE.

ALTITUDE TRAINING

Altitude training is the practice by some endurance athletes of training for several weeks at high altitude, preferably over 2,400 m (8,000 ft) above sea level, though more commonly at intermediate altitudes due to the shortage of suitable high-altitude locations. At intermediate altitudes, the air still contains approximately 20.9% oxygen, but the barometric pressure and thus the partial pressure of oxygen is reduced.

Depending very much on the protocols used, the body may acclimate to the relative lack of oxygen in one or more ways such as increasing the mass of red blood cells and hemoglobin, or altering muscle metabolism. Proponents claim that when such athletes travel to competitions at lower altitudes they will still have a higher concentration of red blood cells for 10–14 days, and this gives them a competitive advantage. Some athletes live permanently at high altitude, only returning to sea level to compete, but their training may suffer due to less available oxygen for workouts.

Altitude training can be simulated through use of an altitude simulation tent, altitude simulation room, or mask-based hypoxicator system where the barometric pressure is kept the same, but the oxygen content is reduced which also reduces the partial pressure of oxygen. Hypoventilation training, which consists of reducing the breathing frequency while exercising, can also mimic altitude training by significantly decreasing blood and muscle oxygenation

Training Regimens

Live-high, Train-low

One suggestion for optimizing adaptations and maintaining performance is the live-high, train-low principle. This training idea involves living at higher altitudes in order to experience the physiological adaptations that occur, such as increased erythropoietin (EPO) levels, increased red blood cell levels, and higher VO_2 max, while maintaining the same exercise intensity during training at sea level. Due to the environmental differences at high altitude, it may be necessary to decrease the intensity of workouts. Studies examining the live-high, train-low theory have produced varied results, which may be dependent on a variety of factors such as individual variability, time spent at high altitude, and the type of training program. For example, it has been shown that athletes performing primarily anaerobic activity do not necessarily benefit from altitude training as they do not rely on oxygen to fuel their performances.

A nontraining elevation of 2,100–2,500 m (6,900–8,200 ft) and training at 1,250 m (4,100 ft) or less has shown to be the optimal approach for altitude training. Good venues for live-high train-low include Mammoth Lakes, California; Flagstaff, Arizona; and the Sierra Nevada, near Granada in Spain.

Altitude training can produce increases in speed, strength, endurance, and recovery by maintaining altitude exposure for a significant period of time. A study using simulated altitude exposure for 18 days, yet training closer to sea-level, showed performance gains were still evident 15 days later.

Opponents of altitude training argue that an athlete's red blood cell concentration returns to normal levels within days of returning to sea level and that it is impossible to train at the same intensity that one could at sea level, reducing the training effect and wasting training time due to altitude sickness. Altitude training can produce slow recovery due to the stress of hypoxia. Exposure to extreme hypoxia at altitudes above 16,000 ft (5,000 m) can lead to considerable deterioration of skeletal muscle tissue. Five weeks at this altitude leads to a loss of muscle volume of the order of 10–15%.

Live-high, Train-high

In the live-high, train-high regime, an athlete lives and trains at a desired altitude. The stimulus on the body is constant because the athlete is continuously in a hypoxic environment. Initially VO_2 max drops considerably: by around 7% for every 1000 m above sea level at high altitudes. Athletes will no longer be able to metabolize as much oxygen as they would at sea level. Any given velocity must be performed at a higher relative intensity at altitude. However, after long periods of training at altitude, highly trained athletes returning to sea level do not exhibit increased red blood cell count or improved performance on 4000 m cycling tests.

Repeated Sprints in Hypoxia

In repeated sprints in hypoxia (RSH), athletes run short sprints under 30 seconds as fast as they can. They experience incomplete recoveries in hypoxic conditions. The exercise to rest time ratio is less than 1:4, which means for every 30 seconds all out sprint, there is less than 120 seconds of rest.

When comparing RSH and repeated sprints in normoxia (RSN), studies show that RSH improved time to fatigue and power output. RSH and RSN groups were tested before and after a 4 week training period. Both groups initially completed 9–10 seconds all out sprints before total exhaustion. After the 4 weeks training period, the RSH group was able to complete 13 all out sprints before exhaustion and the RSN group only completed nine.

Possible physiological advantages from RSH include compensatory vasodilation and regeneration of phosphocreatine (PCr). The body's tissues have the ability to sense hypoxia and induce vasodilation. The higher blood flow helps the skeletal muscles maximize oxygen delivery. A greater level of PCr augments the muscles power production.

Repeated sprints in hypoxia is still a relatively new training method. For it to be fully understood and trusted, more double blind studies must be conducted. To achieve the best results a larger sample size should be used.

Artificial Altitude

Altitude simulation systems have enabled protocols that do not suffer from the tension between better altitude physiology and more intense workouts. Such simulated altitude systems can be utilized closer to competition if necessary.

In Finland, a scientist named HeikkiRusko has designed a 'high-altitude house.' The air inside the house, which is situated at sea level, is at normal pressure but modified to have a low concentration of oxygen, about 15.3% (below the 20.9% at sea level), which is roughly equivalent to the amount of oxygen available at the high altitudes often used for altitude training due to the reduced partial pressure of oxygen at altitude. Athletes live and sleep inside the house, but perform their training outside (at normal oxygen concentrations at 20.9%). Rusko's results show improvements of EPO and red-cell levels.

Artificial altitude can also be used for hypoxic exercise, where athletes train in an altitude simulator which mimics the conditions a high altitude environment. Athletes are able to perform high intensity training at lower velocities and thus produce less stress on the musculoskeletal system. This is beneficial to an athlete who suffered a musculoskeletal injury and is unable to apply large amounts of stress during exercise which would normally be needed to generate high intensity cardiovascular training. Hypoxia exposure for the time of exercise alone is not sufficient to induce changes in hematologic parameters. Hematocrit and hemoglobin concentrations remain in general unchanged. There are a number of companies who provide altitude training system, most notably Hypoxico, Inc. who pioneered the artificial altitude training systems in the mid 1990's.

MOUNTAINEERING

The term *mountaineering* describes the sport of mountainclimbing, including ski mountaineering. Hiking in the mountains can also be a simple form of mountaineering when it involves scrambling, or short stretches of the more basic grades of rock climbing, as well as crossing glaciers.

While mountaineering began as attempts to reach the highest point of unclimbed big mountains it has branched into specializations that address different aspects of the mountain and consists of three areas: rock-craft, snow-craft and skiing, depending on whether the route chosen is over rock, snow or ice. All require experience, athletic ability, and technical knowledge to maintain safety.

Mountaineering is often called *Alpinism*, especially in European languages, which implies climbing with difficulty such high mountains as the Alps. A mountaineer with such great skill is called an *Alpinist*. The word alpinism was born in the 19th century to refer to climbing for the purpose of enjoying climbing itself as a sport or recreation, distinct from merely climbing while hunting or as a religious pilgrimage that had been done generally at that time.

The UIAA or *Union Internationale des Associations d'Alpinisme* is the world governing body in mountaineering and climbing, addressing issues like access, medical, mountain protection, safety, youth and ice climbing.

Technique

Snow

Compacted snow conditions allow mountaineers to progress on foot. Frequently crampons are required to travel efficiently over snow and ice. Crampons attach to a mountaineer's boots to provide additional traction on hard snow (névé) and ice. Using various techniques from alpine skiing and mountaineering to ascend/descend a mountain is a form of the sport by itself, called ski mountaineering. Ascending and descending a snow slope safely requires the use of an ice axe and many different footwork techniques that have been developed over the past century, mainly in Europe (e.g. French technique and German technique). The progression of footwork from the lowest angle slopes to the steepest terrain is first to splay the feet to a rising traverse, to kicking steps, to front pointing the crampons.

The progression of ice axe technique from the lowest angle slopes to the steepest terrain is to use the ice axe first as a walking stick, then a stake, then to use the front pick as a dagger below the shoulders or above, and finally to swinging the pick into the slope over the head. These various techniques may involve questions of differing ice axe design depending on terrain, and even whether a mountaineer uses one or two ice axes. Anchors for the rope in snow are sometimes unreliable, and include the snow stakes, called pickets, deadman devices called flukes which are fashioned from aluminum, or devised from buried objects that might include an ice axe, skis, rocks or other objects. Bollards, which are simply carved out of consolidated snow or ice, also sometimes serve as anchors.

Glaciers

When traveling over glaciers, crevasses pose a grave danger. These giant cracks in the ice are not always visible as snow can be blown and freeze over the top to make a *snowbridge*. At times snowbridges can be as thin as a few inches. Climbers use a system of ropes to protect themselves from such hazards. Basic gear for glacier travel includes crampons and ice axes. Teams of two to five climbers tie into a rope equally spaced. If a climber begins to fall the other members of the team perform a self-arrest to stop the fall. The other members of the team enact a crevasse rescue to pull the fallen climber from the crevasse.

Ice

Multiple methods are used to travel safely over ice. If the terrain is steep but not vertical, then the lead climber can place ice screws in the ice and attach the rope for protection. Each climber on the team must clip past the anchor, and the last climber picks up the anchor itself. Occasionally, slinged icicles or bollards are also used. This allows for safety should the entire team be taken off their feet. This technique is known as Simul climbing and is sometimes also used on steep snow and easy rock.

If the terrain becomes too steep, standard ice climbing techniques are used in which each climber is belayed, moving one at a time.

SHELTER

Tent (Fig. 16.1)

Tents are the most common form of shelter used on the mountain. These may vary from simple tarps to much heavier designs intended to withstand harsh mountain conditions. In exposed positions, windbreaks of snow or rock may be required to shelter the tent. One of the downsides to tenting is that high winds and snow loads can be dangerous and may ultimately lead to the tent's failure and collapse. In addition, the constant flapping of the tent fabric can hinder sleep and raise doubts about the security of the shelter. When choosing a tent, alpinists tend to rely on specialized mountaineering tents that are specifically designed for high winds and moderate to heavy snow loads. Tent stakes can be buried in the snow ('deadman') for extra security.

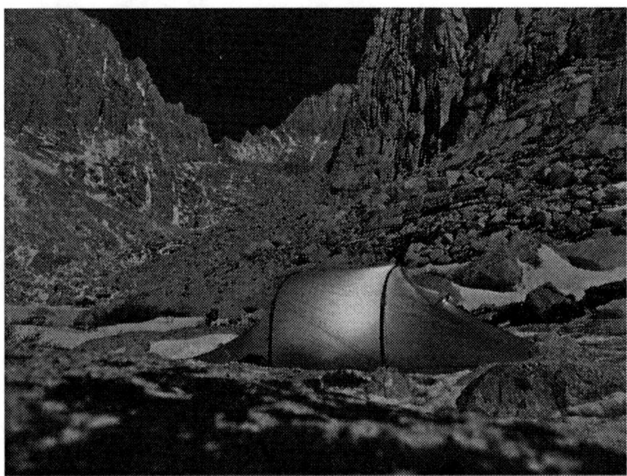

Fig. 16.1 Tent

Snow Cave (Fig. 16.2)

Where conditions permit snow caves are another way to shelter high on the mountain. Some climbers do not use tents at high altitudes unless the snow conditions do not allow for snow caving, since snow caves are silent and much warmer than tents. They can be built relatively easily, given sufficient time, using a snow shovel. A correctly made snow cave will hover around freezing, which relative to outside temperatures can be very warm. They can be dug anywhere where there is at least four feet of snow. The addition of a good quality bivvy bag and closed cell foam sleeping mat will also increase the warmth of the snow cave. Another shelter that works well is a quinzee, which is excavated from a pile of snow that has been work hardened or sintered (typically by stomping). Igloos are used by some climbers, but are deceptively difficult to build and require specific snow conditions.

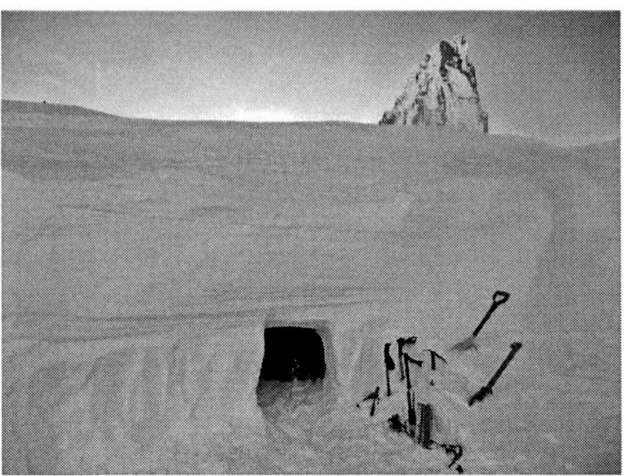

Fig. 16.2 Snow cave

HAZARDS

Mountaineering is considered to be one of the most dangerous activities in the world. Loss of life is not uncommon on most major extreme altitude mountaineering destinations every year. Dangers in mountaineering are sometimes divided into two categories: objective hazards that exist without regard to the climber's presence, like rockfall, avalanches and inclement weather, and subjective hazards that relate only to factors introduced by the climber. Equipment failure and falls due to inattention, fatigue or inadequate technique are examples of subjective hazards. A route continually swept by avalanches and storms is said to have a high level of objective danger, whereas a technically far more difficult route that is relatively safe from these dangers may be regarded as objectively safer.

In all, mountaineers must concern themselves with dangers: falling rocks, falling ice, snow-avalanches, the climber falling, falls from ice slopes, falls down snow slopes, falls into crevasses and the dangers from altitude and weather. To select and follow a route using one's skills and experience to mitigate these dangers is to exercise the climber's craft.

Falling Rocks

Every rock mountain is slowly disintegrating due to erosion, the process being especially rapid above the snow-line. Rock faces are constantly swept by falling stones, which may be possible to dodge. Falling rocks tend to form furrows in a mountain face, and these furrows (couloirs) have to be ascended with caution, their sides often being safe when the middle is stoneswept. Rocks fall more frequently on some days than on others, according to the recent weather. Ice formed during the night may temporarily bind rocks to the face but warmth of the day or lubricating water from melting snow or rain may easily dislodge these rocks. Local experience is a valuable help on determining typical rock fall on such routes.

The direction of the dip of rock strata sometimes determines the degree of danger on a particular face; the character of the rock must also be considered. Where stones fall frequently debris will be found below, whilst on snow slopes falling stones cut furrows visible from a great distance. In planning an ascent of a new peak or an unfamiliar route, mountaineers must look for such traces. When falling stones get mixed in considerable quantity with slushy snow or water a mud avalanche is formed (common in the Himalayas). It is vital to avoid camping in their possible line of fall.

Falling Ice

The places where ice may fall can always be determined beforehand. It falls in the broken parts of glaciers (seracs) and from overhanging cornices formed on the crests of narrow ridges. Large icicles are often formed on steep rock faces, and these fall frequently in fine weather following cold and stormy days. They have to be avoided like falling stones. Seracs are slow in formation, and slow in arriving (by glacier motion) at a condition of unstable equilibrium. They generally fall in or just after the hottest part of the day. A skillful and experienced ice-man will usually devise a safe route through a most intricate ice-fall, but such places should be avoided in the afternoon of a hot day. Hanging glaciers (i.e. glaciers perched on steep slopes) often discharge themselves over steep rock-faces, the snout breaking off at intervals. They can always be detected by their debris below. Their track should be avoided.

Falls from Rocks

A rock climber's skill is shown by their choice of handhold and foothold, and their adhesion to the holds once chosen. Much depends on the ability to estimate the capability of the rock to support the weight placed on it. Many loose rocks are quite firm enough to bear a person's weight, but experience is needed to know which can be trusted, and skill is required in transferring the weight to them without jerking. On rotten rocks the rope must be handled with special care, lest it should dislodge loose stones on to those below. Similar care must be given to handholds and footholds, for the same reason. When a horizontal traverse has to be made across very difficult rocks, a dangerous situation may arise unless at both ends of the traverse there are firm positions. Mutual assistance on hard rocks takes all manner of forms: two, or even three, people climbing on one another's shoulders, or using an ice axe propped up by others for a foothold. The great principle is that of co-operation, all the members of the party climbing with reference to the others, and not as independent units; each when moving must know what the climber in front and the one behind are doing. After bad weather steep rocks are often found covered with a veneer of ice (verglas), which may even render them inaccessible. Crampons are useful on such occasions.

Avalanches

Every year, 120 to 150 people die in small avalanches in the Alps alone. The vast majority of Alpine victims are reasonably experienced male skiers aged 20–35 but also include ski instructors and guides. However, a significant number of climbers are killed in Scottish avalanches often on descent and often triggered by the victims. There is always a lot of pressure to risk a snow crossing. Turning back takes a lot of extra time and effort, supreme leadership, and most importantly there is seldom an avalanche that proves the right decision was made. Making the decision to turn around is especially hard if others are crossing the slope, but any next person could become the trigger.

Ice Slopes

For travel on slopes consisting of ice or hard snow, crampons are a standard part of a mountaineer's equipment. While step-cutting can sometimes be used on snow slopes of moderate angle, this can be a slow and tiring process, which does not provide the higher security of crampons. However, in soft snow or powder, crampons are easily hampered by balling of snow, which reduces their effectiveness. In either case, an ice axe not only assists with balance but also provides the climber with the possibility of self-arrest in case of a slip or fall. On a true ice slope however, an ice axe is rarely able to effect a self-arrest. As an additional safety precaution on steep ice slopes, the climbing rope is attached to ice screws buried into the ice.

Snow Slopes

Snow slopes are very common, and usually easy to ascend. At the foot of a snow or ice slope is generally a big crevasse, called a *bergschrund*, where the final slope of the mountain rises from a snow-field or glacier. Such *bergschrunds* are generally too wide to be stepped across, and must be crossed by a snow bridge, which needs careful testing and a painstaking use of the rope. A steep snow slope in bad condition may be dangerous, as the whole body of snow may start as an avalanche. Such slopes are less dangerous if ascended directly, rather than obliquely, for an oblique or horizontal track cuts them across and facilitates movement of the mass. New snow lying on ice is especially dangerous. Experience is needed for determining the feasibility of advancement over snow in doubtful condition. Snow on rocks is usually rotten unless it is thick; snow on snow is likely to be sound. A day or two of fine weather will usually bring new snow into sound condition. Snow cannot lie at a very steep angle, though it often deceives the eye as to its slope. Snow slopes seldom exceed 40°. Ice slopes may be much steeper. Snow slopes in early morning are usually hard and safe, but the same in the afternoon are quite soft and possibly dangerous; hence the advantage of an early start.

Crevasses

Crevasses are the slits or deep chasms formed in the substance of a glacier as it passes over an uneven bed. They may be open or hidden. In the lower part of a glacier the crevasses are open. Above the snow-line they are frequently hidden by arched-over accumulations of winter snow. The detection of hidden crevasses requires care and experience. After a fresh fall of snow they can only be detected by sounding with the pole of the ice axe, or by looking to right and left where the open extension of a partially hidden crevasse may be obvious. The safeguard against accident is the rope, and no one should ever cross a snow-covered glacier unless roped to one, or even better to two companions. Anyone venturing onto crevasses should be trained in crevasse rescue.

WEATHER

The primary dangers caused by bad weather center on the changes it causes in snow and rock conditions, making movement suddenly much more arduous and hazardous than under normal circumstances.

Whiteouts make it difficult to retrace a route while rain may prevent taking the easiest line only determined as such under dry conditions. In a storm the mountaineer who uses a compass for guidance has a great advantage over a merely empirical observer. In large snow-fields it is, of course, easier to go wrong than on rocks, but intelligence and experience are the best guides in safely navigating objective hazards.

Summer thunderstorms may produce intense lightning. If a climber happens to be standing on or near the summit, they risk being struck. There are many cases where people have been struck by lightning while climbing mountains. In most mountainous regions, local storms develop by late morning and early afternoon. Many climbers will get an 'alpine start'; that is before or by first light so as to be on the way down when storms are intensifying in activity and lightning and other weather hazards are a distinct threat to safety. High winds can speed the onset of hypothermia, as well as damage equipment such as tents used for shelter. Under certain conditions, storms can also create waterfalls which can slow or stop climbing progress. A notable example is the Föhn wind acting upon the Eiger.

Solar Radiation

Solar radiation increases significantly as the atmosphere gets thinner with increasing altitude thereby absorbing less ultraviolet radiation. Snow cover reflecting the radiation can amplify the effects by up to 75% increasing the risks and damage from sunburn and snow blindness.

Chapter 17

IVF Management

INTRODUCTION

Infertility may not be considered a public health problem in many countries, but it is a devastating occurrence in the life of the people who suffer from it. In our country and many others, womanhood remains undefined without motherhood. The social stigma attached to infertility makes it a core issue in the lives of these women. Despite the population explosion in India 10–15% of couples are infertile. The need for assisted reproductive technology (ART) centers in India is on the rise, with increasing incidence of subfertility, advancement in diagnostic and therapeutic technology along with an increase in the sect of population which can afford to avail ART.

In the past decade, developments in the field of ART have intensified the hopes and wishes of infertile people to resolve their infertility and have resulted in an increasing demand for such services in both developed and developing countries. The increasing effort and determination on the part of researchers and clinicians to overpower and eliminate the stigma of infertility and the promise to help every infertile couple experience the reality of parenthood has led to aggressive research providing a therapy for most causes of infertility along with efforts to obviate the complications associated these therapies.

CATEGORIES OF INFERTILITY CARE UNITS

The severity in the cause of infertility varies between couples. Sometimes, simple counseling or minor intervention will be all that is necessary. Others may require more aggressive treatment; such cases should be referred to speciality clinics. It is, therefore, recommended that infertility treatment should be offered at four levels.

Primary (Level 1A) Infertility Care Units

Primary infertility care unit or clinic would be clinics where preliminary investigations are carried out and type and cause of infertility diagnosed.

They could be a doctor's consulting room, such as a gynecologist's or a physician's consulting room, or even a general hospital. Investigations into the cause of infertility by diligent history taking, physical examination and a simple semen analysis that can detect cases of azoospermia, and can determine if the cause of infertility is related to the female or the male or to both the partners. Multifactorial or unexplainable cases should be referred to specialty secondary (Level 2) or tertiary (Level 3) infertility care units.

Primary (Level 1B) Infertility Care Units Engaging in Intrauterine Insemination

Facilities for semen preparation and certification and for intrauterine insemination (IUI), including an appropriate sterile area for IUI. The IUI in such clinics must be done under the supervision of a gynecologist with a postgraduate degree. They have facilities for investigating sperm function, assessment of follicular growth and ovulation by serial transvaginal sonography (TVS), hysteroscopy and laparoscopy.

Secondary (Level 2) Infertility Care Units

These units must have infrastructure for further in-depth investigation and extended treatment of infertility except where oocytes are handled outside the body. Sperm function tests, assessment of follicular growth and ovulation by serial transvaginal sonography (TVS), facilities for semen preparation and intrauterine insemination (IUI), provision for semen collection in men with a vibrator or an electroejaculator in functional erectile and ejaculatory problems, endoscopic surgery and provision for extended treatment of infertility except for oocyte pick up and IVF, ICSI.

Tertiary (Level 3) Infertility Care Units

Such units will have three functions to perform, viz. diagnostic and therapeutic at the highest level of specialization and with the best of facilities, and research. Endocrine assay, karyotyping, color Doppler for checking growing follicles, functional integrity of corpus luteum, and developing endometrium in stimulated or unstimulated cycle can be assessed. All varieties of assisted reproductive technologies, including ICSI, and embryo freezing are included.

THE PROJECT REPORT OF *IN VITRO* FERTILIZATION

This document outlines the details for setting-up a tertiary care infertility unit with the facilities of IVF, ICSI and PGD. A well-designed IVF laboratory is an asset to an IVF program.

Various aspects which need planning are:

- Location of the laboratory area and basic infrastructure
- Laboratory equipment and consumables quality control
- Laboratory maintenance and future expansion.

Feasibility Study

Demand

- *National demand*: Infertility is a common problem occurring in 10–15% of reproductive age groups. In a country with a total population of 10 billion it translates into approximately 250 million people attempting parenthood at a given time and 13–18 million couples requiring these services.
- *Demand in Delhi and surrounding areas*: Delhi and NCT has a population of 20 million. On translating the national demand to a local one for a population of 20 million 5,00,000 people would be attempting parenthood at a given time and 36,000 would be requiring these services.
- *International demand*: There is a huge scope of medical tourism in these cases. The waiting period for IVF is 3 years in the UK. The cost is more than 3 times. A referral system can be evolved to encourage medical tourism. Package deals can be worked out which are inclusive of travel and stay. The following are a sample of the cost of these procedures in the USA.

In vitro fertilization (IVF) (in office)	$5800.00
In office IVF with intracytoplasmic sperm injection (ICSI)	$7300.00
Gamete intra-Fallopian transfer (GIFT) including operating room, anesthesia, and surgeon fees	$6400.00
GIFT to IVF conversion	$1000.00
Zygote intra-Fallopian transfer (ZIFT) including operating room, anesthesia, and surgeon fees	$7600.00
Tubal reanastomosis including operating room, anesthesia, and surgeon fees	$8350.00
Intrauterine insemination (IUI) including sperm preparation and ultrasound	$395.00
Frozen embryo transfer including office visit to plan the transfer, medications, and ultrasound	$2450.00
Screening Laboratories (required unless performed previously on both husband and wife)	
Coagulation studies	$700.00
Immunology studies	$400.00
Endometrial biopsy	$260.00
Dilation/Sounding	$140.00
Semen analysis (Complete with sperm survival)	$180.00
Follicular study ultrasound	$195.00
Follow-up ultrasound to monitor cycle	$175.00
Full pelvic ultrasound	$260.00
Hysterosalpingogram	$250–$500
Sonohysterogram	$445.00

Supply

- *Institutes providing services*: Delhi has about 16 infertility and IVF centers. Noida has only one IVF center. Many of these centers are ill-equipped and do not meet required standards. This really falls short of the requirement. A state of the art ART center is the need of the hour.
- *Lack of trained doctors in the field*: There is a definite lack of trained and dedicated docters in this field. IVF requires complete dedication to the field.

There is a definite deficit between demand and supply, the demand greatly exceeding the supply.

Objectives of IVF Center

- To make a Pan India IVF brand
- To start with one center at Delhi or Noida and expand to multiple centers all over
- To initially target at least 120 IVF cycles per year
- To develop egg donation and freezing programs
- To develop Preimplantation Genetic Diagnosis Programs
- To also develop high level of research facilities which may later be expanded to include stem cell technology.
- To increase awareness of facilities of IVF among general public, practioners and the general gynecologist by organizing talks, seminars, camps and a monthly bulletin compiled by ABC hospital will IVF center which includes awareness of facilities being provided by the center.
- To make IVF center a training center for ART techniques and apply for accreditation of the same.
- To ensure that the laboratory has international standards and ISO recognition, followed by accreditation by other national and international laboratory accreditation agencies.
- Partnerships with a brand name.
  - Academic partnerships with leading practioners across India, using them as hubs for referral to this super specialized service.
  - Create partnerships with leading academic institutes from India and abroad
  - Back to back partnership with medical schools to provide continuous skilled manpower
- To target international population with view of medical tourism.

Organization Chart (Proposed) (Flow chart 17.1)

Flow chart 17.1 Organizational chart of an IVF center

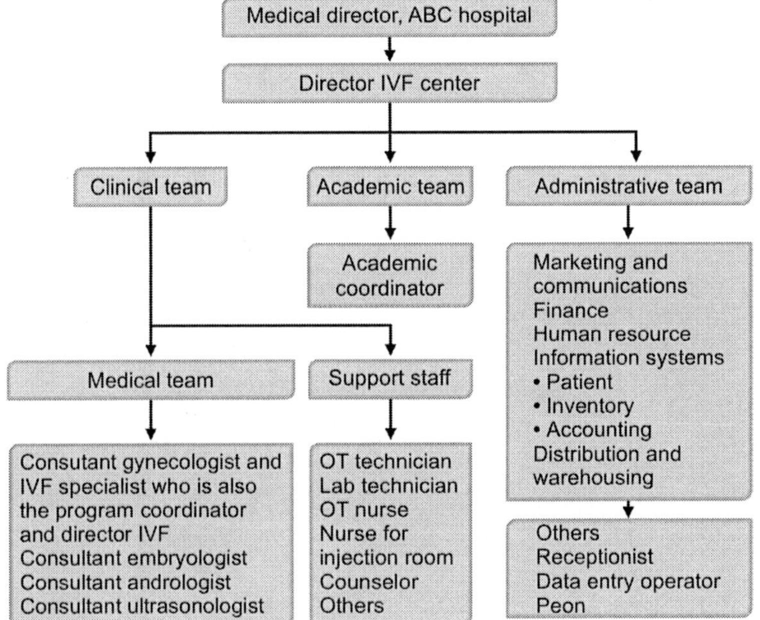

Facilities

ART facilities to be provided.

A variety of ART procedures will be provided:

- Artificial insemination with husband's semen (AIH)
- Artificial insemination with donor semen (AID)
- Intrauterine insemination with either husband's or donor semen (IUI-H or IUI-D)
- *In vitro* fertilization and embryo transfer (IVF-ET)
- IVF-associated techniques
- Intracytoplasmic sperm injection (ICSI) with ejaculated, epididymal or testicular spermatozoa
- Oocyte donation (OD) or embryo donation (ED)
- Cryopreservation
  - Freezing semen
  - Freezing embryos
  - Oocyte cryopreservation.

Other Facilities
- Ultrasonographic follicular monitoring
- Endocrinology workup and tests
- Ovulation induction
- Embryoreduction
- Semenanalysis
- Hysterosonosalpingography.

Targets

Procedure and Targets

Procedure types:
- *Level I*: Intrauterine insemination (Phase 1)
- *Level II*: IVF and ET (Phase 1)
- *Level III*: ICSI (Phase 1)
- *Level IV*: PGD (Preimplantation Genetic Diagnosis)—(Phase 2).

Target:
- 40–50 IUI per month
- 20–25 IVF/ICSI per month.

Cost of procedure to patient:
- IUI—3000/-
- IVF—40, 000/-
- ICSI—45,000/-.

Location of the Laboratory

The laboratory should be away from traffic, dust and pollution, preferably on a higher floor (not ground floor) moisture prone areas like basements must be avoided. Access to laboratory should be restricted. It should be away from the hospital traffic. Bulky instruments need to be moved in and out while setting the laboratory and for maintenance. Hence, access to the laboratory needs to be large enough to accommodate them.

Basic Infrastructure

Electricity

Power points should be made at a regular distances over working benches. They should be provided in a number over and above the estimated requirement. Supply from different electric phases and provision for uninterrupted power supply or a generator will help in case of power supply or a generator will help in case of power failure.

Back-up Power Supply

There should be no interruption in power supply to the incubator and to other essential services in the clinic. Given the power supply situation in India, it is, therefore, imperative that a power back-up in the form of UPS systems and/or a captive power generation system is available in infertility clinics offering ART services.

Apart from the publicly distributed power supply the laboratory would be equipped with adequate provision of:

- Power conditioning equipment
- In-house generator capacity
- Uninterrupted power supply.

Air Conditioning

It has to have a separate air-conditioning unit, which is not common with the rest of the hospital air.

Water Supply

Scrubbing and washing area will need adequate water supply and well concealed drainage.

Clean Air

Filtered air supply with regular air changes will help in maintaining a sterile envoirnment. Comfortable and constant temperature should be maintained by air-conditioning system. It is preferable to have a room with Hepa filters. Coda filters can also be installed. The air of the sterile area should not be mixed with unsterile area and the AC ducting should be such that there is no mixing of air. Different air mixing units for central AC should be used.

Floors, Walls and Ceiling

The floors should not be slippery and should be easily cleaned. Tiles should be as large as possible so that there are minimum joints which may accumulate dust particles. False ceilings are not recommended as it is inaccessible for maintenance. Walls of IVF laboratory and OT should be dark preferable black granite with minimum joints.

Doors

The entry should preferably be with electric eye doors. The doors should be coated or of aluminium which can be cleaned by ethyl alcohol.

Furniture

The working benches should be of correct height. The surfaces should be nonporous and easily cleanable. Chairs and stools with adjustable height add to the comfort of the scientist and reduce fatigue. Easily slidable drawers with adequate capacity for storage should be installed in the laboratory with working benches. It is preferable not to put shelves on the wall as dust can collect on top and they can go unnoticed.

AREA AND PLAN LAYOUT

Area

An IVF/ICSI and PGD laboratory would require an area of 2000 sq feet. This would also take into consideration adding on instruments for ever expanding technology in this sector. The IVF laboratory and the OT occupy the major space.

Nonsterile Area

- A reception and waiting room for patients
- *Office of the gynecologist and program director*: This room would have an adjoining room which could serve as a counseling room and record keeping room equipped with a computer
- Conference room
- *Examination room*: A room with privacy for interviewing and examining male and female partners independently is essential. Adequate measures must be taken to ensure that history taking and examination are carried out in strict privacy, maintaining the dignity of the patients. The room must be equipped with an examination table and gynecological instruments for examining the female per vaginum,

an appropriate ultrasonographic machine with a probe for transvaginal examination of the female and examination of the testes and excurrent male reproductive tract. A color Doppler would be needed.

- *Store room*: A well-stocked store for keeping essential stock of especially those items that have to be imported, precluding the need to be caught short in the middle of treatment. Facilities must be available for storing sterile (media, needles, catheters, petri dishes and such-like items) and nonsterile material under refrigerated and nonrefrigerated conditions as appropriate.
- *Record room*: Record keeping must be computerized as far as possible so that data is accessible retrospectively for analysis or when called upon by the supervisory agency. There are many software programs for this purpose, which are commercially available today. A user-friendly one should be chosen that could be used widely. Besides containing essential details of the patient's records, it must contain history of the cause of infertility as diagnosed earlier, results of new diagnosis if relevant, the treatment option best suited for the particular patient, the treatment carried out and the outcome of treatment, and follow-up if any. Any other noteworthy point such as possible adverse reaction to drugs, must be recorded.
- *Autoclave room*: A separate facility must be available for sterilizing and autoclaving all surgical items as well as some of those to be used in the *in vitro* culture laboratory.
  - *Steps for vermin proofing*: Adequate steps should be taken to make the whole clinic vermin proof, with suitable traps for preventing insects and other forms of unwanted creatures entering the clinic. This essential detail should be planned at an early stage because no pesticide can be used in a fully functional IVF clinic, as it could be toxic to the gametes and embryos.
- *Semen collection room*: This must be a well-appointed room with privacy and an appropriate environment; it should be located in a secluded area close to the laboratory. Such a facility must be available in-house rather than having the patient collect the sample and bring it to the laboratory for analysis as, in the latter case, semen quality and identity is likely to be compromised. This room must have a washbasin with availability of soap and clean towels. The room must also have a toilet and must not be used for any other purpose.

- *Semen processing laboratory*: There must be a separate room with a laminar air flow for semen processing, preferably close to the semen collection room. This laboratory must also have facilities for microscopic examination of postcoital test smears. Good laboratory practice (GLP) guidelines as defined internationally must be followed. Care must be taken for the safe disposal of biological waste and other materials (syringes, glass slides, etc.). Laboratory workers should be immunized against hepatitis B and tetanus.
- *Clean room for IUI*: There must be a separate area/room with an appropriate table for intrauterine insemination (IUI). It could be combined with the Recovery room.
- *Recovery room*: There should be at least 3 beds in the recovery.
- Changing room before the entry into sterile area there should be a changing room which could also incorporate a docters rest room with an attached bathroom.

Sterile Area

The sterile area shall house the operation theater, and an adjoining embryology laboratory and a room to keep the cryocans for freezing. Entry to the sterile area must be strictly controlled by an anteroom for changing footwear, area for changing into sterile garments and a scrub-station. The sterile area must be air-conditioned where fresh air filtered through an approved and appropriate filter system is circulated at an ambient temperature (22–250°C).

- Scrub station.
- *The operation theater*: This must be well equipped with facilities for carrying out transvaginal ovum pick-up under ultrasound guidance. The operation theater must be equipped for emergency resuscitative procedures.
- *Room for intrauterine transfer of embryo*: This room must be a sterile area having an examination table on which the patient can be placed for carrying out the procedure and rest undisturbed for a period of time. It can be done in the same room as OT.
- *The embryology laboratory complex*: The embryology laboratory must have facilities for the control of temperature and humidity and must have filtered air with an appropriate number of air exchanges per hour. Walls and floors must be composed of materials that can be easily washed and

disinfected; use of carpeting must be strictly avoided. The embryology laboratory must have the following:

- A laminar flow bench with a thermostatically controlled heating plate
- A stereo microscope
- A routine high-powered binocular light microscope
- A 'high resolution' inverted microscope with phase contrast or Hoffman optics, preferably with facilities for video recording
- A micromanipulator
- A CO_2 incubator, preferably with a back-up
- A hot air oven
- A laboratory centrifuge
- A refrigerator.

The embryology laboratory must have a daily logbook in which all the day's activities are recorded, including the performance of the equipment. The laboratory must have a separate area for andrology separated by a door.

- *Room for cryocans for freezing*: There should be a door separating it from the main laboratory. Liquid nitrogen cans and equipment for freezing embryo should be present.
- *Area for provision for sterile water*: There must also be the provision of sterile water with Milli-Q filtration to provide clean water to clean the laboratory.

FLOOR PLAN

- *Floor plan*: Overall *in vitro* fertilization (IVF) center plan
  - Floor plan IVF laboratory
  - Floor plan IVF operation theater (OT)
  - Insemination room and recovery floor plan
  - Floor plan intrauterine insemination (IUI) laboratory
  - Changing room and lounge (Optional—Area can be reduced)
  - Semen collection room and injection room
  - Gyne examination room
  - Reception
  - Gyne office and counseling room
  - Endoscopy OT (Optional).

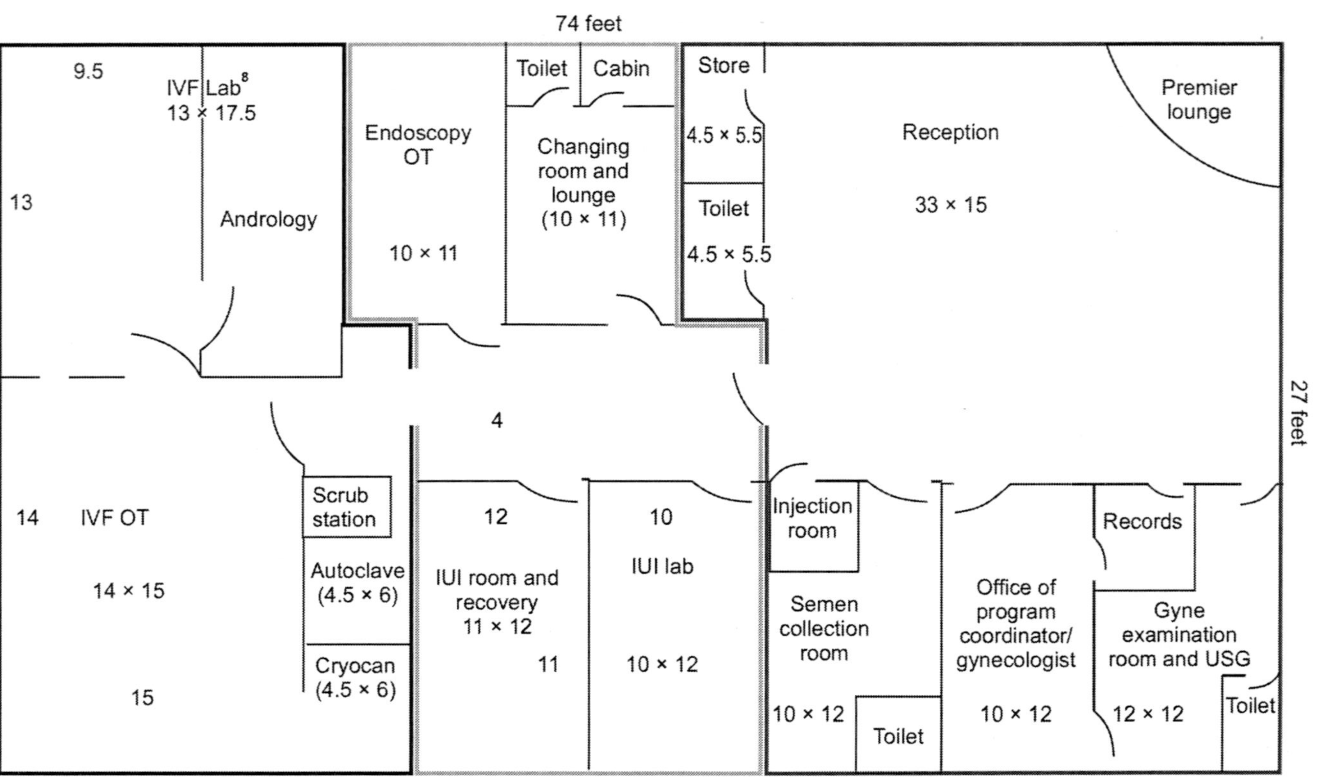
74 feet
27 feet
9.5
IVF Lab8
13 × 17.5
13
Andrology
Endoscopy OT
10 × 11
Toilet
Cabin
Changing room and lounge (10 × 11)
Store
4.5 × 5.5
Toilet
4.5 × 5.5
Reception
33 × 15
Premier lounge
4
14
IVF OT
14 × 15
15
Scrub station
Autoclave (4.5 × 6)
Cryocan (4.5 × 6)
12
IUI room and recovery 11 × 12
11
10
IUI lab
10 × 12
Injection room
Semen collection room
10 × 12
Toilet
Office of program coordinator/ gynecologist
10 × 12
Records
Gyne examination room and USG
12 × 12
Toilet

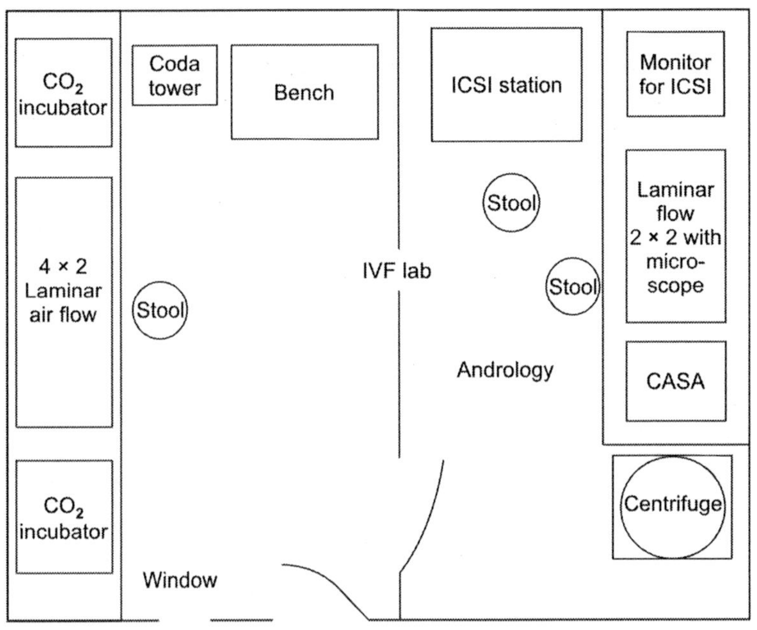
CO_2 incubator
Coda tower
Bench
ICSI station
Monitor for ICSI
Laminar flow 2 × 2 with micro-scope
Stool
IVF lab
Stool
4 × 2 Laminar air flow
Stool
Andrology
CASA
CO_2 incubator
Centrifuge
Window

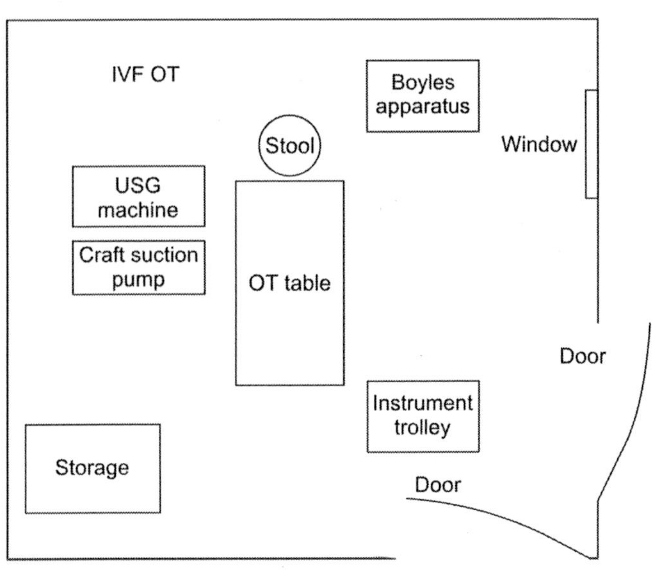
IVF OT
Boyles apparatus
Stool
Window
USG machine
Craft suction pump
OT table
Door
Instrument trolley
Storage
Door

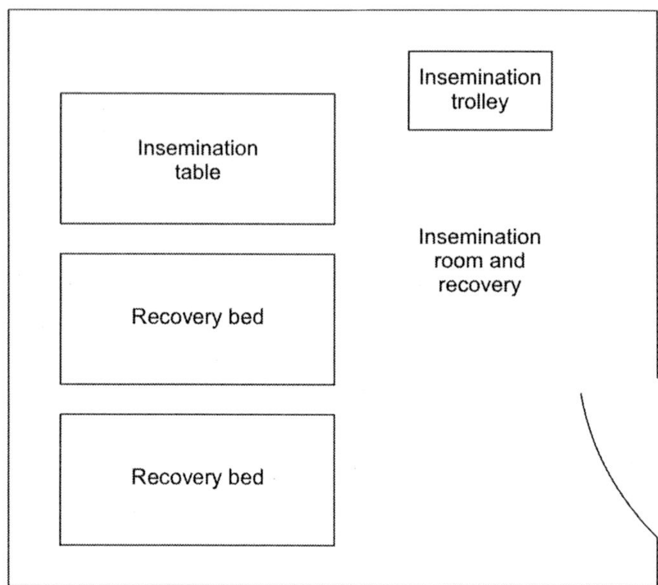

The IUI Laboratory

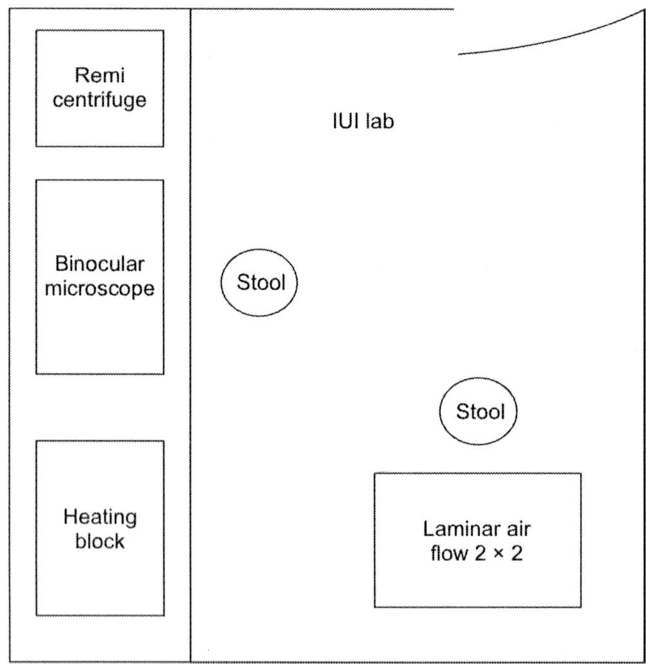

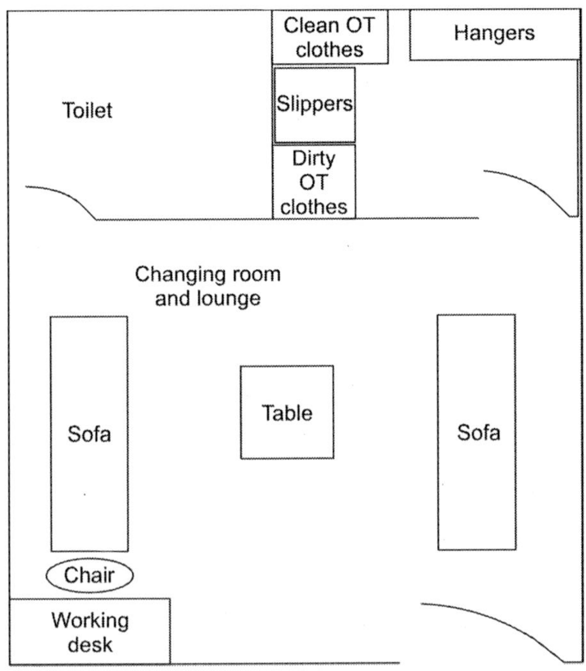
Clean OT clothes
Hangers
Toilet
Slippers
Dirty OT clothes
Changing room and lounge
Sofa
Table
Sofa
Chair
Working desk

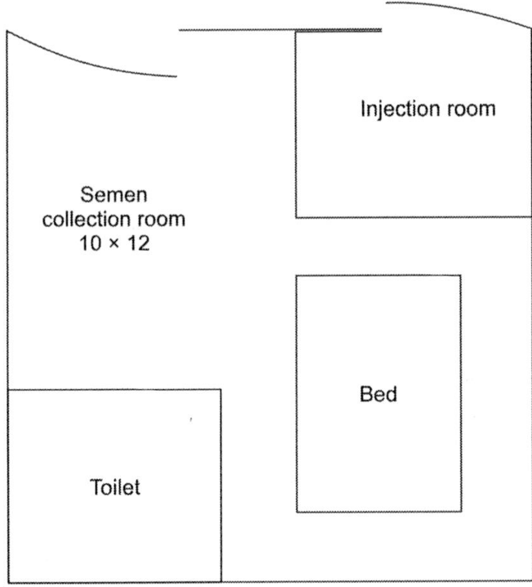
Injection room
Semen collection room 10 × 12
Bed
Toilet

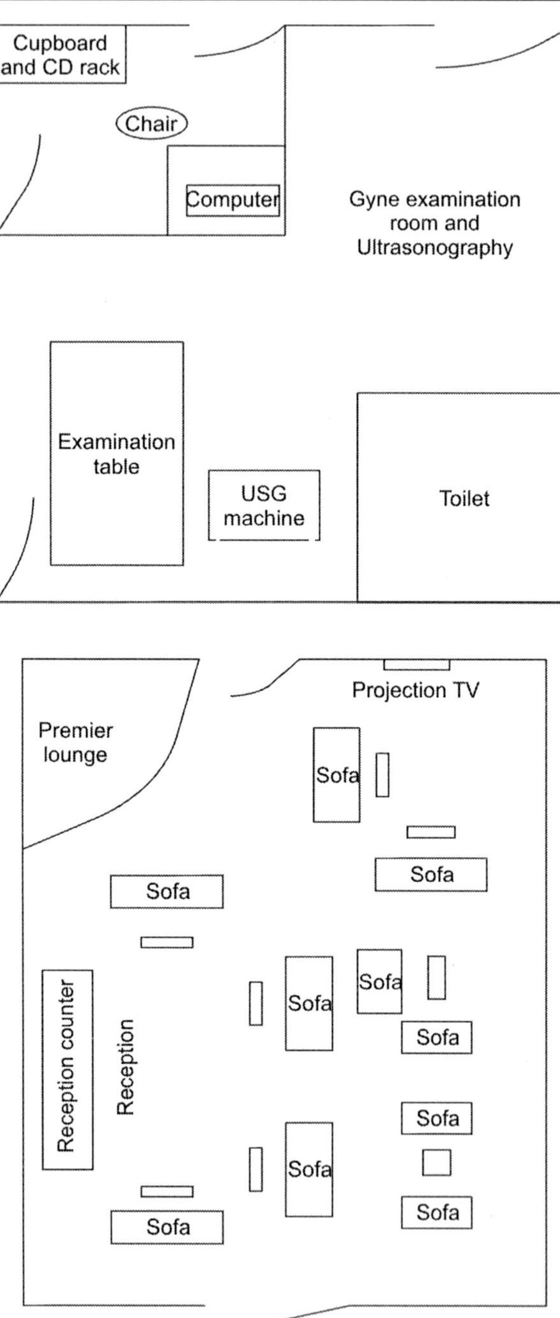
Cupboard and CD rack
Chair
Computer
Gyne examination room and Ultrasonography
Examination table
USG machine
Toilet
Projection TV
Premier lounge
Sofa
Sofa
Sofa
Reception counter
Reception
Sofa
Sofa
Sofa
Sofa
Sofa
Sofa
Sofa
Sofa

THE STAFF

The practice of assisted reproductive technology (ART) requires a well-orchestrated teamwork between the:

- Gynecologist and program coordinator/director
- Andrologist
- Utrasonologist
- Clinical embryologist
- Counselor
- Technicians
- Trained OT nursing sisters.

Other Staff

- Receptionist
- Record keeper and data entry manager cum secretary
- Public relation team
- Marketing team.

Gynecologist and Program Coordinator

The qualification for a gynecologist is a postgraduate degree in gynecology. Additional experience should include understanding the causative factors of male and female infertility. Having adequate knowledge of the practice and use of diagnostic methods for determining the cause of infertility and its treatment such as hormone therapy, IUI, etc.

The responsibilities of the gynecologist would include the following:

- Interviewing of the infertile couple initially
- History taking
- Physical examination of the female
- Recommending appropriate tests to be carried out, interpreting them and treating medical disorders (infections, endocrine anomalies)
- Advising the couple on planned relationship in simple cases
- Carrying out artificial insemination by husband (AIH), artificial insemination by donor (AID), IUI and monitoring the ovulation induction protocols for IVF.

The treating doctor must be responsible for maintaining all records of diagnosis, treatment given and consent forms. It would be the gynecologist's responsibility to see that all equipment and instruments in the operation theater are properly functional and in order, and that a logbook is maintained of their use and operation.

As the program coordinator/director should be able to coordinate the activities of the rest of the team and take care of staff administrative matters, stock keeping, finance, maintenance of patient records, statutory requirements, and public relations. He/she should ensure that the staff are keeping up with the latest developments in their subject, by providing them with information from the literature, making available to them access to the latest journals, and encouraging them to participate in conferences and meetings and present their data. The program coordinator/director should have a postgraduate degree in an appropriate medical or biological science.

Andrologist

A urologist with a postgraduate degree in urology that often takes on the task of treating male infertility. An andrologist may be attached part time to the unit. Such individuals must receive additional training in diagnosis of various types of male infertility covering psychogenic impotence, anatomical anomalies of the penis which disable normal intercourse, endocrine factors that cause poor semen characteristics and/or impotence, infections, and causes of erectile dysfunction. The andrologist must have knowledge of the occupational hazards, infections and fever that cause reversible or irreversible forms of infertility, and knowledge of ultrasonographic or vasographic studies of the reproductive excurrent ducts to detect partial occlusion that can be surgically corrected.

Clinical Embryologist

The clinical embryologist must be knowledgeable in mammalian embryology, reproductive endocrinology, genetics, molecular biology, biochemistry, microbiology and *in vitro* culture techniques. The biologist must also be familiar with ART. He/she must be either a medical graduate or have a postgraduate degree or a doctorate in an appropriate area of life sciences. A person with a BSc or BVSc degree but with first-hand, hands-on experience of the techniques mentioned below and of discharging the responsibilities listed below, would be acceptable for functioning as a clinical embryologist in the particular clinic. Such persons would also be eligible to take a test to be designed and conducted by an appropriate designated authority, to qualify for a position of a clinical embryologist in a new clinic. The responsibilities of the clinical embryologist would be:

- To ensure that all the necessary equipment are present in the laboratory and are functional.
- To perform all the procedures pertaining to processing, handling and culturing of gametes and embryos in the laboratory and hand over the embryo to the gynecologist.
- To maintain records of all the procedures carried out in the laboratory.

Counselors

Counselors are an important adjunct to any infertility clinic. The patients are adequately informed of what and what not to expect from the treatment offered to them. Counseling for ART is not taught as a separate subject anywhere. A person who has at least a degree (preferably a postgraduate degree) in Social Sciences, Psychology, Life Sciences or Medicine, and a good knowledge of the various causes of infertility and its social and gender implications, and the possibilities offered by the various treatment modalities, should be considered as qualified to occupy this position. The person should have a working knowledge of the psychological stress that would be experienced by potential patients, and should be able to counsel them to assuage their fears and anxiety and not to have unreasonable expectations from ART. The counselor must invariably apprise the couple of the advantages of adoption as against resorting to ART involving a donor.

SALARY STRUCTURE OF STAFF

Salary to be decided by the management of the hospital.

Clinical Team

Medical Team

- Gynecologist and IVF specialist
- Embryologist
- Andrologist
- Ultrasonologist.

Support Staff

- Counselor
- OT nursing sister
- OT technician
- Laboratory technician
- Nurse for injection room.

Academic Team

Academic coordinator.

Administrative Team

- Manager finanace
- Manager marketing

- Marketing team
- Manager distribution and warehousing
- Manager human resource
- Manager information systems.

Others

- Receptionist
- Data entry operator
- Peon
- Sweeper.

EQUIPMENT

Incubators

The CO_2 incubators are required to maintain optimum culture conditions. These can come with either thermal conductivity or infrared sensors. Each of them has their own merits. One can choose between a water-jacketed filter and one without. The incubator which maintains the temperature accurately and has minimal CO_2 recovery should be preferred. A second backup incubator is a must. Also a second one decreases the frequency of repeatedly opening the first as samples are distributed. CO_2 supplied to the incubator should be of medical grade. Through a two stage regulator and at ideal pressure to minimize gas consumption without affecting CO_2 recovery time. Metal gas tubing should be avoided in line filter between CO_2 cylinder and incubator eliminates all contamination from the gas.

- Binder (Germanv) CO_2 incubator with hot air sterlization at 187.5°C
  Other standard features include:
  - Data logging
  - Altitude compensation
  - Perma dry humidification system
  - Fan free interiors
  - FP IR sensor
  - Cost: ₹ 5,25,000/-
- Heracell CO_2 incubator 150—One
  Cost: ₹ 5,80,000/-

Laminar Flow Hoods (Clean Air Station)

A vertical laminar flow is preferred. The size of the hood can be according to need. Accessories such as gas ports, burner connections can be added to the flow hood. Some work stations like K systems can be brought in with integrated heating systems. However, independent detachable heating appliances for microscope stage, petri dishes are advisable for maintaining flexibility in operations

- Laminar flow hood 2' × 2' (Andrology work)—Two
  Size: 2' × 2' × 2'
  Cleanliness: Class 100.
  Particle retention: 0.3 micron and above.
  Noise level: 60–65 decibels (A).
  Model no: ATV 0600.
  Power input: 230V Ac/50Hz
  Cost: ₹ 45,000/-
- Laminar flow hood 4' × 2' (K systems) (For IVF laboratory embryology work)—One
  Size: 4' × 2' × 2' (Inner all sides steel body)
  Cost: ₹ 13,00,000

Microscopes

Stereo Zoom Microscope

Good quality optics makes oocyte identification easy and reduces the strain on the eyes. Ergonomically placed zooming and focusing of knobs are useful. Trinocular microscopes makes documentation and teaching possible. Transmitted light source which provides even illumination should be chosen.

Stereozoom microscope Nikon Japan 1 (Model SMZ 645)—One
With diopter adjuster, rubber eye shield, reticle lead.
Diascopic stand (Transmitted light illuminator).
C-Ds diascopic stand S with reflecting mirror supplied with transparent stage glass
A pair of armrests C-DSLS
Lamphouse 6V20W for C-Ds.
Transformer TN (220–240V).
Power Cord BE.
6V–20W Halogen lamp with reflector.
Trinocular version model is SMZ 800 for ₹ 2,50,000 + additional color CCO/ camera for ₹ 25,000.

Inverted Microscope

This is useful for studying the pronucleus stage and embryo morphology. Micromanipulation requires inverted microscope with Hoffman modulation or Varel contrast system making sure, it can be adapted with a micromanipulator and PGD techniques in the future.

Integra Ti micromanipulator for ICSI and PGD from research instruments the UK—One.

Integra Ti stage including:

- 4 channel temperature controller
- Two additional metal heated stage
- Digital help menu
- Pipette home function 1 set TDU5000

Left side single tool holder

Right side single tool holder

SAS 11/2E

MSHD oil syringe

X-Y mechanical stage

with

Nikon Japan inverted research microscope model te2000-s with Hoffman modulation contrast (without rectangular stage).

Lamphouse-2 BL with Precentered 100W halogen.

TE2000-S main body, side port coaxial coarse fine focus

W/tension adjustment, light distribution observation/side port,: 100/0.20/80 vinyl cover type 108.

T-DH 100W Dia illumination pillar (Tiltable) supplied with detachable condenser carrier, diffuser four filter holder and field diaphragm, 45 mm filter slots.

Lamphouser remote cable T-PS 100 W power supply 100–240V for T-DH 100 W Dia illumination pillar.

Halogen lamp l2-100W LL

25 inclination tube D 25 inclination angle, Turret selector incorporated B/2.5x/C/O.

CFI lOX W/Diopter adjustment (FOV 22 mm)

CFI UW eyepiece guard

UV eyepiece cap

C-N6 sextuple nosepiece

Filter 45 mm NCBll, daylight color balance

Filter 45 mm heat absorbing.

Hoffman modulation contrast system

C-mount TV adapter A

SPARES

Halogen lamp l2V -100 W LL

₹ 18,50,000.

Binocular Microscope for IUI and Andrology—Two

Halogen Light: 6V 20W.
Focusing by co-axial coarse and fine focusing controls.
Objectives: 4x, 10x, 20x and 40x Eyepiece: Compensating widefield paired Eyepiece WFI0x
₹ 35,000.

Ovum Aspiration Pump

Ovum aspiration pump craft UK—One
Low Pressure: 0–550 mm
Hg = 0–666 mbar
Volume of overflow vessel: 2 × 100 mL
Connecting for aspiration tubing: 2–4 mm
Power supply: 230V
Power frequency: 50/60 Hz
Power point 50VA
Nominal current: 220 mA
Power line isolation: 0.315 AT 5
₹ 1,10,000.

Laboratory Purification System

CODA tower unit—One
With 4 separate filters and about 18-air changes per hour
₹ 5,50,000.

Heating Appliances

Maintaining temperature of the gametes all along the procedure in laboratory is of prime importance. The microscope stage warmer maintains temperature of the culture dish during identification and manipulation of oocyte. A dry bath for test tube will maintain temperature of follicular fluid during oocyte retrieval. The petri plate warmer maintains the temperature of the dishes before they are actually placed on the microscope stage:

- Dry bath—Two
  Digital cell transporter with steel body
  Heating block (Dry bath) for heating of test tubes in removable, autoclavable anodized aluminum blocks for maintenance of required temperature

Digital display and control of temperature With ± 0.2°C accuracy from ambient to 110°C, 3 anodized blocks of 75 × 50 × 50 mm to accommodate 12 × 13 mL and 12 × 6 mL tubes
₹ 22,500

- Petri dish warmer—One
  Steel body for preheating of slides, petri dishes, pipettes, etc. of desired temperature
  Anodized aluminum heating plate (Approx dimension 300 × 100 × 40 mm). Temperature range: from ambient to 110°C with accuracy of ± 0.2°C
  ₹ 22,500
- Stage warmer —Two
  Steel body for preheating of slides, petri dishes, pipettes, etc. of desired temperature anodized aluminium heating plate (Approx dimension 300 × 100 × 40 mm). Temperature range: from ambient to 110°C with accuracy of + 0.2°C
  ₹ 22,500.

MedeaLAB CASA

Computer-assisted semen analysis
₹ 9,50,000
Requires a PC Pentium IV with 64 MB Ram.

Programmable Biological Freezer

Embryo and sperm cryopreservation is an essential part of an IVF program. With ICSI, where the chances of getting more embryos has increased, cryobanking really plays an important role in reducing costs and enhancing success of the program.

Programmable embryo freezer—One
Cryologic Australia model CL 2200
Controlled rate preprogrammed freezer for freezing sperms, oocytes, embryos completely with 8 preprogrammed controllers
Vertical freezing of straws
Standard cryochamber
LN2 bath (Capacity 1.5L)
Carry case
Temperature sensor: Platinum resistance element
Temperature display: Digital, LCD, 0.1°C resolution
Timing: Digital, quartz crystal.
Weight: 2.2 kg.
₹ 4,50,000.

Cryocan—One
Capacity can 35 liters—45,000
Capacity can 26 liters—29,500.

Laser

Laser system for assisted hatching and embryo biopsy, from RI UK
Control box, hand held control unit, collimator, mirror, fiber optic cable, Pilot laser targeting system and laser objective, to be mounted on inverted Microscope with software for embryo analysis.
₹ 25,00,000.

Spindle Imaging System

Spindle imaging system for oocyte imaging for routine operation.
For noninvasive imaging of the spindle and zona pellucida in living oocyte with facility of color overlay.

From Cambridge Research Instruments USA specifications:
Optical:
Wavelength of operation: 546 run
Spatial resolution: Diffraction limited
Relay optics: 0.65 × (requires 1 × c-mount attachment)
Electrical controls:
Power source: Universal serial bus 2.0 (USB 2.0) to CPU
Image acquisition: Image
Output format: BMP or TIFF camera: CCD chip dimensions: 2 (3" diagonal
Image size: 1392 × 1040, 8-bit Pixel dimensions: 8.98 × 6.71 mm
₹ 30,00,000.

Sperm Counting Chamber

Makler sperm counting chamber—One
For accurate method of sperm counting with cover slip. From Makler (Israel)
₹ 35,000.

Centrifuge

Centrifuge with digital speed and time indicator. Remi (India)—Two
With all accessories to accommodate 15 mL tubes and swing out rotor with 8 × 15 mL places
₹ 15,000.

Ultrapure Water Systems

Milli-Q—Two
It is useful to provide water for washing the laboratory One requires two Milli-Q systems.
Cost as per company specifications.

Miscellaneous

Hot Air Oven—One—Cost as per company specifications.
Heat sealing machines (For polybags and heat sealing straws).

Consumables

Semen collecting containers—25
6 mL test tubes—100
14 mL tube—100
Graduated conical tubes—100
5 ml sterile serological pipettes—100
IUI cannulas—25
1 mL syringe—25
5 mL syringe with needle—25
Glass slides—1 Box
Frosted glass slides—1 Box
Cover slip square 22 × 22 mm—2 Box
pH paper—10 pkts
Stainless steel trays—1
Stainless steel discard bowls—1
Forceps—1
Glass marking pencil—1
Plastic 15 mL test tube stand—1
Gloves—1
Semen diluting fluid
Eosin
Ethanol 1
Tissue culture grade plastic tubes
Petri dishes, four well dishes
Pasteurs pipette
Serological pipette
Pipette stands
Total cost: ₹ 22,000.

Ovum Pick-up and Embryo Transfer

Pick-up needle, embryo transfer catheter—Recurring cost per procedure.

Culture Media

Flushing medium—Recurring cost per procedure
Sperm preparation medium
Universal IVF medium
Toxin free liquid paraffin
Embryo freezing package.

IVF Management Software

It is designed to cover important areas in a fertility clinic. It can be used in a LAN environment with multiple users. Degree of access to individual user can be predefined by the administrator.
With Hardware Lock (Dongle)
System requirements: Minimum requirement is Pentium II or higher computers with 64 MB RAM.
20 MB of free hard space Windows operating system LAN connection if multiple user
Cost: ₹ 55,000.

All costs are exclusive of sales tax, octroi, packing, forwarding and insurance charges.

Annual Maintenance Contract

Annual maintenance for 3 years to be taken.

The AMC will be required for the equipment of IVF/IUI laboratory which is available on a consolidated basis @ 10% of the total project value per annum for the first year after the expiry of warranty. For subsequent years, the annual increment on the AMC value shall be to the tune of 5%.

The AMC will start after expiry of the first 12 months after installation.

The AMC would cover routine visits and would include calibrations/diagnostic protocols/cleaning, etc. The cost for the spares, however, will have to be paid at actual.

Website

₹ 50,000 with an ongoing cost of 6,000 per year.

Other Equipment

- Ultraound machines:
  - Phillips HD-3 black and white—One
    Two probes
    ₹ 8,00,000
  - Philips envisor color Doppler
    Two probes
    ₹ 16,00,000
- Endoscope
  - Bettocchi office hysteroscope (2.9 mm)—Karl Storz
    ₹ 3,43,000
  - Basic gynelaparoscope—Karl Storz
    ₹ 4,73,000
  - TRICAM SL II camera control unit—Karl Storz
    Camera
    ₹ 3,75,000
  - Tricam camera head color system—Karl Storz
    ₹ 3,00,000
  - Thermoflator set—Karl Storz
    ₹ 3, 41,000
  - Xenon light source
    ₹ 1,30,000
  - 19" Flat screen monitor
    ₹ 2,00,000
  - Examination sheath
    ₹ 19,000
  - Hysteromat
    ₹ 3,00,000

  Operative instruments will be added as required. Prices subject to confirmation from equipment manager.
- Boyles apparatus—Two
  ₹ 80,000
- OT table—Two
  ₹ 50,000
- OT light—Two
  ₹ 50,000.

Computers—Four

Desktop office PC—Two
₹ 40,000

Office imaging PC—Two
₹ 80,000

HP-AIO network ready laser jet—One
₹ 22,000

Laser printer color—One
₹ 25,000

Ethernet network cables and switches
₹ 20,000

Internet connection
DSL router
₹ 2000
Prices subject to confirmation from equipment manager.

Furniture

OT table—2
Examination table—2
Beds—3
Chairs
Sofas
Tables
Desks
Stools
Cupboards.

MARKETING

The success of any venture is dependent on marketing it.

Marketing consists of:

- Creating an awareness of need in the general public and practitioners
- To make aware of existence of the Ojjus Goodwill IVF center
- To introduce them to the procedures being offered by the laboratory
- To include practitioners as a part of the team by arranging visits to the laboratories and arranging CME courses on basic infertility and IUI
- To have monthly lectures with invited audience
- To create awareness outside Delhi of the services of Ojjus Goodwill IVF center
- To give feedback on all patients referred to the center

- To provide infertility consultation services to all general gynecologists in and near Delhi under the brand name of Ojjus Goodwill
- To have a tie up with international names for medical tourism
- To Project the services and work done in the form of a monthly bulletin compiled by the Director of the IVF center—Monthly recurring expenditure ₹ 20,000
- To project the institution as a training center for ART with partnership with other institutes.

A separate budget should be kept aside for marketing.

TIME FRAME

Time frame—6 months.

The essence of successful project execution lies in understanding the scope of work to be done, risks to be incurred, resources to be required, tasks to be accomplished, milestones to be tracked and schedule to be followed. The methodology for undertaking the work would be designed to take care of all such aspects.

THE FUTURE PERSPECTIVE

The Future

The future includes:

- Plans for future expansion are to open more centers all over India under the brand name of ABC Hospital making it a brand name.
- To make it an Internationally recognized training center for ART.
- Expand facilities to newer horizons.

With the fast changing technology in ART, ABC Hospital-IVF should stand out as a center which keeps-up with the recent and provides the latest technology.

Chapter 18 Electronic Medical Records

INTRODUCTION

Electronic medical records (EMRs) are a longitudinal electronic record of patient health/medical information generated by one or more encounters in any care delivery setting. This information contains patient demographics, progress notes, problems, medications, vital signs, past medical history, immunizations, laboratory data, radiology reports, and more. EMRs automate and streamline clinicians' workflow, they have the ability to generate a complete record of clinical patient encounters, as well as support other care-related activities directly or indirectly via interface—including evidence-based decision support, quality management, and outcomes reporting.

Historically, the deployment of EMRs can be divided into two major time periods. First, the early efforts began in the 1960s and '70s, when academic medical centers developed their own systems. Second, beginning in the 1980s, leaders saw benefits to industry-wide standards and began forming organizations to tackle the broader issues that would facilitate the widespread use of electronic medical information. The first EMR systems were known as clinical information systems in the mid-1960s. After then, EMRs have appeared in the national political forum, indicating widespread concerns about record keeping's effect on public health.

A simple example benefit of EMRs is they can store all records pertaining to patients, and multiple providers can access the data depending upon the requirements, request, and reference. So, paper storage becomes virtually obsolete, fewer medical errors occur, and each provider can see the patient history of medication and, hence, prescribe accordingly.

An electronic medical record (EMR) is a systematic collection of electronic health/medical information about an individual patient or population. It is a record in digital format that is theoretically capable of being shared across different healthcare settings. In some cases, this sharing can occur by way of network-connected, enterprise-wide information systems and other information networks or exchanges. EMRs may include a range of data, including demographics, medical history, medication and allergies, immunization status, laboratory test results, radiology images, vital signs, personal statistics like age and weight, and billing information.

The system is designed to represent data that accurately captures the state of the patient at all times. It allows for an entire patient history to be viewed without the need to track down the patient's previous medical record volume and assists in ensuring data is accurate, appropriate and legible. It reduces the chances of data replication as there is only one modifiable file, which means the file is constantly up to date when viewed at a later date and eliminates the issue of lost forms or paperwork. Due to all the information being in a single file, it makes it much more effective when extracting medical data for the examination of possible trends and long-term changes in the patient.

An EMR contains the standard medical and clinical data gathered in one provider's office. An electronic medical record (EMR) is a digital version of a paper chart that contains all of a patient's medical history from one practice. An EMR is mostly used by providers for diagnosis and treatment.

The electronic medical records (EMRs) are a digital version of the paper charts in the clinician's office. An EMR contains the medical and treatment history of the patients in one practice. EMRs have advantages over paper records.

For example, EMRs allow clinicians to:

- Track data over time.
- Easily identify which patients are due for preventive screenings or checkups.
- Check how their patients are doing on certain parameters—such as blood pressure readings or vaccinations.
- Monitor and improve overall quality of care within the practice.

But the information in EMRs does not travel easily out of the practice. In fact, the patient's record might even have to be printed out and delivered by mail to specialists and other members of the care team. In that regard, EMRs are not much better than a paper record.

Five key criteria for ascertaining EMR value are:

1. Can EMRs improve quality and convenience of patient care?
2. Can EMRs increase patient participation in their care?
3. Can EMRs improve accuracy of diagnoses and health treatments?
4. Can EMRs improve care coordination?
5. Can EMRs increase efficiency of practice and cost savings?

EMRs allows physicians and staff members to:

- View medical histories and insurance information.
- Document interactions with patients.

- Perform and manage referrals.
- Order laboratory tests and view test results.
- Send electronic prescription requests to pharmacies (reducing the risk that hard-to-read handwriting will lead to medical errors).
- Flag potentially harmful drug interactions.

Tragic events like those that occurred in the US on September, 11, Hurricane Katrina, and the California fires have showcased the benefits of electronic record keeping. Those injured or affected by any of those events were more easily treated and may have found better outcomes than those for whom no medical records were available. Large scale EMR systems replicate their stored records in several places across the country so that one tragic event would not destroy them.

However, with all the benefits described above, one should note that implementing an EMR is not like buying a new copy machine; it takes time, effort and resources—both financially and physically to implement one successfully. Providers considering implementation typically also have questions such as, "What is in it for my patients? What is in it for me? Will it be worth it?"

Insights to these questions can be found below:

- *For providers:*
  - Quick access to patient records from inpatient and remote locations for more coordinated, efficient care.
  - Enhanced decision support, clinical alerts, reminders, and medical information.
  - Performance-improving tools, real-time quality reporting.
  - Legible, complete documentation that facilitates accurate coding and billing.
  - Interfaces with laboratories, registries, other EMRs, and health information exchanges (HIEs).
  - Safer, more reliable prescribing.
  - Meaningful use incentives.
- *For patients:*
  - Less requirement to fill out the same forms at each office visit.
  - Reliable point-of-care information and reminders notifying providers of important health interventions.
  - Convenience of e-prescriptions electronically sent to the pharmacy.
  - Patient portals for online interaction with providers.
  - Electronic referrals allowing for easier access to follow-up care with specialists.

ASSESSING RETURN ON INVESTMENT

Two main results from implementing EMRs are that users gain a secure and reliable environment with more data access options among staff; and second, workflow is improved gaining greater efficiency among staff thus slowing down the need to add more staff even as the practice grows while increasing the amount of quality time spent with patients. The majority of physicians report data access as the top safety benefit. The key to any of these benefits is effective management of the transition from a paper-based system to electronic health records: administratively, financially, culturally, and technologically.

SECURITY RETURN ON INVESTMENT

Internal control: With EMRs, providers can track who accesses all files. Anyone working in a paper-based practice could potentially access, view, and copy the protected health information undetected.

Encryption: Encrypted files require a specific code key to read data. If EMRs are appropriately encrypted, then if data are accessed not according to procedure, the information is unreadable.

Disaster recovery: Back-up is one of the biggest advantage of digital records, while papers are likely to be destroyed due to natural disasters, fires, etc. web-based EMRs utilize remote back-ups to allow doctors secure access to critical data from anywhere they have internet access. Practices can save hours previously spent on manual back-ups and improve reliability due to the high rate that tape back-ups are inaccessible due to unreadable tape.

OTHER AREAS FOR RETURN ON INVESTMENT

Reduced storage: Paper records require a substantial amount of space compared to digital records; providers have to keep information on file for the treatment of their patients and also have to keep those files on hand due to healthcare regulations for at least 6 years.

Access anytime, anywhere: The EMR users enjoy the relatively new luxury of access to their data from wherever they want, whenever they want, whiles still remaining Health Insurance Portability and Accountability Act (HIPAA) compliant. Multiple departments can add clinical information to the health record, too, and view the same file even when another user has it open with some EMRs.

Improved accuracy: Malpractice is possible in paper-based medical records due to incomplete documentation and unreadable handwriting, while electronic systems come with features that make sure all information-related patient care is included on the form are proper.

Reduced costs: Overall costs of implementing an electronic health records are less than the paper record, as paper-based records have higher costs due to the necessity of more manpower to manage, access, file, and maintain.

Improved risk management: With all patient information in digital form, providers are able to track clinical issues more effectively allowing them to more easily identify areas of risk. These areas include easier access to patient histories, drug information, decision support, proper coding, and more.

Five Key Areas for Return on Investment Summary

Regardless of how familiar one's paper-based systems are, it is clear that EMRs can improve quality and convenience of patient care, increase patient participation in their care, improve accuracy of diagnoses and health treatments, improve care coordination, and increase efficiency of practice and cost savings. Implementations require careful care and planning, but as outlined, can offer providers myriad benefits.

- Hours saved generating reports.
- Medical record staff working hours decrease.
- Paper medical record forms printing and binder costs savings.
- Nursing and front office staff hours saved.
- Training the staff for manual documentation hours saved.
- Chart audit and assembly hours saved.
- Less time on documentation and more time to treat more patients.
- Costs for long-term and on-site storage of medical records eliminated.
- Immediate retrieval of medical records.
- Greater employee satisfaction gaining efficiency in the workplace.
- No lost (and easy to audit) medical records.
- Decision support and coding tools including prescriptions.

BENEFITS OF ELECTRONIC MEDICAL RECORDS

An EMR is more beneficial than paper records because it allows providers to:

- *Track* data over time.
- *Identify* patients who are due for preventive visits and screenings.
- *Monitor* how patients measure up to certain parameters, such as vaccinations and blood pressure readings.
- *Improve* overall quality of care in a practice.

Adoption of EMRs will facilitate access to medical records across and within clinics and will allow rapid and continuous assessments of patients' characteristics and service provision. It has been consistently pointed out that medical practice can be improved by reducing the medical errors that occur during treatment. Commonly, errors occur due to incomplete medical records, transcription mistakes or failure to correlate medical histories with current treatment decisions. Further, it was reported that although paper-based records are easier to create, they prove difficult to search, as in one of the studies where physicians could not find relevant information about the patient in traditional paper-based records in 80% of outpatient visits. Thus, the effective use of automation gives chance to practitioners to make decisions at every level and treat patients to the best of their abilities. An EMR environment is a complex and sophisticated environment, with its foundation being the clinical data repository (CDR) along with a real-time transaction processing database of patients' clinical information for practitioners. Because the retrieval of data is easy, analysis can be done quickly and rapid assessment of a health program or policy can be done in no time. In one study, the authors showed this benefit by analyzing the records based on EMR maintained in STD clinics. The STD electronic medical record system, due to its flexibility of design and control over enhancements, was made to register, store and retrieve information in a highly clinically usable format. This enabled presentation of legible, completed and uniform data for easy analysis and decision making. Enabling staff to view and edit patient charts from multiple work locations improved information sharing and regular monitoring of clinical quality outcomes. Computerized clinical decision support system, alerts and reminders about individual patient and access to both recommended and alternate treatments ensured best of the provider's practice in interest of patient care. Further, confidentiality of the information was maintained by installing various security features in the form of automatic log out of inactive sessions and agency-wide network security systems to prevent access by unauthorized individuals.

The EMRs provide access to unprecedented amounts of clinical data for research that can accelerate the level of knowledge of effective medical practices. The evidence-based medicine will get the much needed boost. It is cost-effective as well. In a systematic review of PubMed and EBSCO business, looking for cost indicators of electronic health record (EHR) implementations and their associated benefit indicators, the authors discovered the rapid capital-recovering process. On an average, the annual benefits were 76.5% of the first year costs and 308.6% of the annual costs.

EMR AND CLINICAL TRIAL

An EMR has immense role in each step of a clinical trial, right from designing of the trial to evidence-based clinical care. EMR helps in identifying the eligible patients from a list of patients suffering from a particular disease. It provides easy access to detailed clinical care data, which helps in formulating new clinical trial hypotheses.

There are challenges for the use of EMR in clinical trials. The investigator, who chooses to enrol the patients based on the record has access to the whole medical history of the subject. There is no scope of blinding. Incorporating the information collected and interventions introduced during the clinical trial into routine EMR of the subject is another area of debate.

Issues in EMR

Following EMR is a debatable issue. Many doctors are reluctant in this system as they feel that it will reduce the clinical productivity. Some software uses strictly formatted or categorical fields to promote uniformity. This has been widely criticized for its restrictive framework, conveying limited or sometimes altered information due to structured approach and being resource intensive because of the demand of standardized and up to date clinical set of terms. Besides, this form of data entry is predicted to pose extraburden on caregivers as they will be required to extract precoded information from narratives. The other drawback of the system is absence of any account of the clinician patient experiences of electronic record use in clinical setting. This provides important insights regarding adaptability of an automated system's rigidity to suit the fluid process of patient management. An important issue is the privacy of the patients. Because the health record of each patient on EMR is widely available, it can be misused. Proper system should be in place to deal with this very important disadvantage of the EMR.

ELECTRONIC MEDICAL RECORD VERSUS PAPER MEDICAL RECORD

Many providers have been hesitant to take on the task of converting from the paper-based medical record system to the electronic medical record. Making the change can be time-consuming and costly. Also, physicians and staff may have a difficult time transitioning to a new way of collecting and handling patient information. However, the benefits of highly outweigh the challenges.

Reduced Storage

In comparison to digital records, paper records require a substantial amount of space. Not only do providers have to keep information on.

Ease of Access

With a digital record, access is virtually unlimited. Physicians can have access to test results almost immediately. Multiple departments can add clinical information to the medical record without having to locate or checkout a paper medical record chart.

Improved Accuracy

Medical errors in a paper-based medical record system can sometimes be related to incomplete documentation and illegible handwriting. Electronic systems come with features that make sure all information necessary for patient care is included on the form. Some EMR software packages have edits in place that require the user to add additional information as needed.

Reduced Costs

Although, providers may have the initial costs of implementing an electronic medical record system, the overall costs are less than those associated with the paper record. Paper medical records have higher costs due to the necessity of more personnel to manage, access, file, and maintain paper charts.

Increased Risk Management

With all patient information in digital form, providers are able to track clinical issues more effectively allowing them to easily identify areas of risk. Processes can quickly and accurately be put in place in order to improve patient care.

Paper-based records require a significant amount of storage space compared to digital records. The costs of storage media, such as paper and film, per unit of information differ dramatically from that of electronic storage media. When paper records are stored in different locations, collating them to a single location for review by a healthcare provider is time consuming and complicated, whereas the process can be simplified with electronic records. This is particularly true in the case of person-centered records, which are impractical to maintain if not electronic. When paper-based records are required in multiple locations, copying, faxing, and transporting costs are significant compared to duplication and transfer of digital records. Because of these many 'after-entry' benefits, large medical institutions are heavily promoting the adoption of electronic medical records.

One study estimates electronic medical records improve overall efficiency by 6% per year, and the monthly cost of an EMR may (depending on the cost of the EMR) be offset by the cost of only a few 'unnecessary' tests or admissions.

However, the increased portability and accessibility of electronic medical records may also increase the ease with which they can be accessed and stolen by unauthorized persons or unscrupulous users versus paper medical records.

Handwritten paper medical records can be associated with poor legibility, which can contribute to medical errors. Preprinted forms, the standardization of abbreviations, and standards for penmanship were encouraged to improve reliability of paper medical records. Electronic records help with the standardization of forms, terminology and abbreviations, and data input (Table 18.1). Digitization of forms facilitates the collection of data for epidemiology and clinical studies.

In contrast, EMRs can be continuously updated. The ability to exchange records between different EMR systems would facilitate the coordination of healthcare delivery in nonaffiliated healthcare facilities. In addition, data from an electronic system can be used anonymously for statistical reporting in matters such as quality improvement, resource management and public health communicable disease surveillance.

Table 18.1 Differences between paper-based and electronic-based record systems

Paper-based systems	Electronic health records
Paper charts can be easily misplaced	Electronic files can be easily searched and backed-up, available on server
Time consuming to pull charts and re-file	Charts are updated and e-filed easily
Appointment reminders have to be sent manually	Automatic appointment reminders are sent from the EMR
Scheduling is done manually	Scheduling is much more automated
Manual filing of insurance cards	Insurance cards are scanned and instantly put into the system
Manual communication about billing	The EMR system sends billing reminders
Drug recalls are difficult to communicate and cross-reference with affected patients	Patient files can be flagged for drug recalls and updates
Difficult and time consuming tasks include identification of patient characteristics	Patient characteristics are fully searchable and linked to patient histories
Difficult to manage chronic diseases	Patient groups can be set-up and managed
Human error can occur in clinical information	Reduced risks due to human errors

Ambulance Services

Ambulance services have introduced the use of EMR systems. The benefits of EMR in ambulances include the following: better training for paramedics, review of clinical standards, better research options for prehospital care and design of future treatment options.

Automated handwriting recognition of ambulance medical forms has also been successful. These systems allow paper-based medical documents to be converted to digital text with substantially less cost overhead. Patient identifying information would not be converted to comply with government privacy regulations. The data can then be efficiently used for epidemiological analysis.

Technical Features

- Digital formatting enables information to be used and shared over secure networks.
- Track care (e.g. prescriptions) and outcomes (e.g. blood pressure).
- Trigger warnings and reminders.
- Send and receive orders, reports, and results.

Health Information Exchange

- Technical and social framework that enables information to move electronically between organizations.
- Reporting to public health.
- e-prescribing.
- Sharing laboratory results with providers.

Using an EMR to read and write a patient's record is not only possible through a workstation but, depending on the type of system and healthcare settings, may also be possible through mobile devices that are handwriting capable, tablets and smartphones. Electronic medical records may include access to personal health records (PHRs) which makes individual notes from an EMR readily visible and accessible for consumers.

Some EMR systems automatically monitor clinical events, by analyzing patient data from an electronic health record to predict, detect and potentially prevent adverse events. This can include discharge/transfer orders, pharmacy orders, radiology results, laboratory results and any other data from ancillary services or provider notes. This type of event monitoring has been implemented using the Louisiana Public Health Information Exchange linking state wide public health with electronic medical records. This system alerted medical providers when a patient with HIV/AIDS had not received care in over 12 months. This system greatly reduced the number of missed critical opportunities.

QUALITY

Several studies call into question whether EMRs improve the quality of care. However, a recent multiprovider study in diabetes care, published in the New England Journal of Medicine, found evidence that practices with EMR provided better quality care.

Ekectronic medical records (EMRs) do help improve care coordination. Since anyone with that EMR can view the patients chart, it cuts down on guessing histories, seeing multiple specialists, smoothing transitions between care settings, and better care in emergency situations. EMRs may also improve prevention by providing doctors and patients better access to test results, identifying missing patient information, and offering evidence-based recommendations for preventive services.

Electronic medical record (EMR): Titles such as automated medical record; computer-based patient record; electronic medical record, and electronic health record have been used by hospitals/countries over recent years with varying definitions. For instance, in some countries, the term Electronic Medical Record or EMR is used to describe a system based on document imaging or an electronic record system developed within a general medical practice or community health center. It has also been referred to as an electronic version of the traditional paper record.

In a number of countries, however, the term EMR also refers to a fully automated electronic medical record, including all clinical data.

The ultimate goal in the development of health information systems, however, is one that has not been fully reached in most countries to date. It is a longitudinal health record with entries by multiple providers of health-care in multiple sites where care is provided. That is:

A medical record that reflects the entire health history of an individual across his or her lifetime including data from multiple providers in a range of contexts.

If considering an EMR, it is important to understand the definitions used by organizations/countries and to define, if required, what your institution/country would like to implement. The questions which need to be answered are:

- Is a fully integrated health record, including all clinical data, the ultimate goal? That is, will data be entered by all health professionals at the time the patient is seen in a hospital, health center or clinic, with all data held in the one electronic record and accessed by multiple providers at multiple sites?

- Or will it be limited to a fully electronic health record within one hospital or healthcare facility setting? Will it be called an 'electronic health record'? An 'electronic medical record', or by another name?

When people refer to what they have been using as an electronic health record, it may not be the same as other electronic health records developed in different institutions/countries.

The point to remember is that the term Electronic Health Record is widely used in many countries with some variation in definition.

Ideally an electronic health record should be able to:

- Collect clinical, administrative and financial data at the point of care.
- Exchange data more easily between health professionals to facilitate continuing care.
- Measure clinical improvement and health outcomes, compare the outcomes against benchmarks and facilitate research and clinical trials.
- Provide valuable statistical data in a timely and efficient manner to public health and government ministries (such reporting of health data is important in the detection and monitoring of disease outbreaks, as well as providing meaningful and accurate statistics to measure the health status of the population).
- Support management in administrative and financial reporting and other processes (Mon, 2004).

The introduction of an electronic health record in an institution/country must be carefully planned, have complete backing and support of the administration, medical and nursing staff, and clerical personnel. Current problems identified in healthcare documentation in the patient's health record and health record services, as well as privacy and confidentiality issues, must be addressed and quality control measures introduced before a successful change can be implemented. As for a manual system, an electronic health record must also meet legal, confidentiality, and retention requirements of the patient, the attending health professional and the healthcare institution/country.

Whether a manual or electronic health record is maintained, there is still the need to ensure that the information generated by healthcare data is accurate, timely, and available when needed.

Database technology has proven to be extremely valuable in the development of the EMR. Although document imaging will remain a valuable part of the EMR, it will play a reduced role and decisions will need to be made as to whether previous health records will be included in the EMR.

Before planning an electronic health record system, other administrative questions must be addressed, such as:

- What type of system would be required to meet perceived needs of an electronic health record for your healthcare facility/country?
- Is there available funding?
- What type and size of computers would be required to meet the needs within the funds available?
- Does the hospital/country have an adequate and reliable electricity supply?
- Does the hospital/country have sufficient trained staff and the provision for training new staff?

The introduction of an EMR can be a mammoth undertaking. It is important that MROs develop and maintain an effective and efficient manual medical record system to ensure that a future move to an EMR will go smoothly.

AN ELECTRONIC HEALTH RECORD IS NOT A SIMPLE REPLACEMENT OF THE PAPER RECORD

If there are problems associated with a manual medical record system which are not resolved, automating health record content and procedures will only perpetuate the problem.

Before an EMR can be introduced, detailed discussion is required to address a number of perceived problems such as: the cost involved, available funding for healthcare, which is limited in most countries; lack of computer skills and expertise of medical and clerical staff; and resistance by some medical practitioners and health professionals generally to a change from manual to electronic documentation.

The move to a fully electronic health record is a major undertaking and cannot be entered into lightly. Over the years, a number of countries have made attempts to introduce some form of electronic medical record. Some have been successful and others have not yet reached their goal. In addition, some countries are planning the introduction of a nation-wide electronic health record while a small number have actually implemented what they describe as a national EMR. Definitions, however, vary and what one country means by an electronic health record may not be the same as defined by another country.

The computerization of a number of hospital applications such as pathology, biochemistry, etc. have been most successful as have the computerization of the MPI, ATD, etc. Also in some hospital departments such as hematology, cardiology, and intensive care, computerized clinical systems have been introduced and have been most successful.

The computerization of all clinical data in a medical/health record, however, is not yet widespread.

Some of the early attempts at automation referred to an automated medical record, which was a collection of computer-stored images of traditional health record documents, consists mainly of administrative and clinical support systems such as laboratory tests, X-ray reports, etc.

This form of automation addressed aspects such as access to, space for, and control of problems related to the current paper-based records but did not address data input/output deficiencies.

How to Implement Electronic Medical Records?

1. *Assess your practice readiness*: The first step in EMR implementation is to conduct an assessment of your current practice and its goals, needs, and financial and technical readiness. With an accurate view of your level of preparedness, your practice can design an implementation plan that meets the specific needs of your practice.
2. *Plan your approach*: Planning draws on the information gathered during the assessment phase, to outline the practice's EMR implementation plan.
3. *Select or upgrade to a certified EMR*: There are a number of steps involved in choosing the right EMR system for your practice. Eligible healthcare professionals and eligible hospitals must use certified EMR technology in order to achieve meaningful use and qualify for incentive payments. Looking to make your current EMRs meaningful use compliant? Start here.
4. *Conduct training and implement an EMR system*: EMR implementation involves the installation of the EMR system and associated activities, such as training, mock "go-live," and pilot testing.
5. *Achieve meaningful use*: The final phase of EMR implementation includes successfully attesting to demonstrating meaningful use of EMRs, and reassessing what you have learned from training and everyday use of the system.
6. *Continue quality improvement*: Emphasizes continuous evaluation of your practice's goals and needs post-EMR-implementation to continue improving workflows that achieve the individual practice's goals while leveraging the functionality of electronic medical records (EMRs).

Step 1: Assess Your Practice Readiness

The assessment phase is foundational to all other EMR implementation steps, and involves determining if the practice is ready to make the change from paper records to electronic medical records (EMRs), or to upgrade their current system to a new certified version.

Why Implement EMRs?

More importantly, the assessment phase should address the following question: "WHY" implement EMRs? This EMR implementation step should help practice leadership evaluate their current state to determine what is working well and what can be improved. Some of the question providers ask themselves during this phase include:

- "Am I accomplishing what I thought, I would be doing when I decided to go to medical school?"
- "Are we providing the best possible care to our patients, or are we simply trying to make it through the week?"
- "If I had more time, what would I do differently?"
- "What would it be like to leave the office yet stay connected to my practice?"

At this stage, practice leadership and staff should consider the practice's clinical goals, needs, financial and technical readiness as they transition.

Assess Your Current Practice

The assessment should look at the current state of the practice:

- Are administrative processes organized, efficient, and well-documented?
- Are clinical workflows efficient, clearly mapped out, and understood by all staff?
- Are data collection and reporting processes well-established and documented?
- Are staff members computer literate and comfortable with information technology?
- Does the practice have access to high-speed internet connectivity?
- Does the practice have access to the financial capital required to purchase new or additional hardware?
- Are there clinical priorities or needs that should be addressed?
- Does the practice have specialty specific requirements?

Through the regional extension centers (RECs), we have learned that these questions and assessment tools provide a good understanding of the current state of the practice and can help identify key goals for improvement. Often, these goals relate to patient quality, patient satisfaction, practice productivity and efficiency, improved quality of work environment, and most important to the overall goal—improved healthcare.

Envision the Future

The next EMR implementation step is to envision the future state of the practice. What would the practice leadership like to see different in the future? More specifically:

- What will be different for the patients?
- What will be different for the providers?
- What will be different for the staff?

Set Goals

Goals and needs should be documented to help guide decision-making throughout the implementation process. And they may need to be re-assessed throughout the EMR implementation steps to ensure a smooth transition for the practice and all staff.

We recommend that you set goals in areas that are important and meaningful to your practice. These may be clinical goals, revenue goals, or goals around work environment. Goals in all three areas will help assure balanced processes after the implementation. Goals that are important to you will help you and your staff through the change process. We recommend you follow the "SMART" goals process. This process includes setting objectives and goals that meet the following criteria:

- *Specific*: Achieving the goal would make a difference for our patients and our practice.
- *Measurable*: We can quantify the current level and the target goal.
- *Attainable*: Although the goal may be a stretch, we can achieve it.
- *Relevant*: This is worth the effort.
- *Time bound*: There are deadlines and opportunities to celebrate success!

These goals become the guide posts for an EMR implementation project, and achieving these goals will motivate providers and practice staff to make necessary changes and attain new skills.

Critical outcomes of the assessment process include:

- *A designated leadership team* for the EMR implementation process (clinical and practice management staff, or for small practices, the entire team). Having strong and positive advocate(s) for change can be one of the strongest tools to guide the transition.
- *A unified vision,* where each member of the practice team understands how they will be affected by the change and understands the roadmap to success.
- *Measureable, quantifiable, realistic goals,* which are the key to the assessment phase.

National Learning Consortium Resources
Over the coming months, the national learning consortium (NLC) will continue to share experiences from the field and the resulting leading practices and tools that can be used throughout the all phases of the EMR implementation life cycle.

Learn more about the National Learning Consortium
The material in these guides and tools was developed from the experiences of Regional Extension Center staff in the performance of technical support and EMR implementation assistance to primary care providers. The information contained in this guide is not intended to serve as legal advice nor should it substitute for legal counsel. The guide is not exhaustive, and readers are encouraged to seek additional detailed technical guidance to supplement the information contained herein.

Reference in this website to any specific resources, tools, products, process, service, manufacturer, or company does not constitute its endorsement or recommendation by the US Government or the US Department of Health and Human Services.

Step 2: Plan your Approach

Clarify and Prioritize
Building an EMR implementation plan becomes critical for identifying the right tasks to perform, the order of those tasks, and clear communication of tasks to the entire team involved with the change process. One effective first step in the planning process is for the team to segment tasks into three categories:

1. What new work tasks/process are we going to *start* doing?
2. What work tasks/process are we going to *stop* doing?
3. What work tasks/process are we going to *sustain*?

The start/stop/sustain exercise helps clarify what the new work environment will be like after the change and help the team prioritize tasks in the overall EMR implementation plan.

Steps in the Planning Phase
Here are some tactical steps that typically occur during the EMR implementation planning phase. You may collaborate and use tools provided by your Regional Extension Center (REC), IT vendor, and/or EMR vendor (if you already have an existing EMR product) to complete these activities.

- Analyze and map out the practice's current workflow and processes of how the practice currently gets work done (the current state).

- Map out how EMRs will enable desired workflows and processes, creating new workflow patterns to improve inefficiency or duplicative processes (the future state).
- Create a contingency plan—or back-up plan—to combat issues that may arise throughout the implementation process.
- Create a project plan for transitioning from paper to EMRs, and appoint someone to manage the project plan.
- Establish a chart abstraction plan, a means to convert or transform, information from paper charts to electronic charts. Identify specific data elements that will need to be entered into the new EMR and if there are items that will be scanned.
- Understand what data elements may be migrated from your old system to your new one, such as patient demographics or provider schedule information. Sometimes, being selective with which data or how much data you want to migrate can influence the ease of transition.
- Identify concerns and obstacles regarding privacy and security and create a plan to address them. It is essential to emphasize the importance of privacy and security when transitioning to EMRs. Get started using this Health Information Privacy and Security: 10 Step Plan.

National Learning Consortium Resources

The following resources are examples of tools that are used in the field today, and that are recommended by "boots-on-the-ground" professionals for use by others who have made the commitment to implement or upgrade to certified EMR systems.

Learn more about the National Learning Consortium

The material in these guides and tools was developed from the experiences of Regional Extension Center staff in the performance of technical support and EMR implementation assistance to primary care providers. The information contained in this guide is not intended to serve as legal advice nor should it substitute for legal counsel. The guide is not exhaustive, and readers are encouraged to seek additional detailed technical guidance to supplement the information contained herein.

Reference in this website to any specific resources, tools, products, process, service, manufacturer, or company does not constitute its endorsement or recommendation by the US Government or the US Department of Health and Human Services.

Step 3: Select or Upgrade to a Certified EMR

Selecting an EMR system is a critical decision and a significant planning task. There are different opinions regarding when the selection of an EMR system should be made in the planning phase. Some practices go through the planning process and develop the selection criteria they wish to use. Other practices begin by selecting an EMR system and then conduct planning to support the selected EMR system. Most practices develop an initial plan to identify their key goals, select an EMR system that supports these goals, and then finalize their plan after the selection.

After establishing the practice's objective(s) and planning how EMRs will affect workflows, the leadership team and staff can determine what to look for when considering and selecting an EMR system. The following are several considerations for EMR software comparison that the Regional Extension Centers (RECs) have found useful over the past several months:

- Understand if and how a vendor's product will accomplish the key goals of the practice. Essentially, a test drive of your specific needs with the vendor's product. Provide the vendor with patient and office scenarios that they may use to customize their product demonstration.
- Clarify start-up pricing before selecting an EMR system [hardware, software, maintenance and upgrade costs, option of phased payments, interfaces for labs and pharmacies, cost to connect to health information exchange (HIE), customized quality reports].
- Define implementation support (amount, schedule, information on trainer(s) such as their communication efficiency and experience with product and company).
- Clarify roles, responsibilities, and costs for data migration strategy if desired. Sometimes, being selective with which data or how much data to migrate can influence the ease of transition.
- Server options [e.g. client server, application service provider (ASP), software as a service (SAS)].
- Ability to integrate with other products (e.g. practice management software, billing systems, and public health interfaces).
- Privacy and security capabilities and back-up planning.
- Linking payments and EMR incentive rewards to implementation milestones and performance goals.
- Vendor's stability and/or market presence in region.
- Cost to connect to HIE.
- Consider costs of using legal counsel for contract review verses open sources through medical associations.

National Learning Consortium Resources

The following resources are examples of tools that are used in the field today, and that are recommended by "boots-on-the-ground" professionals for use by others who have made the commitment to implement or upgrade to certified EMR systems.

Learn more about the National Learning Consortium
The material in these guides and tools was developed from the experiences of Regional Extension Center staff in the performance of technical support and EMR implementation assistance to primary care providers. The information contained in this guide is neither intended to serve as legal advice nor should it substitute for legal counsel. The guide is not exhaustive, and readers are encouraged to seek additional detailed technical guidance to supplement the information contained herein.

Reference in this website to any specific resources, tools, products, process, service, manufacturer, or company does not constitute its endorsement or recommendation by the US Government or the US Department of Health and Human Services.

Step 4: Conduct Training and Implement an EMR System

The EMR implementation involves the installation of the EMR system and associated activities, such as training, mock 'go-live,' and pilot testing. The EMR implementation plan and schedule (developed during the planning phase) should be followed and executed during this phase, in addition to execution of the following:

- Chart abstraction plan and other data migration plans in conjunction with your EMR vendor.
- Execution of an EMR implementation training plan that includes practice specific goals and needs, as well as compliance with meaningful use objectives.
- Privacy and security risk management mitigation plan.

National Learning Consortium Resources
Over the coming months, the NLC will continue to share experiences from the field and the resulting leading practices and tools that can be used throughout all phases of the EMR implementation life cycle.

Learn more about the National Learning Consortium
The material in these guides and tools was developed from the experiences of Regional Extension Center staff in the performance of technical support and EMR implementation assistance to primary care providers. The information contained in this guide is not intended to serve as legal advice nor should it substitute for legal counsel. The guide is not exhaustive, and readers are encouraged to seek additional detailed technical guidance to supplement the information contained herein.

Reference in this website to any specific resources, tools, products, process, service, manufacturer, or company does not constitute its endorsement or recommendation by the US Government or the US Department of Health and Human Services.

Step 5: Achieve Meaningful Use

The Medicare and Medicaid EMR Incentive Programs provide a financial incentive for achieving 'meaningful use,' which is the use of certified EMR technology to achieve health and efficiency goals. This section provides an overview of the Stage 1 and Stage 2 EMR meaningful use core and menu objectives for eligible professionals (EPs) as outlined by CMS—which are intended to set a baseline for electronic data capture and information sharing.

The meaningful use objectives are grouped into five patient-driven domains that relate to health outcomes policy priorities. As depicted in the dashboards below, each core and menu objective is aligned to one of the following domains:

- Improve quality, safety, efficiency
- Engage patients and families
- Improve care coordination
- Improve public and population health
- Ensure privacy and security for personal health information.

Step 6: Continue Quality Improvement

This final phase refers to reassessing what you have learned from training and everyday use of the system. It emphasizes continuous evaluation of your practice's goals and needs post-EMR implementation to continue improving workflows that achieve the individual practice's goals and needs while leveraging the functionality of electronic medical records (EMRs):

- Were the goals and needs met?
- Do workflow processes need to be re-evaluated?
- Is additional training required?
- Are you capturing the required data elements needed for internal clinical priorities, as well as for reportable quality measures?
- Do staff roles and responsibilities need adjustments?
- Is the technology in the appropriate locations?
- Is the technology reliable?
- Is the technology 'fast enough'?
- Is additional hardware needed?

A post-EMR implementation evaluation will help shape both the practice and its evolution. Often, what happens during the implementation phase is very different from what was planned. The practice needs to continuously evaluate its processes to ensure that the practice is functioning efficiently to ensure staff and patient satisfaction. To learn more about quality improvement, read about meaningful use clinical quality measures.

LONG-TERM PRESERVATION AND STORAGE OF RECORDS

An important consideration in the process of developing electronic medical records is to plan for the long-term preservation and storage of these records. The field will need to come to consensus on the length of time to store EMRs, methods to ensure the future accessibility and compatibility of archived data with yet-to-be developed retrieval systems, and how to ensure the physical and virtual security of the archives.

Additionally, considerations about long-term storage of electronic medical records are complicated by the possibility that the records might one day be used longitudinally and integrated across sites of care. Records have the potential to be created, used, edited, and viewed by multiple independent entities. These entities include, but are not limited to, primary care physicians, hospitals, insurance companies, and patients. It was noted that "choices about the structure and ownership of these records will have profound impact on the accessibility and privacy of patient information.

The required length of storage of an individual electronic health record will depend on hospital policy and on national or state regulations, which are subject to change over time.

While it is currently unknown precisely how long EMRs will be preserved, it is certain that length of time will exceed the average shelf-life of paper records. The evolution of technology is such that the programs and systems used to input information will likely not be available to a user who desires to examine archived data.

CHALLENGES IN IMPLEMENTING EMR

Utility of EMRs, in spite of being widely acknowledged, pose several challenges in its adoption by both developed and emerging economies, including India. In India, information and communication technologies are increasingly becoming an integral part of inpatient, outpatient and administrative areas of healthcare. Standardization of interfaces to ensure interoperability and exchange of useful and clinically understandable health information is one of the potential issues. Although some form of clinical automation in health informatics has started, it is yet to be implemented in major ancillary departments like laboratory, pharmacy and radiology in most healthcare facilities. The pressing need of revolutionizing the health information system in India, in spite of being well-recognized, is not backed by any assessment of proportion of doctors enthusiastic about embracing this form of technology. Several software packages are currently available in the Indian market that offer EMR along with Hospital Information System, but, unfortunately, there are only few takers as no serious effort is being made for educating the medical community about its benefits. Other nontechnical concerns are poor sociological conceptualization, fear of reducing the semantic richness of narratives to limited codes and weakly connected phrases and increased possibility of communication errors between clinicians in acquiring, presenting and using information. All these demands, substantial informatics effort to overcome the current paucity of a fully integrated, clinically useful electronic records system. An important challenge in implementing EMR on a broad basis is 'customization', although it has its own share of disadvantages, like high cost of maintenance. Each healthcare environment functions differently, often in significant ways. It is difficult to create a 'one-size-fits-all' EMR system.

Chapter 19

Green Buildings in Healthcare

INTRODUCTION

Green building (also known as *green construction* or *sustainable building*) refers to a structure and using process that is environmentally responsible and resource-efficient throughout a building's life cycle: from siting to design, construction, operation, maintenance, renovation, and demolition. This requires close cooperation of the design team, the architects, the engineers, and the client at all project stages. The Green Building practice expands and complements the classical building design concerns of economy, utility, durability, and comfort.

Although new technologies are constantly being developed to complement current practices in creating greener structures, the common objective is that green buildings are designed to reduce the overall impact of the built environment on human health and the natural environment by:

- Efficiently using energy, water, and other resources.
- Protecting occupant health and improving employee productivity.
- Reducing waste, pollution and environmental degradation.

WHAT IS LEED?

The Leadership in Energy and Environmental Design (LEED) Green Building Rating System, developed by the US Green Building Council (USGBC), provides a suite of standards for environmentally sustainable construction.

Purpose of LEED

- Define "Green building" by establishing a common standard of measurement.
- Promote integrated, whole-building design practices.
- Recognize environmental leadership in the building industry.
- Stimulate green competition.
- Raise consumer awareness of green building benefits.
- Transform the building market.

LEED RATING SYSTEM

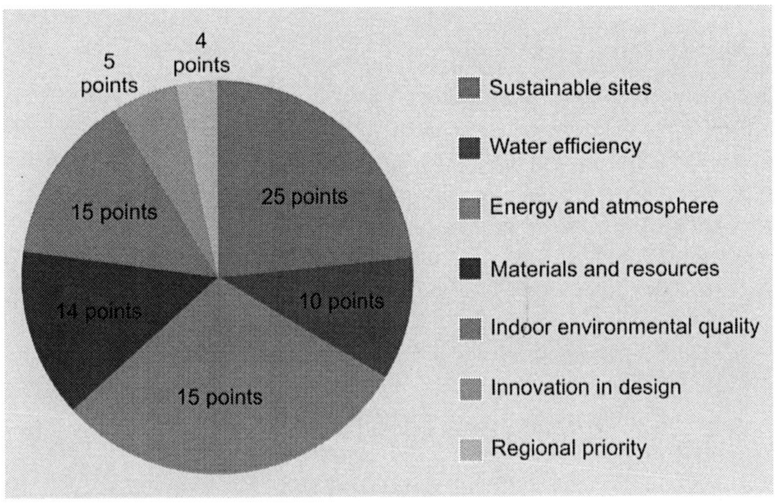

(For color version see Plate 1)

The rating system addresses six major areas:

1. Sustainable sites
2. Water efficiency
3. Energy and atmosphere
4. Materials and resources
5. Indoor environmental quality
6. Innovation and design process.

Advantages of LEED?

- LEED certified buildings are supposed to use resources more efficiently when compared to conventional buildings.
- LEED certified buildings often provide healthier work and living environments, which contributes to higher productivity and improved employee health and comfort.
- A long list of benefits of implementing a LEED strategy is there which ranges from improving air and water quality to reducing solid waste, benefiting owners, occupiers, and society as a whole.

LEED Levels of Certification?

- *Certified:* 26–32 points
- *Silver:* 33–38 points

- *Gold:* 39–51 points
- *Platinum:* 52–69 points.

Rating System

Sustainable Sites 26 Possible Points

- *Prerequisite 1:* Construction Activity Pollution Prevention
- *Credit 1:* Site Selection
- *Credit 2:* Development Density and Community Connectivity
- *Credit 3:* Brownfield Redevelopment
- *Credit 4.1:* Alternative Transportation—Public Transportation Access
- *Credit 4.2:* Alternative Transportation—Bicycle Storage and Changing Rooms
- *Credit 4.3:* Alternative Transportation—Low-emitting and Fuel-efficient Vehicles
- *Credit 4.4:* Alternative Transportation—Parking Capacity
- *Credit 5.1:* Site Development—Protect or Restore Habitat
- *Credit 5.2:* Site Development—Maximize Open Space
- *Credit 6.1:* Storm Water Design—Quantity Control
- *Credit 6.2:* Storm Water Design—Quality Control
- *Credit 7.1:* Heat Island Effect—Nonroof
- *Credit 7.2:* Heat Island Effect—Roof
- *Credit 8:* Light Pollution Reduction.

Water Efficiency 10 Possible Points

- *Prerequisite 1:* Water Use Reduction
- *Credit 1:* Water-efficient Landscaping
- *Credit 2:* Innovative Wastewater Technologies
- *Credit 3:* Water Use Reduction.

Energy and Atmosphere 35 Possible Points

- *Prerequisite 1:* Fundamental Commissioning of Building Energy Systems
- *Prerequisite 2:* Minimum Energy Performance
- *Prerequisite 3:* Fundamental Refrigerant Management
- *Credit 1:* Optimize Energy Performance
- *Credit 2:* On-site Renewable Energy
- *Credit 3:* Enhanced Commissioning
- *Credit 4:* Enhanced Refrigerant Management
- *Credit 5:* Measurement and Verification
- *Credit 6:* Green Power.

Materials and Resources 14 Possible Points

- *Prerequisite 1:* Storage and Collection of Recyclables
- *Credit 1.1:* Building Reuse—Maintain Existing Walls, Floors and Roof

- *Credit 1.2:* Building Reuse—Maintain Existing Interior Nonstructural Elements
- *Credit 2:* Construction Waste Management
- *Credit 3:* Materials Reuse
- *Credit 4:* Recycled Content
- *Credit 5:* Regional Materials
- *Credit 6:* Rapidly Renewable Materials
- *Credit 7:* Certified Wood.

Indoor Environmental Quality 15 Possible Points
- *Prerequisite 1:* Minimum Indoor Air Quality Performance
- *Prerequisite 2:* Environmental Tobacco Smoke (ETS) Control
- *Credit 1:* Outdoor Air Delivery Monitoring
- *Credit 2:* Increased Ventilation
- *Credit 3.1:* Construction Indoor Air Quality Management Plan—During Construction
- *Credit 3.2:* Construction Indoor Air Quality Management Plan—Before Occupancy
- *Credit 4.1:* Low-emitting Materials—Adhesives and Sealants
- *Credit 4.2:* Low-emitting Materials—Paints and Coatings
- *Credit 4.3:* Low-emitting Materials—Flooring Systems
- *Credit 4.4:* Low-emitting Materials—Composite Wood and Agrifiber Products
- *Credit 5:* Indoor Chemical and Pollutant Source Control
- *Credit 6.1:* Controllability of Systems—Lighting
- *Credit 6.2:* Controllability of Systems—Thermal Comfort
- *Credit 7.1:* Thermal Comfort—Design
- *Credit 7.2:* Thermal Comfort—Verification
- *Credit 8.1:* Daylight and Views—Daylight
- *Credit 8.2:* Daylight and Views—Views.

Innovation in Design 6 Possible Points
- *Credit 1:* Innovation in Design
- *Credit 2:* LEED Accredited Professional.

Regional Priority 4 Possible Points
- *Credit 1:* Regional Priority.

LEED INDIA

LEED India certification is obtained after submitting an application documenting compliance with the requirements of the rating system as well as paying registration and certification fees.

Certification is granted solely by the Indian Green Building Council (IGBC) responsible for the third party verification of project compliance with LEED requirements.

A few innovations onwards Green building (Figs 19.1 to 19.7):
It is a common observation that maximum and unnecessary wastage of the most important resource *water* takes place in the lavatories of any commercial/open to public building, to prevent it there are a few out of the blue thoughts depicted above-using waste water after washing hands to flush of the human excreta, similarly using water extracted postwashing clothes for the same purpose.

Now days to save water urinals are made flushless, it contains an antimicrobial aromatic mesh instead to keep the toilets clean.

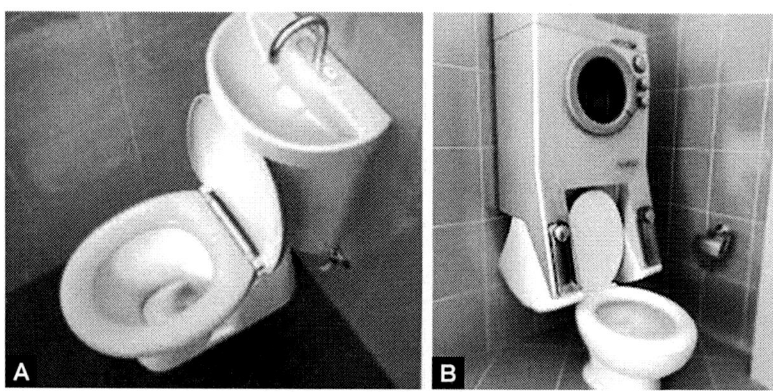

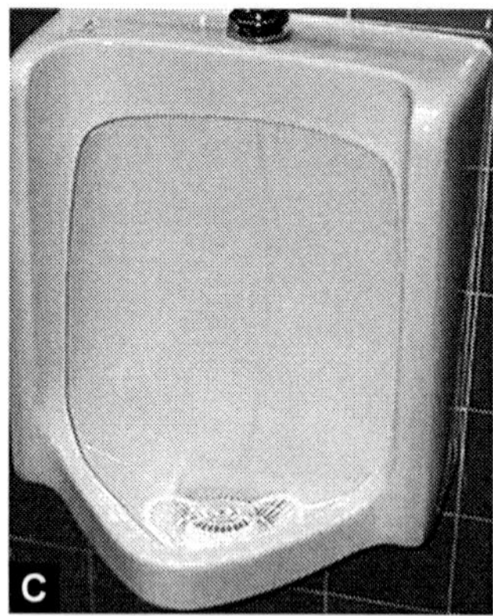

Figs 19.1A to C: Bio toilet

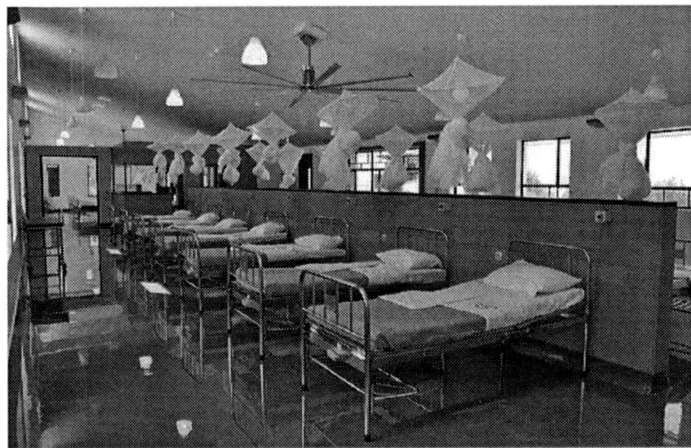

Fig. 19.2: Natural light-friendly wards *(For color version see Plate 1)*

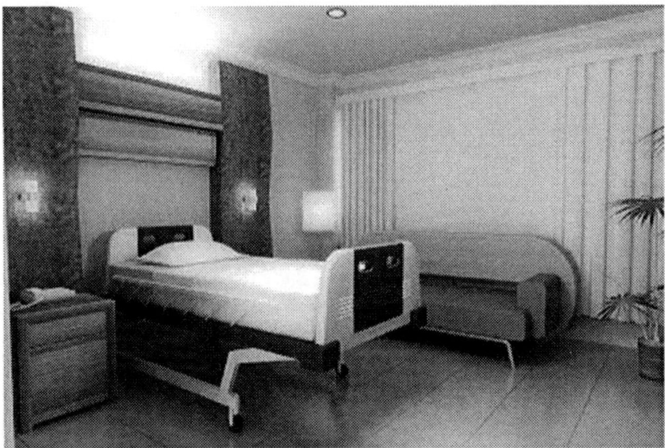

Fig. 19.3: Super deluxe room

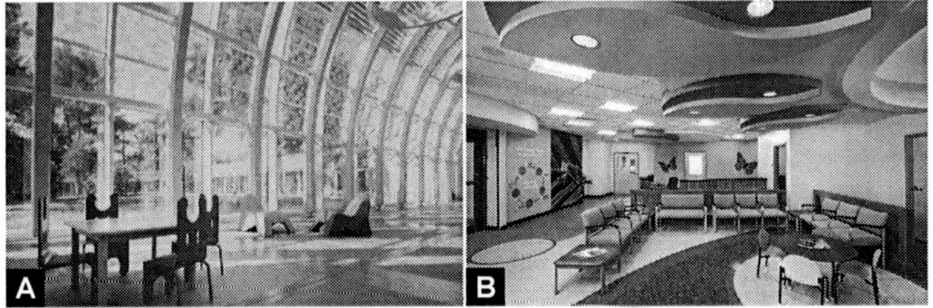

Figs 19.4A and B: Environment-friendly patient area *(For color version see Plate 2)*

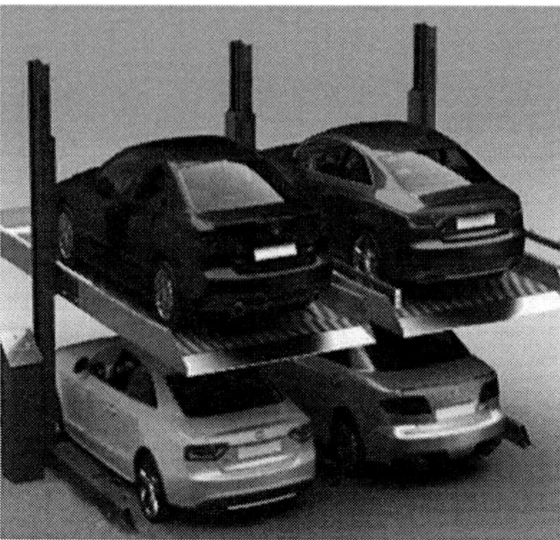

Fig. 19.5: Multi-level parking

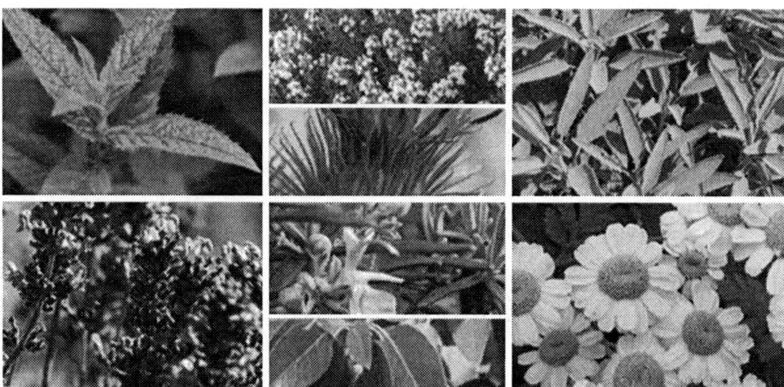

Fig. 19.6: Eco-friendly environment *(For color version see Plate 2)*

To choose vibrant colors for the general ward, so that it gives a pleasant feel and provides a better environment for patient recovery. The huge windowpanes are also helpful as far as preventing usage of electricity in the day time is concerned.

The private rooms can have a small balcony along with a tinge of colorful antimicrobial paint and a huge window, it all combines together and enhances the quality of treatment course, it improves the patient compliance and redices the ammount of actual medicine intake.

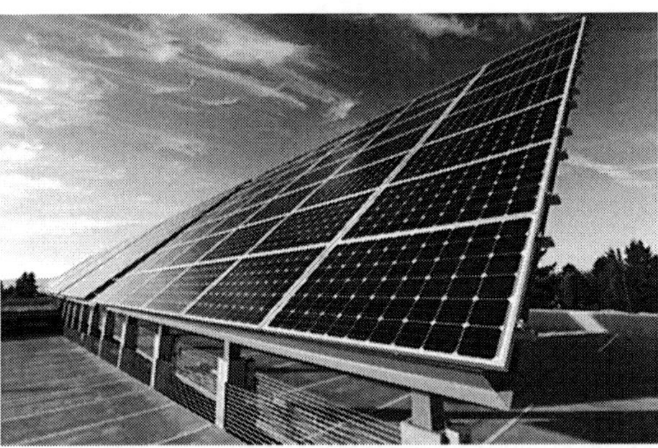

Fig. 19.7: Solar system

Atria is the call of the hour to prevent huge electricity usage during the day hours (supposedly to be the busiest) in modern architecture, an *atrium* (plural: *atria* or *atriums*) is a large open space, often several stories high and having a glazed roof and/or large windows, often situated within a larger multistorey building and often located immediately beyond the main entrance doors. Atria are a popular design feature because they give their buildings a feeling of space and light.

Mechanical lift parking are a common site in a few malls and metro stations, but are yet to be seen in hospitals, it can do wonders as less space is required to accommodate double the number of vehicles, rest of the space can be used for landscaping and promoting greenary and trees.

In landscaping, focus has been in using native plants like *Rhoeo, Chlorophytum, Bauhinia purpurea, Bauhinia blakeana, Plumeria alba, Pisonia alba, Polyalthia longifolia,* etc. that require less water for survival.

The most preffered source of energy in a public building should be solar energy as we completely make use of the sun's energy to cook food, use it to make warm water available, etc., it emencely reduces the cost of production.

Chapter 20 Hospital Architecture: Importance and Management

INTRODUCTION

Architecture plays a very important role in delivery of healthcare. It not only lets one decide upon the type of building and infrastructure in the hospital but also goes a long way in planning space requirements of not only the patients and healthcare professionals in different settings but also for various functions/categories of activities and traffic movement of patients, attendants, materials and service providers. It is a key factor in the infection control in any hospital. It caters for not only the patient's comfort but also the layout of various departments and services. The layout of the departments within a hospital goes a long way in making the department more efficient, effective and functional. Due care has to be given to the interplay of various departments in a hospital.

Architecture would have a very significant impact upon the operational and maintenance expenditure in the years ahead. It has to provide a congenial, safe, secure and infection free environment with ample scope for expansion. Architecture of any hospital and the departments has not only to specifically cater to the disciplines for which it has been designed but also for general areas such as, the approach and entrance from the road to the parking. The ambience of the hospital and the various departments would depend upon the designs and layouts chosen.

The architecture has to ensure that the buildings blend with the surroundings and has to cater for the prevailing weather conditions throughout the year which not only temperature and humidity but also the direction and speeds of the wind during various seasons. This is necessary for the proper orientation of the buildings.

It has to ensure that the above requirements are optimally addressed but also that the stipulations of the legal and statutory requirements such as, safety, security, structural strengths, etc. are fully complied with.

It has to cater for all that within the strict constraints of the financial budget and implications.

PLANNING PUBLIC SPACES FOR HEALTHCARE FACILITIES

During the industrial age when it was learned that germs cause illness and that pollution can trigger disease in immune-stressed patients, public spaces for healing were replaced with private spaces. The sick were separated from the healthy and buildings became more compartmentalized.

Today, the assumption that patients should be separated and isolated is evaluated in the interests of safety and best practices. And there is also much more emphasis on the patient as a customer with rights and desires for self-direction, family inclusiveness and participation in caregiving and healing.

Clearly, healthcare's consumer-driven agenda has architectural implications, not the least of which centers on the total experience. Healthcare public spaces have a role in forming that experience.

Memorable and Positive

Healthcare public spaces have been examined at least since 2007, when a group of healthcare design professionals thought it worthy of exploration. In the ensuing years, healthcare architects have come to view public space as a vital player in the overall healthcare experience.

Healthcare public space can create a memorable and positive experience by providing orientation, instilling pride, building confidence and helping the healing process.

A public space is defined as one that provides access to all. It is a place where people can congregate and engage in multiple activities, a place of movement and flow, and a place of cultural collectiveness. Favorite public spaces might be described as grand or intimate, quiet or loud, public or private, but in all cases they are memorable and enhance the human experience.

So, how might general public space relate to healthcare public space? What is similar and what is different? Both general public space and healthcare public space share the same characteristics, but healthcare public spaces also have their own special patterns.

Typologies

The unique functions of healthcare public spaces can be categorized over the following formal typologies:

- *Collector spaces:* These are accepting and orienting spaces with high populations. They are active and have increased noise levels.
- *Introspective spaces:* These are accepting but calming spaces. They also feature high populations, but are personal, quieter and highly passive.

- *Purpose spaces:* These are spaces with specific functions. They are service-based and feature various user volumes. Noise levels are usually moderate in these dynamic spaces.
- *Mover spaces:* These spaces feature constant movement as well as ebb and flow of user volumes. These highly dynamic spaces are characterized by moderate noise levels.
- *Switchboard spaces:* These are spaces of orientation and wayfinding with consistently high populations. These dynamic spaces feature moderate noise levels and organizational clarity.
- *Attributes:* Once the typology is defined, the following unique identity attributes of healthcare must be considered for each space:
  - *Environmental factors:* These include the healing powers of natural light and air quality.
  - *User groups:* These include diverse user groups and healthcare-focused user groups.
  - *Public and private relationships:* There are public and private boundaries that must be respected and clearly defined for best care practices.
  - *Context of body health:* People needing care for a diversity of ailments are the norm in these spaces.
  - *Passage of time:* Time is often perceived differently in the healthcare environment by patient, family and staff.
  - *Emotional disposition:* Patients in a healthcare setting can feel uncertainty and vulnerability, and experience emotional highs and lows.

A number of conclusions can be drawn from these elements. First is a heightened awareness and appreciation of the relevance of healthcare public space in the healing process. Second is the knowledge that healthcare public space can take different forms, serve different functions and express different patterns of use. Healthcare public space can be a primary space, such as a lobby, or a background or support space. But, most importantly, it also can be clinical space.

Another lesson is that healthcare public spaces do not exist in isolation. Instead, they stitch together the entire healthcare experience, which includes the five different healthcare public space typologies. Some of these spaces constitute seams of human interaction while others constitute a formal stage for this interaction.

How should designers build on the power of the public space experience in the design process? The answer is to look beyond just physical metrics like the square footage of the space and consider the emotional content of space. One way to do this is to assign one of the five typologies to a healthcare public space, and then determine which attributes should apply to the design of that space.

Defining healthcare public space and using it to enhance the design of healthcare facilities present challenges, but given the importance of the healthcare experience to patients and their families, it is worth the effort.

Let us explain the approach of an experienced architect in meeting the technical requirements of some important areas of a hospital such as operation theater (OT) complex, to start with—while designing the same.

OPERATION THEATER COMPLEX

An operation theater complex is the "heart" of any major hospital providing surgical services. An operating theater, operating room, surgery suite or a surgery center is a room within a hospital within which surgical and other operations are carried out. Operating theaters were so-called in the United Kingdom because they traditionally consisted of semicircular amphitheaters to allow students to observe the medical procedures. The old operating theater in London is one of the oldest, dating back to 1822 (Oxford English Dictionary and Wikipedia.com).

The patient is the center point of a functioning OT complex. He/she is in isolation for varying times, away from his near and dear ones and is physically sick. Efforts are directed to maintain vital functions, prevent infections/promote healing with safety, comfort and economy.

The establishment and working of the operation theater (OT) needs specialized planning and execution and is not a simple civil engineering work. A "civil-mechanical-electrical-electronic-biomedical" combo effort driven and coordinated by the needs, preferences and safety of the medical/surgical team forms the basis for starting and maintaining an operation theater. Anesthesiologists, by virtue of their knowledge of the intricacies of physiology, physics and biomedical aspects of medicine and constant proximity to the operation theater should preferably be involved from the early stages of planning of operating theaters.

On an average, operation theaters cater to 50% of the needs of total healthcare seekers. Anesthesia-controlled time typically represents a small fraction (10–20%) of the total case time, the remainder (>80%) being surgeon and nurse-controlled.

In this Chapter, we will discuss the various considerations while planning an operation theater complex to explain the importance of architecture in hospitals. [Functioning of an OT complex including scheduling, administration, staffing, sterilization techniques and data/audit management are out of purview of this topic].

Purpose of Operation Theater Complex

Operation theater complexes are designed and built to carry out investigative, diagnostic, therapeutic and palliative procedures of varying degrees of invasiveness. Many such set-ups are customized to the requirements based on size of hospital, patient turnover and may be specialty specific. The aim is to provide the maximum benefit for maximum number of patients arriving to the operation theater. Both the present as well as future needs should be kept in mind while planning.

Different Zones of Operation Theater Complex

The location and flow of the patients, the staff and the materials form the three broad groups to be considered during all stages of design.

Four zones can be described in an OT complex, based on varying degrees of cleanliness, in which the bacteriological count progressively diminishes from the outer to the inner zones (operating area) and is maintained by a differential decreasing positive pressure ventilation gradient from the inner zone to the outer zone.

1. *Protective zone:* It includes:
   - Change rooms for all medical and paramedical staff with conveniences
   - Transfer bay for patient, material and equipment
   - Rooms for administrative staff
   - Stores and records
   - Pre- and postoperative rooms
   - ICU and PACU
   - Sterile stores
2. *Clean zone:* Connects protective zone to aseptic zone and has other areas also like:
   - Stores and cleaner room
   - Equipment store room
   - Maintenance workshop
   - Kitchenette (pantry)
   - Firefighting device room
   - Emergency exits
   - Service room for staff
   - Close circuit TV control area.
3. *Aseptic zone:* Includes operation rooms (sterile).
4. *Disposal zone:* Disposal areas from each operation room and corridor lead to disposal zone.

Types of Operation Theater Complexes

There are three main categories of operating theaters:

1. The single theater suite with OT, scrub area (and gowning), anesthesia room, trolley preparation, utility and exit bay plus staff change and limited ancillary accommodation.
2. The twin theater suite with facilities similar to 1, but with duplicated ancillary accommodation immediate to each OT, sometimes sharing a small postanesthesia recovery area.
3. OT complexes of three or more OTs with ancillary accommodation including postanesthesia recovery, reception, porter's desk, sterile store and staff change.

Principles to be taken into Consideration While Planning an Operation Theater (Physical/Architecture)

- *Location:* Low rise buildings limited to two or three storeys high are preferred because of maximum advantage of natural light and ventilation as appropriate can be derived. The OT should be separate from general 'traffic' and air movement of rest of the hospital, OT, surgical wards, intensive care units (ICU), accident and emergency (A and E) department, radiological department (X-ray) should be closely related and access is also required to sterilizing and disinfecting unit (SDU) and laboratory facilities. The location of the operation complex in a multistorey building is planned on the first floor, connecting to surgical and other wards on the same floor. Adequate electric lift is planned for vertical movement from casualty on the ground floor and ENT, orthopedics, ophthalmology and other wards on the floors above.
- Zone wise distribution of the area, so as to avoid crisscross movements of men and machines.
- Adequate and appropriate space allotted as per utility of the area.
- Provision for emergency exit.
- Provision for ventilation and temperature control, keeping in mind the need for laminar flow, HEPA filter air-conditioner, etc.
- *Operation rooms:* The number and size can be as per the requirement but recommended size is 6.5 m × 6.5 m × 3.5 m. Glass windows can be planned on one side only.
  - *Doors:* Main door to the OT complex has to be of adequate width (1.2–1.5 m). The doors of each OT should be spring loaded flap type, but sliding doors are preferred as no air currents are generated. All fittings in OT should be flush type and made of steel.

The surface/flooring must be slip resistant, strong and impervious with minimum joints (e.g. mosaic with copper plates for antistatic effect) or joint-less conductive tiles/terrazzo, linoleum, etc. the recommended minimum conductivity is 1 m Ohm and maximum 10 m Ohms.

Presently the need for antistatic flooring has diminished as flammable anesthetic agents are no longer in use.

- *Walls:* Laminated polyester or smooth paint provides seamless wall; tiles can break and epoxy paint can chip out. Collusion corners to be covered with steel or aluminum plates, color of paint should allow reflection of light and yet soothing to eyes. Light color (light blue or green) washable paint will be ideal. A semi-matt wall surface reflects less light than a highly gloss finish and is less tiring to the eyes of OT team.
- *Operation table:* One operation table per OT.
- *Electric point:* Adequate electric points on the wall (at < 1.5 m height from the floor) (discussed later).
- *X-ray illuminators:* There should be X-ray film illuminators preferably recessed into the wall.
- *Scrub area:* May be planned for at least for 2–3 persons in each OT.

- There has to be a preparation room in clean zone.
- Corridors not less than 2.85 m width for easy movement of men, stretcher and machines.
- Separate corridors for uses other than going into OT.
- Rooms for different persons working in OT and for different purpose (it should be as per zone and size).
- Gas and suction (control, supply and emergency stock) for all OTs and areas where patients are retained. Oxygen gas and suction pipe to be connected with central facility and standby local facility should also be available.
- *Provision for adequate and continuous water supply:* Besides normal supply of available water at the rate of 400 liters per bed per day, a separate reserve emergency over head tank should be provided for operation theater. Elbow taps have to be 10 cm above wash basins.
- Proper drainage system.
- Preoperative area with reception with separate designated area for pediatric patients is desirable.
- Adequate illumination with shadow less lamps of 70,000–120,000 lumens intensity, for assessing patient color and tissue visibility (discussed under "lighting").

- The safety in working place is essential, and fire extinguishers have to be planned in appropriate zone.
- Provision for expansion of the OT complex should be borne in mind during planning stages itself.

Recommendations on the Number of OTs Required

It is observed that out of all surgical beds of the hospital, 50% of patients are expected to undergo surgery. Thus, for 100 beds, with average length of stay of 10 days for each patient, 10 operations per day can be performed.

In general, multiuse OTs, instead of multiple OTs offer advantages of efficient manpower utilization, economical maintenance and better training of supporting staff.

Thus, in a 300 bedded hospital (with 150 surgical beds), one OT complex with three OTs for general surgery, gynecology, orthopedics/ENT, one for endoscopy and one for septic may have to be catered for.

The OT will be required, generally, with 8 hours a day working duration.

Ventilation

Ventilation should be on the principle that the direction of airflow is from the operation theater towards the main entrance. There should be no interchange air movement between one OT and another. Efficient ventilation will control temperature and humidity in OT, dilute the contamination by microorganisms and anesthetic agents.

There are two types of air-conditioning systems: (i) recirculating and (ii) nonrecirculating.

Nonrecirculating systems heat/cool the air as desired and convey it into the operating room with ideally 20 air exchange per hour. Air is then exhausted to outside. Anesthetic agents in the OT air are also automatically removed. These are thus ideal but are expensive.

The circulating system takes some or all of the air, adjusts the temperature and circulates air back to the room.

The broad recommendations include:

- 20–30 air exchanges/hour for recirculated air
- Only up to 80% recirculation of air to prevent build-up of anesthetic and other gases
- Ultraclean laminar airflow—the filtered air delivery must be 90% efficient in removing particles more than 0.5 mm
- *Positive air pressure system in OT:* It should ensure a positive pressure of 5 cm H_2O from ceiling of OT downwards and outwards, to push out air from OT

- Relative humidity of 40–60% to be maintained
- Temperature between 20°C and 24°C. Temperature should not be adjusted for the comfort of OT personnel but for the requirement of patient, especially in pediatric, geriatric, burns, neonatal cases, etc.

Pendant Services

Two ceiling pendants for pipeline services should be designed; one for surgical team and one for anesthetist. Anesthetic pendant should be retractable and have limited lateral movement and provide a shelf for monitoring equipment. It should have oxygen, nitrous oxide, four bar pressure medical compressed air, medical vacuum, scavenging terminal outlets and at least four electric sockets.

Piped Gases in the Operation Theater

- Automatic/semiautomatic fail safe manifold room to be designed
- Two outlets for O_2 and suction and one for N_2O are a minimum in each OT
- Pipeline supply system should be able to cut off from mainline if the problem occurs anywhere along the delivery hosing/tubing.

Scavenging

The method of scavenging should be decided during planning stage of OT. The US and the international standards are available for scavenging but it is ideal to plan the type of system (active/passive) and number and location of scavenging outlets beforehand.

Electrical

All electrical equipment in the OT will need proper grounding. In the past, isolated power systems were preferred when explosive agents were being used. They have the advantage of a transformer using grounded electricity and there is no risk to the patient or machines if a machine gets faulty.

The grounded systems as used at homes offer protection from macro-shock but devices may lose power without warning. Life support systems, if in use, could be disturbed.

Following criterias are ideal with respect to electricity in OT complex:

- Use of circuit breakers/interrupters is desirable if there is an overload or ground fault
- Power line of 220 volts

- Suspended ceiling outlets should have locking plugs to avoid accidental disconnection
- Insulation around ceiling electrical power sources should withstand frequent bendings and flexings. They should not develop cracks and should not damage wires. Wires inside rigid or retractable ceiling service column can help to some extent
- Wall outlets to be installed 1.5 m above ground (as already mentioned)
- Use of explosion proof plugs
- Multiple outlets from different electrical line sources should be available
- Electrical load calculation should be based on, equipment likely to be used and appropriate current carrying capacity cords to be used
- *Emergency power:* OT electrical networks need to be connected to the emergency generators with automatic two way changeover facility.

Lighting

Some natural daylight is preferred by staff. Wherever possible, high level windows which give a visual appreciation of the 'outside world' should be considered in the OT.

- *General lighting:* Color corrected fluorescent lamps (recessed or surface ceiling mounted) to produce even illumination of at least 500 lux at working height, with minimal glare are preferred. Means of dimming may be needed during endoscopies. To minimize eye fatigue, the ratio of intensity of general room lighting to that at the surgical site should not exceed 1:5, preferably 1:3. This contrast should be maintained in corridors and scrub areas, as well as in the room itself, so that the surgeon becomes accustomed to the light before entering the sterile field. Color and hue of the lights also should be consistent
- About 2000 lux light is needed to assess the patients color
- White and glistening/shiny body tissues need less light than dark and dull tissues
- *Operating area:* Overhead light should be shadow less and give 25,000–125,000 lux of light (50,000–100,000 lux at the center and at least 15,000 lux at the periphery)
- About 10–12 inch of focus of light gives adequate illumination both at depth as well as surface of body
- Lights should be freely movable both in horizontal and vertical ranges. Pendant systems are preferred. OT light should produce blue white color of daylight at spectral energy range of 50,000 K (35,000–67,000 Kelvin acceptable)

- Halogen lights produce less heat and hence preferred. OT light should not produce more than 25,000 mw/cm^2 of radiant energy. Elimination of heat by dichroic reflectors (cold mirrors) with heat absorbing reflectors or filters should be available along with the luminaire
- An auxiliary light for a second surgical site is often beneficial
- UPS of adequate capacity to be installed after considering OT light, anesthesia machine, monitors, cautery, etc. until the backup generator takes over.
- In endoscopic OTs, a reduced lighting is sometimes recommended. A grazing light over the floor can be helpful.

Anesthesia Equipment and Monitoring Needs

At least one anesthesiologist should be in the team involved in planning an OT. It is imperative that certain mandatory considerations with respect to the anesthetic equipment and monitors be planned during the planning and design stage itself. Personal, practice and cost preferences may influence the plans.

The other important issues to be addressed would be communications, catering, cleaning, data management, OT pharmacy, accommodation for different categories and status of personnel working in the OT complex, sterile department (TSSD), waiting areas for patients preparation before operation, postoperative recovery and attendants and the statutory requirements.

Statutory Requirements

The design and planning of an OT complex will need compliance with mandatory regulations related to local administration such as Government Municipal Corporation, Pollution Control Board, Fire Safety Department, Water Supply and Drainage Department, etc.

THE AUTHORITY FOR STANDARDIZATION

Recommendations are available in various surgical, anesthesia and nursing manuals with regard to the planning and establishment of operation theaters/complexes. The hospital can get accredited by the National Board for Accreditation for Hospitals and Healthcare providers (NABH), Joint Commission Internationale (JCI), having professionally sponsored programs that stimulate a high quality of patient care in healthcare facilities.

CONCLUSION

In the present era of evidence-based medicine, it becomes imperative to give maximum importance to architectural planning any facility like an operation theater complex. Within the limitations of finance and space, the best results can be obtained and anesthesiologist with multiple roles inside the operation theater complex, should be consulted in the process. Efforts should be made to conform to the standards laid down by local bodies and international agencies, as healthcare facilities in India are now catering to more and more international clientele. However, new OTs and hospitals that are being established cannot be expected to fulfill all theoretical requirements as new ideas are constantly being developed. By the time they are incorporated into buildings, fresh ones take their place on the drawing board.

Chapter 21 Knowledge Process Outsourcing: The Next Big Opportunity in Healthcare

After the success of business process outsourcing (BPO) in India, it is now the turn of knowledge process outsourcing (KPO) to make its presence felt. KPOs deliver high value to organization by providing domain-based processes and business expertise rather than just process expertise.

The BPO success in India is encouraging overseas companies eyeing Indian market for outsourcing their high-tech knowledge-based jobs. Operational cost saving, pool of talented workforce, infrastructure improvement and favorable government policies are the major factors responsible for driving KPOs in India. This is coupled with a shortage of talent able to provide KPO services in the US. India fills this gap with its cadre of trained professionals in the field of education, law, finance, science, medicine, IT, engineering and various other competitive fields.

INDIA: PREFERRED DESTINATION

The Indian workforce is highly literate and they are well-versed with English language, thanks to Indian educational system. Every year, India is producing hundreds and thousands of English-speaking trained professionals in the fields of IT, engineering, education, law, science, finance, architecture and other competitive fields.

Survey reveals that 45% of Indian KPOs have the highest quality certification like Six Sigma.

BUYERS OF HEALTHCARE KPO SERVICES

The healthcare outsourcing market can be primarily divided into three major blocks:

1. Providers (hospital and physical groups).
2. Payers (Healthcare Insurance Companies and TPAs).
3. Drug manufacturers and clinical research.

KPO SERVICES IN HEALTHCARE

- Medical transcription
- Medical coding
- Medical billing
- Healthcare insurance verification
- E-marketing
- E-learning
- Legal services
- Healthcare training and consultancy
- Healthcare knowledge management
- Patient research.

KPO IN MEDICAL TRANSCRIPTION

Medical transcription services are offered through KPOs, which connect and manage with an advanced internet-based workflow monitoring system. KPO is dedicated to provide timely, accurate medical transcription services with guaranteed turnaround times.

Reports handled through KPOs are:
- Operative note
- Progress note
- Discharge summary
- Independent medical evaluation
- Telephone consultancy
- Consultation history
- Physical exam note.

KPO IN MEDICAL CODING

In healthcare KPOs, most of the coders are certified by the American Association of Professional Coder (AAPC) and have to have a minimum four-year experience. A certified coder is extremely careful while coding for patient records. The coder determines the code to be used following each patient disease processes. Utmost attention is paid to quality to get reimbursement from the insurance company/TPA for the service rendered by the physician.

KPO medical coder are proficient with CPT, ICD-9 coding, insurance/TPA and Government regulations requirement and software like ENCODERPRO, CODERITTE and HCPCS.

Benefits

Why should your company invest in KPOs? The fundamentals of outsourcing apply to knowledge-based services as well. A shortage of trained professionals shoots up the cost of maintaining such services in the host country when the same job can be done with similar precision and quality and at less than half the cost abroad. The major KPO benefits are described below.

Outsourcing to KPO firms can provide the following benefits:

- Valuable cost savings that can be utilized elsewhere
- Standard operational efficiency
- Trained professionals at work
- Savings in time and management energy for maintaining in house services
- Increase in profits
- Option to recruit a larger work force without raising costs.

KPO Skills Defined

The following skills form the basis of knowledge-based firms and their workforce.

- Analyzing data and information to produce meaningful documents
- Researching information from various sources
- Converting raw technical data into presentable documents
- Use of high levels of conceptualization and theoretical knowledge
- Proficiency with various advanced software and hardware devices
- Maintaining workflow, meeting deadlines, and applying quality controls.

What KPO can Deliver to you?

With a good firm, you get the following:

- Good quality work
- Lower costs
- On-time delivery of services
- Uninterrupted services.

KPO Company Advantages

- KPO company guarantees 95–98% accuracy and compliance with all government regulations
- Clean claims and fewer denials
- Experience and technological innovations ensure optimal revenue
- Clients receive regular feedback on coding changes, front-office documentation practices, and periodic reports, such as utilization reviews, case-mix review, and coding-related denial analysis.

KPO in Medical Billing

Medical billing include the following:

- Patient personnel detail entry
- Charge entry
- Claim submission
- Payment reconciliation.

KEY BENEFITS

- Improved hospital collection and cash flow
- Faster payment recovery
- Higher customer satisfaction
- Quick response
- Can easily handle new clients without adding staff or new infrastructure
- Minimize claim denials
- Accurately set patients coverage expectation.

Outsourcing KPO services provide:

- Trained professionals at work
- Possibility to appoint a larger work force without raising costs
- Save time and management energy for maintaining in house services
- Standard operational efficiency
- Valuable cost saving that can be utilized elsewhere
- An increase in profits.

Challenges in KPO

KPOs present substantial opportunities for players in the outsourcing business.

- Maintaining higher quality standards as the stakes for the clients are higher
- Investment in KPO infrastructure
- The lack of good talent pool for the execution of projects
- Requirement of higher level of control
- Higher level of confidentiality
- Enhanced risk management
- KPO operations are difficult because of difficulty in finding highly trained professionals and imparting continuous training
- Identification of performance criteria.

Continuous monitoring, assessment, feedback appropriate coaching, mentoring and identification of the right career path are also challenging assignments for KPOs.

ROAD AHEAD

According to a report by Global Sourcing, the global knowledge process outsourcing industry is expected to reach US$ 17 billion by 2010, of which US$ 12 billion would be outsourced to India.

India will be a leader in this race. According to a report by Evalueserve, India will capture more than 70% of the KPO territory by 2010. The number of KPOs professionally in India, which at present is 25,000, will increase to more than 25,00,000 by the year 2010. Apart from India, countries like Russia, China, Iceland and Israel are also expected to join the KPO industry.

Chapter 22 Opportunities in Healthcare Administration and Alternative Therapies

"This is the right and exciting time to ensure an international future in the world's largest and fastest growing hospital and healthcare industry.

Be a healthcare professional with a sharp Managerial and Administrative prospective".

Hospital administration is one of the most competitive and challenging career you can embark on and one of the most rewarding. Doctors as Consultant, write prescriptions, diagnostic tests and perform surgery, right? Well, who take care of doctors, nurses, technicians, paramedicals, administrative staff, the patient and countless other things that go into running a successful management and administration of the hospital and providing effective healthcare of superior quality at low cost?

These important tasks are responsibility of a *Hospital Administrator or Health Administrator.*

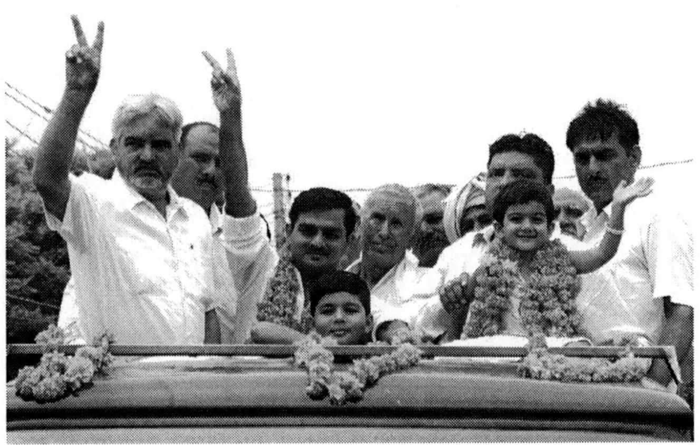

Public Welcome of India's Top Hospital Administrator

The Indian hospital and healthcare industry has the potential to become a global hub for healthcare services. An increasing number of global players in healthcare are focusing on the Indian market. The healthcare industry is expected to grow rapidly over the next decade to reach ₹ 4.9 trillion by 2012. The size of the Indian hospital industry is presently estimated at ₹ 2.7 trillion. This industry is growing at an annual rate of 13%. According to a WHO report, India needs to add 80,000 hospital beds each year for the next five years to meet the demands of its growing population.

The private sector accounts for nearly 86% of the healthcare market while the public sector accounts for the rest. With over a 350 million strong middle class demanding quality healthcare, the Indian hospital industry is poised to grow at an even faster pace. The number of medical tourists visiting India is also increasing every year.

Corporate hospitals, which came into existence with Apollo Hospitals in the 1980s, are now being set-up in almost every Indian city. Corporate groups such as Max, Fortis, Escorts, and Wockhardt have aggressive expansion plans. Furthermore, corporates such as the Tata Group, Birla Group, Larsen & Toubro, and Reliance have established hospitals. With the entry of corporate players into the Indian hospital industry, there has been an improvement in the infrastructure and the quality of services. Increasing lifestyle diseases and the rising demand for quality healthcare services have led to the emergence of specialty clinics.

Hospital Administrators and Managers in the Hospital and Healthcare industry would have to be well-versed in developing the appropriate pricing, branding, operations and promotional strategies. They would be required to understand the quality of healthcare delivery process and suggest improvements. They would have to have a thorough knowledge of all costs and work towards improving profitability of the healthcare sector.

CONCEPT OF HOSPITAL ADMINISTRATION AND MANAGEMENT

Hospital administration is concerned with planning, organizing, staffing, coordinating, controlling and evaluating health services for the community to provide maximum patient care of superior quality at low cost. Hospital administrator is responsible for overall management of the hospital and healthcare services. Hospital administrator act as a liaisons between doctors, patients, staff and health insurance companies. Administrators see that hospital operate efficiently and provide adequate medical care to patient with a human touch. Hospital administrator run the hospital on a day-to-day basis to render better patient care, with a prime objective of patient satisfaction.

Health management is now an area for professional managers. Healthcare is a sunrise sector in India. It is a ₹ 73,000 crore industry with great growth potentials within a decade. India's healthcare industry is wroth ₹ 73,000 crore, i.e. *roughly 4% of the gross domestic* product (GDP). *The industry is expected to grow by around 13%* per year by the next four years. The healthcare service growth involves the entire gamut of operations like healthcare delivery, health insurance, third party administrators, healthcare software, medical equipment and health education.

HOSPITAL ADMINISTRATION IN A NUTSHELL

The hospital administrator plays vital a role in saving lives, without having to take scalpel in hand. Hospital administrators manage hospitals, outpatient clinics, hospices, and drug-abuse treatment centers. Hospitals are open round the clock—24/7—and administrators may be called in at any hour to make decisions and resolve disputes. In large hospitals, there may be several administrators, one for each department. In smaller facilities, they oversee the day-to-day operations of all departments. Administrators make sure hospitals operate efficiently and provide adequate medical care to patients. Their responsibilities are numerous and sometimes require the assistance of the medical and support staff. They act as liaisons between governing boards, medical staff, and department heads and integrate the activities of all departments, so they function as a whole. Following policies set by a governing board of trustees, administrators plan, organize, direct, control and coordinate medical and health services. Administrators recruit, hire, and sometimes trained doctors, nurses, interns, and assistant administrators. Administrators plan budgets and set rates for health services. In research hospitals, administrators develop and expand programs and services for scientific research and preventive medicine. In teaching hospitals, they aid in the education of new doctors. Administrators plan departmental activities, evaluate doctors and other hospital employees, create and maintain policies, help develop procedures for medical treatments, quality assurance, patient services, and public relations activities such as active participation in fund-raising and community health planning. Hospital administrators work long or irregular hours. Administrators also attend staff meetings, participate in health planning councils, go to fund-raising events, and travel to professional association conventions. A hospital administrator's job is difficult and demanding. They need to keep-up with advances in medicine, computerized diagnostic and treatment equipment, data processing technology, government regulations, health insurance changes, and financing options. While doctors strive to keep—the blood flowing and the heart beating, the hospital administrator is doing his job in keeping the hospital alive and healthy.

According to the Frost & Sullivan—Hospital Management is among the TOP TEN, Millennium Professions.

Table 22.1 shows differences between hospital management and administration.

Table 22.1 Differences between management and administration

	Management	Administration
1.	Management is an executive function involving the direction of human effort towards the realization of the basic objectives of the organizations	Administration is a determinative function concerned with laying down of basic objectives and broad policies of an organizations
2.	Management is more popular to business enterprises where economic performance is of prime importance	It is preferred in Government departments, hospitals and other nonbusiness organizations
3.	Management is a doing function concerned with of implementation policies largely done and is influenced by the objectives of organizations and is done usually at middle level management	Administration is a thinking process concerned with determination of policies done mainly at top level management and is influenced by outside forces and public opinion
4.	Management—You order others	Administration—You order yourself

The Hospital Administrator population Ratio in India is 1: 2,65,000.

UNIQUENESS OF THE HOSPITAL ADMINISTRATION

Hospital administration is a serious business since it covers a large number of activities. The profession of hospital and healthcare administration is unique because hospitals involve highly qualified professionals dealing with the question of life and death. *Hospital administration is more complex than administration of any other business institute/organization because:*

- Hospital involve 24 hours, 365 day, years after years works.
- Hospital services involve high-risk and quick services.
- Hospital deal with human beings.
- Hospital is a medical and social institution.
- Hospital service is of emergency nature.
- Hospital work within the framework of ethical and legal issues.
- Hospital employs different categories of people with widely varying technical and highly qualified educational background.
- Hospital work is highly stressful since it deal with *a 'Question of life and death'*.

FUTURE TRENDS IN HOSPITAL AND HEALTHCARE MANAGEMENT

Hospital administrators are in great demand. In fact, they are the most sought professionals in healthcare sector today. Hospitals are becoming a highly scientific and complex medical center and are becoming hub of whole system of healthcare. Medical sector becoming increasingly competitive and capital intensive, the need for managing hospitals has become even more acute.

In today's, world of advancing technology healthcare delivery represents an extremely complex collection of diagnostic, operational and administrative processes. Management skills in planning, operation, marketing, materials, telemedicine, HIS and human resource management are the need of the hour. Today, we have about 3.5 lakh health institution in India (large, medium, small). Our health system is unique as compared to other countries—there are government, private, religious, industrials, MNCs, allopathy, ayurveda, homeopathy, paramedicals and nature cure hospitals and institutions. There are newer diseases, newer diagnostic technologies, etc. All these factors will required trained hospital administrators. So , we are on the road to professionalize healthcare services.

HOW TO SERVE HOSPITAL AND HEALTHCARE WITH POWER AND STATUS?

Hospital administration is a challenging profession. The qualities of head and heart that hospital administrator seeks:

- *Keen observer:* 360 degree of vision, should be able to step back and look at the bigger picture and then devise solution. Should possess ability to have both macro- and microperspective on any issue before him.
- *Effective communicator:* Good administrator should be able to convey the things with clarity and as simply as possible without patronizing or scaring other with the command of his vast knowledge or intellect.
- *Good listener:* Hospital requires a lot of patience and sympathy. At times, people only need a good listener, e.g. though their problems cannot be solved—at times, they may also realize this—but all that they need is to know that people in authority are aware of their frustrations and anxieties. He should be able to understand this.
- *Respect for fact and intellectual honest:* Administrator should not speak without facts and should have patience to find the whole truth.
- *Should behave gracefully:* Administrator should never loose temper even under stress.
- *Transparently honest:* He should not be bluff. Truth is always more convenient in today's busy world. He should know how to say no if that is what situation demands, without hurting people as far as possible.
- *Good leader:* A hospital administrator must have leadership skill. Nowadays almost all corporate are realizing the importance of

leadership in the management. He should be able to influence people to act with zeal and enthusiasm to achieve the target goal. He should be able to lead people and not seek directions from them in difficulty. He should inspire confidence—encourage them to give suggestions. Take responsibility for the mistakes of your juniors if committed without motive, i.e. you should be able to know your men.

- *Should not panic:* In the face of problems or difficulties, he should be able to keep cool even in scary situations. When chips are down he should be able to stand, i.e. hold his ground and be counted. Should be able to cope with change effortlessly in today's ever changing environment and should not feel rattled by change. Should react proportionately to the degree of change. Change is the currency of times we are living in.
- *Good judge:* This is the most essential quality for any administrator, you would need it all the time.
- *Should be sensitive:* He should be sensitive to other's suffering and problems even if they are self-inflicted or you are not able to help much.
- *Should be habitually objective:* He should be habitually objective with a deep sense of fair play and justice. You should not be hesitant to give credit where it is due and share honor if the situation rightfully demands so.
- *Time management:* Time and tide waits for none. Once the time is lost it is lost forever. So, a particular task should be completed in the allotted time frame.

In final analysis: He is a nice guy, who does not mind even if he finishes second and lets somebody else win if that could bring cheer to someone's life. At times, a gesture is all that you can do. But remember, sometimes even a gesture goes a long way.

Some Other Attributes and Qualities of a Good Hospital Administrator

Ability to deal with people from diverse background is an essential quality of hospital administrators. They should, hence, be sympathetic, tactful and patient listeners. Problem solving is required at all times, hence, the ability to be a team leader with a positive approach is essential. Hospital administrators must understand organizational development, financial budgeting, material management, medical purchasing and maintenances, building regulations and above all must have good public relation skills. Interest in service, in healthcare and in welfare is at the core of this profession. Hospital administrators convene meetings at various levels and, hence, need good communication skills.

- Hospital administrator must be diplomatic, tactful and infinitely patient.
- He must have strong analytical and decision-making abilities.
- He must have excellent interpersonal and communication skills.
- Administrator must have good organizing capacity and must be firm but considerate while handling people.
- He must have a sense of responsibility and take his job seriously.
- He must be an intelligent judge of human nature which quality is essential while selecting personnel.
- He must be expert at educating and providing direction to his subordinates.
- He must be a man with a fine business sense, so that he can secure value for money for the hospital.
- He must be capable of working with everyone cordially, regardless of their position of status in the hospital.
- He must have strong time management skill (Beat the Clock).
- He must review performance and speak with power.

HEALTHCARE ADMINISTRATION: CAREER OVERVIEW

The growth of healthcare service sector has increased the need for management professionals to manage hospitals' affairs. Hospital management has become the need of the hour today. Aspirant should be able to make difficult decision and possess strong time management skills and a very high degree of personal commitment. Therefore, there is a huge demand for professionals with right education and the appropriate skills.

Hospitals in India depend on doctors only. This has been a major roadblock in improving the efficiency and productivity of healthcare sector. The old trend of 'most experienced and bureaucratic medical professionals' has become back dated in the changing scenario of hospital and healthcare sector. Because of consumerism, TQM, emergency medical units, HIS, e-health venture, credit rating firms, NGO, medical tourism, telemedicine, bar coding and asset management, materials management, health insurance, TPA & IT revolution now require trained manpower specialized in hospital management and administration.

For effective management of hospital and healthcare delivery system in India, hospital administrators are in great demand.

Some Facts

Today, 90% of the hospitals in USA and 100% hospitals in UK are headed by the 'Nonmedical Administrators' trained in hospital administration and management.

Sensing better opportunity in hospital and healthcare sector, more and more people from nonmedical background are enrolling for healthcare administration and management courses.

EDUCATION AND TRAINING

The most accepted professional educations in the arena of hospital management is:

- *PhD:* Health management.
- *MPhil:* Management/hospital and health system management.
- Master in Doctorate (*MD—Hospital Administration*).
- Master of Hospital Administration (*MHA*).
- Master of Hospital Management (*MHM*).
- *MBA:* Hospital Management/Healthcare Services (*MBA*).
- Postgraduate Diploma in Hospital Administration (*PGDHA*).
- Postgraduate Diploma in Hospital and Healthcare Management (*PGDHHM*).
- Bachelor of Hospital Management (*BHM*).
- Certificate Level Courses.

AREAS OF SPECIALIZATION

- Medicolegal management.
- Materials management.
- Nursing administration.
- Pharmaceutical management.
- Public health management.
- Healthcare marketing.
- Quality management.
- Finance management.

CAREER PROSPECTS

Healthcare is the world's largest and fastest growing industry. Healthcare professional with a sharp managerial and administrative perspective are in great demand. Healthcare service market is being taken over by the private sector industry bigwigs like—Apollo Hospitals Group, Escort, Ganga Ram Hospital, Fortis Healthcare, Max Healthcare, Wockhardt Hospitals, Tata and other healthcare players coming up!!

Significant potential for employment exists in the management of healthcare in our country. Evidently employment opportunities in healthcare are increasing day-by-day. Many hospitals and pharmaceutical firms are looking for managers who have an in-depth understanding of Hospital and Healthcare Management principles and their applications to health-care delivery systems. If you wish to work for a healthcare organization as a manager or a consultant, or set-up a nursing home or hospital, courses in healthcare management will provide the needed training. So, India has a huge potential for hospital and healthcare growth and, hence, need for more and more healthcare managers/administrator is the need of the hour.

MONEY MATTERS!

Starting salaries per month (Approximate)

The Chief Executive Officer (CEO)	₹ 60,000–1,50,000
Chief Operating Officer	₹ 60,000–1,50,000
Chief Administrative Officer	₹ 60,000–1,50,000
Director—Administration	₹ 50,000–1,50,000
Director—Medical	₹ 50,000–1,50,000
Director—Marketing	₹ 50,000–1,50,000
Director—Materials Management	₹ 50,000–1,00,000
Director—HR	₹ 50,000–1,00,000
Vice President—Medical/Marketing	₹ 50,000–1,00,000
Medical Director/Medical Suptd.	₹ 50,000–1,00,000
Additional Medical Superintendent	₹ 40,000–80,000
Joint/Dy. Medical Superintendent	₹ 30,000–70,000
Assistant Medical Superintendent	₹ 20,000–55,000
Medical Administrator	₹ 22,000–45,000
Dy. General Manager	₹ 25,000–50,000
Hospital Administrator	₹ 25,000–50,000
Manager Administration	₹ 15,000–45,000
Manager—Marketing	₹ 15,000–45,000
Manager—Materials	₹ 15,000–45,000
Manager—Operations	₹ 15,000–45,000
Asst. Manager Level	₹ 12,000–30,000
Manger—HR	₹ 15,000–45,000
Executive Level	₹ 10,000–35,000
Assistant Executive	₹ 8,000–20,000

SOME TOP RECRUITERS

- Indian Spinal Injuries Centre.
- All India Institute of Medical Science.

- Fortis Healthcare Limited.
- Max Healthcare Limited.
- Wockhardt Hospitals.
- Rockland Hospital Balaji Hospital.
- Batra Hospital, Escorts Hospitals.
- Apollo Hospitals.
- Bombay Hospital.
- PD Hinduja Hospital.
- Tata Memorial Centre (TMC).
- Sir Ganga Ram Hospital.
- All Multispeciality Hospitals.
- Public Health Institutes.
- All Hospital Management Colleges/University.
- All Govt. Healthcare Institutes/Agencies.
- All Healthcare Organizations & Institutes.

EDUCATIONAL INSTITUTIONS

Professional training in hospital management is open to qualified doctors and any graduates. The job opportunities available to graduate will obviously be in general administration (Table 22.2).

Course in Hospital Administration are offered at the postgraduate level. Some courses, however, are offered at the graduate level in health management. Medical graduates (graduates from other disciplines are admitted in some courses) are admitted in the course. Duration of courses vary from one to three years, both part time and full time courses are available. Healthcare Management Courses are open to graduates in any discipline (in some cases, only medical/nursing graduates are eligible).

In addition to course work, candidates are required to undertake a project in a specific area of health management and undergo a period of internship in a hospital organization.

Table 22.2 Hospital and health management institutes/university at a glance

Institute/University	Course/Duration	Eligibility/Selection
All India Institute of Medical Sciences Ansari Nagar, New Delhi – 110029 www.aiims.ac.in	Masters in Hospital Administration—2/3 years	MBBS with 3 years experience in a hospital/sponsored graduates with 7 years experience in Hospital Administration 5 years in general practice theory/clinical test/interview

Contd...

Contd...

Institute/University	Course/Duration	Eligibility/Selection
University Centre for Distance Learning, Chaudhary Devi Lal University, Sirsa, Haryana Ph. 01666-248203 www. Cdlu.edu.in	MBA—Hospital Administration—2 years	Any graduate
National Institute of Health and Family Welfare, Munirka, New Delhi – 110067 www.nihfw.org	PG Certificate in Health and Family Welfare Management/Distance mode—1 year	MBBS, 3 years experience course In-service candidates
Delhi University, Faculty of Management Studies, Delhi – 110007 www.fms.edu	MBA (PT) (Healthcare Administration)—3 years	Sponsored MBBS degree holder with 5 years, experience in Hospital Administration
IGNOU, Maidan Garhi, New Delhi – 110068 www.ignou.ac.in	PG Diploma in Hospital and Health Management—1 year	Graduate from Medical, Dental Nursing Pharmacy and related health area with 2.5 years experience
Jawahar Lal Nehru University New Delhi – 110057	Master of Community Health (MCH)	MBBS with 50% and 1 year work experience after internship or MSc in Nursing with 50% and 1 year experience in Community Health Nursing
Devi Ahilya Vishwavidyalaya, Institute of Management Studies, Takshashila Campus, Khandwa Road, Indore – 452001 Ph. 0731-2527532	MBA (Hospital Administration)—2 years	Graduation, Entrance test conducted by professional Examination Board
Punjab University, Sector – 14, Chandigarh – 160014	Diploma in Hospital Administration—2 years	Degree, exam with 50% and 2 years experience
Department of Health Services Studies, Tata Institute of Social Sciences, Sion – Trombay Road, Deonar, PB 8313 Mumbai – 400088	Masters in Hospital/Health Administration—2 years Diploma (PT in Hospital Administation)—1 year	MBBS/BSc Nursing/BA/BCom/ BSc (Any faculty) with 50% (40% SC/ST) age below 45 years Admission Test GD, Interview MBBS/BSc Nursing or working graduates in hospital
International Institute for Population Sciences, Deonar, Mumbai – 400088	Diploma in Health Education—1 year	Graduation

Contd...

Contd...

Institute/University	Course/Duration	Eligibility/Selection
Shivaji University Vidyanagar, Kolhapur, 416004	Diploma in Hospital Administration—1 year	Graduation
SNDT Women's University, Nathibai Thackersey Road, Mumbai – 400 020	PG Diploma in Hospital Management—1 year	Graduation
University of Pune Ganeshkhind, Pune – 411 007	BSc (Hospital Administration) 1 year PG Diploma in Health Education—1 year Diploma in Hospital Management 2 years	Appropriate first degree BPED Graduation
Symbiosis Centre of Health Care Management, Senapati Bapat Road, Pune – 411 004 www.fms.edu	PG Diploma in Hospital and Health Management PG Diploma in Medico Legal Systems—1 year correspondence MBA—2 years	Graduates with 50% written test, group discussion and interview
Birla Institute of Technology and Science, Pilani in collaboration with CMC, Vellore Bombay Hospital and Tulane University Medical Center, New Orlean USA	MPhil Hospital and Health Systems Management (Distance Program)—3 Semesters	MBBS and 1 year experience/ sponsored. Some seats for BE/B Pharma/MSc/MBA with 1 year experience
Indian Institute of Health Management Research, 1, Prabhu Dayal Marg, Sanganer Airport, Jaipur – 302011 www.iihmr.com	Master of Public Health, Master of Health Care Administration—2 years	Graduates with 50% marks AIMAT
Karnataka State Open University, Manasagangotri, Mysore – 570 006	Diploma in Health and Hospital Management—2 years	Graduation
Manipal Academy of Higher Education, Manipal – 576119	DHA 2 years, Bachelor of Health Information, Administration (BHIA)—3 years	MBBS, 10+2 from any Arts/SC/ Commerce group with 50%
Rajiv Gandhi University of Health Sciences, 4th T-Block, Jayanagar, Bengaluru – 560041	MSc (Hospital Administration)—2 years	Graduates in Science
Father Muller Medical College Kankanady, Mangalore – 575002	MSc (Hospital Administration)—2 years	Graduation in relevant discipline
Bharathidasan University Palkalaiperur, Tiruchirappalli Tamil Nadu – 620024	PG Diploma in Rehabilitation Management—1 year	Graduation in relevant discipline

Contd...

Contd...

Institute/University	Course/Duration	Eligibility/Selection
Madurai, Kamraj University, Palkalai Nagar, Madurai – 625021	MHM (Health/Hospital) 2 years Diploma in Medical Records Management, Total Quality Management in Hospital, Ward Management, Dialysis Management, Intensive Care Management, Medical, Imaging Management, Blood Bank Management 1 year	Graduation with 50% after BSc Chem/Botany/Zoology
Sri Ramachandra Medical College and Research Institute, Porur, Chennai – 600116	MBA (Hospital and Health Systems Management) 2 years	Graduates/MBBS Entrance exam on All India Basis
Tamil Nadu Dr MGR Medical University, No. 69 Anna Salai, Chennai – 600 032	PG Diploma in Hospital Administration—1 year PG Diploma in Health Education—1 year	MBBS of MA/MSc/Med/M Nursing/BA/BSc/Edn Nursing with 2 years Standing
Christian Medical College, Therapudi PO Vellore – 632002	Diploma in Hospital Administration—1 year	Graduates and Diploma Holder
Apollo Institute of Hospital Administration. Apollo Hospital Campus, Jubilee Hills, Hyderabad – 500033	Master of Hospital Management—2 years	Graduates in any discipline with 50% marks. Entrance exam/group discussion/interview held in the months of July
ASCI Hinduja Institute of Healthcare Management, ASCI College Park, Banjara Hills, Hyderabad - 500034	Master of Hospital Administration and Master of Healthcare Administration—2 years residential	Graduation Written test, interview/group discussion
University of Calcutta Senate House Kolkata – 700 073	Diploma In Health Education—9 months	MBBS
Birla Institute of Science and Technology, Pilani	MPhil Hospital and Health System Management	MBA/MHA, MBBS
New Delhi YMCA IMS Jai Singh Road, New Delhi Ph. 23361915	PGDHA	Any Graduate
IGNOU, New Delhi www.ignou.ac.in	PGDHHM	Medical Graduate
Alagappa University Tamil Nadu	MBA—Hospital Management	Any Graduate
Jamia Hamdard, New Delhi www.jmi.ac.in	MBA—Healthcare	Any Graduate

Contd...

Contd...

Institute/University	Course/Duration	Eligibility/Selection
Tata Institute of Social Science, Mumbai www.tiss.edu	PhD and MPhil MHA	Any Graduate
Madurai Kamraj University, Madurai	PGDHHM	Any Graduate
All India Institute of Local Self-Government, New Delhi, Mumbai www.aiilsg.org	PGDHA/MBA	Any Graduate
Sikkim Manipal University	MBA—Healthcare	Any Graduate

Note: Please check recognition before taking admission.

SUGGESTED HOSPITAL AND HEALTHCARE MANAGEMENT JOURNAL/NEWSPAPER/MAGAZINES

- Modern Medicare.
- Harvard Business Review.
- Business Today.
- Pharmabiz Hospital Review.
- AHA News.
- American Journal of Managed Care.
- American Journal of Medical Quality.
- Clinical Leadership and Management Review.
- Hospice Management Advisor.
- Medico Legal Times by Symbiosis.
- Health.
- Health Facility Management.
- Health Forum Journal.
- Hospital Practice.

INDIA'S MAJOR HOSPITAL AND HEALTHCARE CONSULTANCY FIRMS

- Six Sigma Hospital and Healthcare Management Consultancy, New Delhi.
- Apollo Hospital Enterprises, Chennai.
- NOUS Hospital Consultancy.
- Hospic, Mumbai.

- Medicontrivers India, Mumbai.
- Ace Vision Health Consultant.
- Professional Health Planner, Delhi.
- KSA Technopak, Delhi.

USEFUL INDIAN HEALTHCARE SITES

Hospitals

- **Indian Spinal Injuries Centre**
  www.isiconline.org
- **Apollo Hospital, Delhi**
  http://www.apollohospdelhi.com
- **Fortis Healthcare Limited, Delhi**
  http://www.fortishealthcare.com
- **Max Healthcare Ltd.**
  http://www.maxhealthcare.com
- **Express Healthcare**
  http://expresshealthcare.com
- **Escort Hospital**
  http://www.ehirc.com
- **Rockland Hospital, Delhi**
  http://www.rocklandhospital.com
- **All India Institute of Medical Sciences (AIIMS)**
  http://www.aiims.edu
- **Government Medical College and Hospital, Chandigarh**
  http://gmch.nic.in
- **Guwahati Medical College and Hospital**
  http://gmchassam.nic.in
- **Institute of Child Health and Hospital for Children**
  http://ich.tn.nic.in
- **Jawaharlal Institute of Postgraduate Medical Education and Research (JIPMER)**
  www.jipmer.edu
- **Jawaharlal Nehru Cancer Hospital and Research Centre, Bhopal**
  http://www.jnch.nic.in

- **Lala Ram Swarup Institute of Tuberculosis and Respiratory Diseases**
  www.lrsitbrd.nic.in
- **National Institute of Mental Health and Neuro Sciences (NIMHANS)**
  www.nimhans.kar.nic.in
- **North Eastern Indira Gandhi Regional Institute of Health and Medical Sciences (NEIGRIHMS)**
  http://neigrihms.nic.in
- **Rajasthan Mobile Surgical Unit**
  http://rajmobileunit.nic.in
- **SGS Medical College and KEM Hospital, Mumbai**
  http://www.kem.edu
- **Tata Memorial Centre (TMC)**
  http://www.tatamemorialcentre.com

Medical Institutions

- **All India Institute of Medical Sciences (AIIMS)**
  http://ww.aiims.edu
- **Chhatrapati Shahuji Maharaj Medical University**
  http://www.kgmcindia.edu
- **Government Medical College and Hospital, Chandigarh**
  http://gmch.nic.in
- **Guwahati Medical College and Hospital**
  http://gmchassam.nic.in
- **Institute of Child Health and Hospital for Children**
  http://ich.tn.nic.in
- **Institute of Human Behaviour and Allied Sciences (IHBAS)**
  http://ihbas.delhigov.nic.in
- **Jawaharlal Institute of Postgraduate Medical Education and Research (JIPMER)**
  www.jipmer.edu
- **Kidwai Memorial Institute of Oncology (KMIO)**
  http://www.kar.nic./kidwai
- **Lala Ram Swarup Institute of Tuberculosis and Respiratory Diseases**
  http://lrsitbrd.nic.in

- **National Institute of Ayurveda**
  http://nia.nic.in
- **National Institute of Homoeopathy (NIH)**
  http://nih.nic.in
- **National Institute of Mental Health and Neuro Sciences (NIMHANS)**
  http://www.nimhans.kar.nic.in
- **National Institute of Pharmaceutical Education and Research (NIPER)**
  http://www.niper.nic.in
- **National Tuberculosis Institute (NTI)**
  http://ntindia.kar.nic.in
- **North Eastern Indira Gandhi Regional Institute of Health and Medical Sciences (NEIGRIHMS)**
  http://neigrihms.nic.in
- **Post Graduate Institute of Medical Education and Research**
  http://pgimer.nic.in
- **Sanjay Gandhi Post Graduate Institute of Medical Sciences**
  http://www.sgpgi.ac.in
- **SGS Medical College and KEM Hospital, Mumbai**
  http://ww.kem.edu
- **Sher-i-Kashmir Institute of Medical Sciences**
  http://www.skims.ac.in/default1.htm
- **Tamil Nadu Dr MGR Medical University**
  http://www.tnmmu.ac.in

Research Councils/Centers

- **Central Council for Research in Ayurveda and Siddha (CCRAS)**
  http://www.ccrag.org
- **Central Council for Research in Homeopathy (CCRH)**
  http://www.ccrhindia.org
- **Central Council for Research in Unani Medicine (CCRUM)**
  http://www.unanimedicine.org
- **Central Drug Research Institute (CDRI)**
  http://www.cdriindia.org

- **Central Institute of Medicinal and Aromatic Plants (CIMAP)**
  http://www.cimap.org
- **Delhi Medical Council**
  http://www.delhimedicalcouncil.nic.in
- **Indian Council of Medical Research (ICMR)**
  http://icmr.nic.in
- **Institute of Genomics and Integrative Biology (IGIB)**
  http://www.igib.res.in
- **Jawaharlal Nehru Cancer Hospital and Research Centre, Bhopal**
  http://jnch.nic.in
- **Kidwai Memorial Institute of Oncology (KMIO)**
  http://www.kar.nic.in/kidwai
- **Malaria Research Centre (MRC)**
  http://www.mrcindia.org
- **National Institute of Pharmaceutical Education and Research (NIPER)**
  http://www.niper.nic.in
- **Post Graduate Institute of Medical Education and Research, Chandigarh**
  http://pgimer.nic.in
- **Tata Memorial Centre (TMC)**
  http://www.tatamemorialcentre.com

MANAGEMENT OF ALTERNATIVE THERAPIES

INTRODUCTION

The term Alternative Therapy or Alternative Medicine means any form of medicine that is outside the mainstream of Western medicine or conventional medicine as practiced a majority of doctors today. This term is loosely used to over all forms of medicine except allopathy. In 1973, the Medical Faculty of the University of Rome convened the first World Congress of Alternative Medicines and the provisional program contained no less than 135 therapies. Some alternative therapies, including traditional Chinese medicine (TCM) and Ayurveda, have antique, non-Western origins and are entirely alternative medical systems; others, such as homeopathy and chiropractic, are native to the West and emerged in the eighteenth and nineteenth centuries. Some, such as osteopathy and chiropractic, employ manipulative physical methods of treatment; others, such as meditation and prayer, are based on mind-body interventions. Treatments considered alternative in one location may be considered conventional in another. Thus, chiropractic is not considered alternative in Denmark and likewise osteopathic medicine is no longer thought of as an alternative therapy in the United States.

Alternative medicine exists in all cultures to some degree and terms such as traditional medicine, indigenous medicine or folk medicine, etc. are used to describe such practices. These medicines date back hundred or even thousand of years depending on the country and culture concerned.

There are more than 100 systems of alternative medicines still in practice all over the world. Every country, region or area has its own traditional system of health and medical cares such as for the Chinese, it is acupuncture; for the French, magnetic healing; for the Germans, Heilpraxis; for the English, Herbalism; for India, Ayurveda with Siddha being widely practice in the southern part of the country; for Japan, Shiatsu, etc.

The most popular forms of alternative medicine are Ayurveda, Homeopathy, Naturopathy, Yoga, Acupuncture, Acupressure, Magneto therapy, Shiatsu, Herbalism, Meditation, Aromatherapy, Bach Flower Remedies, Chromo therapy, Diet therapy, Hydropathy and Reiki.

India is responsible for giving the world a large number of alternative therapies. Apart from the well known Yoga and Ayurveda. There are a number of lesser known therapies that ancient India has gifted the world.

Today, worldwide, alternative health science therapies are gaining ground. Together with the modern system of medicine, alternative health sciences and therapies offer cheaper and easily adaptable solutions to various ailments for positive health. Neither all alternative therapies are equally effective nor are all backed by equally sound research. Here, we present a survey of various alternative therapies along with the claims made for them by their practitioners and adherents.

Yoga Therapy

Yoga therapy tries to re-establish the inner balance by various means, working from the gross to the subtle. On the physical level it uses:

Asanas: They energize the organism, create awareness of the body and its function and stabilize the mind.

Kriyas: These are simple hygienic procedures which support the body's own cleansing mechanisms and draw the attention of the mind towards the affected area.

Pranayamas: These are breathing techniques which have very subtle influences on the whole organism.

Diet: Many diseases are directly or indirectly linked with wrong food habits. A change in diet can stimulate the whole system.

Simple nature cure techniques: The elements water, air, Sun and simple procedures like massaging or steam inhalation are used as a support.

The second line of therapy is the work on the mind. Mental disturbances —anxieties, confusion, and unsteadiness are the most important factors which can cause a disease condition. Therefore, various techniques have been developed to create positive mind states.

Among others there are:
Relaxation: Both physical and mental.

Conditioning: Sitting in a meditative posture one tries to calm down and center oneself.

Bhavanas: Contemplation on certain basic ideas like the transitoriness of all things can stimulate a change of attitude towards life.

Yoga has claimed that tension is disease and relaxation is health. To this end the whole eightfold path of yoga is to purify the body-mind complex.

Mantra Therapy

Mantras work directly upon our karma: the accumulated latencies and tendencies with which we are born. The vibrations of these ancient formulas work through the chakras to increase the flow of beneficial energy throughout the subtle body where these latencies and tendencies are stored. Mantra therapy starts by increasing the total amount of energy available for all of our activities. Certain mantras used singly or in combination can greatly accelerate the quality and quantity of energy used in the healing process. However, if the karmic propensity for a given condition is overwhelming, mantra therapy will not remove the difficulty any more than conventional therapy will. However, it will reduce the karmic baggage you take into future lives.

The energy created through mantra practice may lead one to forms of therapy quite different from the ones used initially. Thus, some unexpected new form of treatment may appear as the result of mantra practice.

Investigate it. Ultimately, we do not know through which door the route to recovery might manifest, and it may be in some form of conventional or traditional care of which we had been previously unaware.

Pranic Healing

Pranic healing is a highly developed and tested system of energy-based healing techniques that utilizes prana to balance, harmonize and transform the body's energy processes. Prana is a Sanskrit word that means life-force.

Pranic healing is a simple yet powerful and effective no-touch energy healing. It is based on the fundamental principle that the body is a 'self-repairing' living entity that possesses the innate ability to heal itself. Pranic healing works on the principle that the healing process is accelerated by increasing the life-force or vital energy on the affected part of the physical body.

Pranic healing is currently being taught to doctors, nurses, massage therapists, acupuncturists, chiropractors, the clergy, homemakers, engineers and many others in all walks of life. It has allowed them to heal confidently and consistently in the shortest learning time possible. They find pranic healing very effective and easy to apply.

In the palm of your hands are energy centers called chakras. Through a simple exercise these chakras will be activated. Once activated, these chakras will become sensitive to feeling others' energy. You can scan that energy field to locate blockages and be able to cleanse, energize and revitalize the area with new prana. You will also learn techniques to stop the drain of energy on your body that many health practitioners experience while working on others. You will actually energize yourself while you are healing someone else!

Colon Hydrotherapy

Do you experience any of these health problems? Constipation, diarrhea, frequent headaches, backaches, fatigue, bad breath, body odor, irritability, confusion, skin problems, abdominal gas and bloating, lower back pain, sciatic pain, low resistance to colds and infections, low energy and vitality. These are all indicators that you may need to cleanse your body's elimination system. Colon hydrotherapy is an excellent way to accomplish this objective.

Benefits accomplished by colon hydrotherapy:

- *Cleansing:* Toxic material is broken down so it can no longer harm your body or inhibit assimilation and elimination. Fecal debris built-up over a long period is gently removed over a series of irrigations.

- *Exercises:* The build-up of toxic debris weakens the colon and impairs its functions. Gentle filling and emptying of the colon can improve peristaltic (natural muscular contraction) activity, which aids efficient removal of waste material.
- *Reshapes:* Over time, the natural shape of a problematic colon will become distorted...causing even more problems. The gentle water action and massage techniques of the therapist will help eliminate protruding pockets of waste and narrow, spastic constrictions.
- *Stimulation of reflex points:* Every system and organ of the body is connected to the colon by reflex points. A colon hydrotherapy session stimulates these reflex points, thereby affecting the corresponding body parts...in a beneficial way, similar to reflexology.

Urine Therapy

Urine is not, as many believe, the excess water from food and liquids that goes through the intestines and is ejected from the body as "waste".

Medical researchers have discovered that many of the elements of the blood that are found in urine have enormous medicinal value, and when reintroduced to the body, they boost the body's immune defenses and stimulate healing in a way that nothing else does.

In 1975, one of the founders of Miles Laboratories, Dr AH Free, published his book, Urinalysis in Clinical Laboratory Practice, in which he remarked that not only is urine a sterile body compound (purer than distilled water), but that it is now recognized that urine contains literally thousand of compounds.

Researchers have discovered that allergic responses are caused by 'renegade' white blood cells that inappropriately attack substances even when they may be no threat to the body. So, it is the activity of these renegade white blood cells, called antigen receptors, that needs to be corrected in order to cure the allergy.

Realising that the urine of allergic individuals contains the allergy causing antigen receptors, researchers thought that to re-introduce the urine back to the allergic individual would mean antibodies would be produced which would then stop the allergic response. And that is exactly what happens. Allergies have been completely turned around with urine therapy.

Multiple sclerosis, colitis, lupus, rheumatoid arthritis, cancer, hepatitis, hyperactivity, pancreatic insufficiency, psoriasis, eczema, diabetes, herpes, mononucleosis, adrenal failure, allergies and so many other ailments have been relieved through use of this therapy.

Laughter Therapy

The experience of Dr Madan Kataria, pioneer of *Hasya Yoga*, with laughter clubs worldwide, taught him that people were definitely deriving health benefits from laughter yoga exercises. But there was no scientific proof that Dr Kataria could offer to satisfy logical minded people especially in the West. "I had no problems in India as more than 100,000 people laughed every morning without asking me for any proof but when it came to the West everybody asked, do you have the data?"

Finally, in 2003–04, the first authentic research was completed by Dr Ilona Papousek from the University of Graz in early fall 2004. According to the news release by Ananova—March, 2004, a new study shows that laughter really is the best therapy for stroke patients, according to scientists. A study was conducted at a computer company where Mr Thomas Flindt led a session of laughter yoga in the beginning of the day throughout the month of May, 2004. This project shows clearly the effect that a regular practice of laughter yoga has on the stress levels. On an individual level, the results are remarkable. The body stress levels are significantly reduced.

Past Life Therapy

"Past life regression therapy includes the mental act of going back to a time prior to this life in order to retrieve memories that may still negatively influence a person's present life. They are probably the source of symptoms running the gamut from phobias to addictions," avers R Chandran, a past life therapist.

Dr Francis Menezes, who has regressed using hypnosis states, says, "To be able to go to your past life, most therapists take you back to yesterday, two days ago, last week, five years ago, ten years back, finally to your mother's womb and beyond. To be born you have to die." "In a hypnotherapy session, your master is in control of you, your blood count level is low, and your heartbeat is slow. It is almost a dreamless state, which is extremely emotionally draining once you wake-up," says Dr Menezes. Interestingly all those who practise past life therapy do not feel the need to prove it. "What is of value here is the outcome which is certainly effective. Besides, how can I try to convince someone who does not want to be convinced?" opines R Chandran.

People who are healed through past life therapy are people who remember names, dates and geographic details. But perhaps, even more important than curing of physical and emotional symptoms, is the knowledge that we do not die even if our bodies do. We are immortal!

There are a number of publications and internet sources that will tell you more about these therapies. Go on, read about them. If do find yourself itching to try a new therapy, be sure to contact an experienced practitioner prior to trying anything new.

Because two-thirds of the world's population (mainly in the third world countries) relies entirely on the traditional medical therapies. The World Health Organization has declared its intention actively to encourage the traditional medicines worldwide in order to that their goal of health for all by the year 2000 AD can be attained. The WHO has pledged itself a realistic approach to traditional medicines in the lights of modern science. In order to discourage harmful practices and encourage useful ones and to promote the integration of proven valuable knowledge and the traditional and Western medicines. The expert of the WHO have identified more than 150 systems of alternative medicines such as Homeopathy, Biochemic, Naturopathy, Acupuncture, Shiatsu therapy, Magneto therapy, Yoga, Osteopathy, Chiropractic, Herbalism, etc. still into practice in the various parts of the world.

EXAMPLES

Alternative therapies based on electricity or magnetism use verifiable electromagnetic fields, such as pulsed fields, alternating-current, or direct-current fields in an unconventional manner rather than claiming the existence of imponderable or supernatural energies.

Substance-based practices use substances found in nature such as herbs, foods, nonvitamin supplements, megavitamins, and minerals, and includes traditional herbal remedies with herbs specific to regions in which the cultural practices arose. Nonvitamin supplements include fish oil, Omega-3 fatty acid, glucosamine, Echinacea, flaxseed oil or pills, and ginseng, when used under a claim to have healing effects.

Mind-body interventions, working under the premise that the mind can affect "bodily functions and symptoms", include healing claims made in hypnotherapy, and in guided imagery, meditation, guided imagery, progressive relaxation, qi gong, tai chi and yoga. Meditation practices including mantra meditation, mindfulness meditation, yoga, tai chi, and qi gong have many uncertainties. According to an AHRQ review, the available evidence on meditation practices through September, 2005 is of poor methodological quality and definite conclusions on the effects of meditation in healthcare cannot be made using existing research.

Naturopathy is based on a belief in vitalism, which posits that a special energy called vital energy or vital force guides bodily processes such as metabolism, reproduction, growth, and adaptation. The term was coined in 1895 by the "father of US naturopathy". Today, naturopathy is primarily practiced in the United States and Canada. Naturopaths in unregulated jurisdictions may use the Naturopathic Doctor designation or other titles regardless of level of education.

Traditional Chinese medicine is based on a concept of vital energy, or Qi flowing in the body along specific pathways. These purported pathways consist of 12 primary meridians. TCM has many branches including, acupuncture, massage, feng shui, herbs, as well as Chinese astrology. TCM diagnosis is primarily based on looking at the tongue, which is claimed to show the condition of the organs, as well as feeling the pulse of the radial artery, which is also claimed to show the condition of the organs.

ALTERNATIVE THERAPIES GUIDANCE

The following is a guide to some alternative therapies:

Acupressure

Similar to acupuncture, but using finger pressure rather than fine needles on specific points along the body to treat ailments such as tension and stress, aches and pains, menstrual cramps, arthritis.

Acupuncture

Fine needles are inserted at specific points to stimulate, disperse, and regulate the flow of vital energy, and restore a healthy energy balance. In addition to pain relief, acupuncture is also used to improve well being and treat acute, chronic, and degenerative conditions in children and adults.

Aromatherapy

Using 'essential oils' distilled from plants, aromatherapy treats emotional disorders such as stress and anxiety as well as a wide range of other ailments. Oils are massaged into the skin in diluted form, inhaled, or placed in baths. Aromatherapy is often used in conjunction with massage therapy, acupuncture, reflexology, herbology, chiropractic, and other holistic treatments.

Astrology

Astrology is a humanistic attempt at trying to understand the cycles that we share with the forces in the Universe. The planets have corresponding rulership to certain vitamins, minerals, cell salts, herbs, metals, colors and parts of the body. Through the chart, one can look to see what natal health conditions exist. Through these precepts, we can then look at the present and into the future to see what areas of our lives are being affected and potentially how we can head off ill health and promote wellness.

Atlas Orthogonal

Atlas orthogonal is a chiropractic program to evaluate and correct subluxation based on scientific and biomechanical procedures. By incorporating the latest advancements in scientific technology, chiropractors can calculate, in precise detail, the vectors specific to an individual subluxation pattern, and program their instrument with the specific correction vectors to deliver the adjustment without any manipulation at all.

Ayurvedic Medicine

Practiced in India for more than 5,000 years, ayurvedic tradition holds that illness is a state of imbalance among the body's systems that can be detected through such diagnostic procedures as reading the pulse and observing the tongue. Nutrition counseling, massage, natural medications, meditation, and other modalities are used to address a broad spectrum of ailments.

Auricular Therapy

Ancient Egyptian writings state that pain can be relieved by stimulating certain points on the ear. In the 1800's, several publications indicated that there were several techniques of cauterization and manipulation of the ears to aid certain disorders. Many benefits can be achieved by massaging and palpating specific points on the ear.

Alexander Technique

The Alexander technique is a method that works to change (movement) habits in our everyday activities. It is a simple and practical method for improving ease and freedom of movement, balance, support and coordination. The technique teaches the use of the appropriate amount of effort for a particular activity, giving you more energy for all your activities. It is not a series of treatments or exercises, but rather a re-education of the mind and body.

Autogenic Training

It is a century-old European method for achieving relaxation-based upon passive concentration and body awareness of specific sensations.

Its effectiveness has been shown in relieving many stress-related disorders including anxiety, tension, insomnia, and examination stress. Persons with chronic medical conditions ranging from migraine, colitis, irritable bowel syndrome, diabetes, high blood pressure, to thyroid disease and many other conditions have also been shown to benefit from the practice of autogenic training.

Anthroposophical Medicine

Anthroposophical medicine involves an internationally organized group of people who think that Rudolf Steiner (an Austrian physician, 1861-1925) found the ultimate truth—the anthroposophy. Steiner said: By anthroposophy, I mean a scientific investigation of the spiritual world which will bring to light the weaknesses and half-truths not only of science but also of modern mysticism. It is a method which, before attempting to investigate the spiritual worlds, first develops psychic powers not normally used in daily life or in current scientific research.

Autourine Therapy

This practice comes from Yoga and is the use of one's own urine as food, medicine, restorative, transforming agent and immune system booster. It is sometimes called 'Your Own Doctor'.

Holotropic Breathwork

It is a simple yet powerful technique for self-exploration and healing, based on combined insights from modern consciousness research, depth psychology and perennial spiritual practices. The method activates non-ordinary states of consciousness which mobilize the spontaneous healing potential of the psyche. Sustained effective breathing, evocative music, focused energy work and mandala drawing are components of this subjective journey. 'Holotropic' literally means 'moving towards wholeness'.

Biofeedback

A method of monitoring minute metabolic changes in one's own body with the aid of sensitive machines. The technique is used especially for stress-related conditions such as asthma, migraines, insomnia, and high blood pressure. Clients learn to make subtle adjustments to move toward a more balanced internal state by consciously visualizing, relaxing, or imagining while observing light, sound, or metered feedback.

Bach Flower Remedies

A system of herbal remedies devised by Edward Bach, these floral remedies can supposedly alter the disharmonies of personality and emotional state that trouble us all from time to time. These remedies are mostly aimed at curing emotional states rather than physical ones.

Cellular Therapy

Cellular therapy also called live cell therapy, cellular suspensions, glandular therapy, fresh cell therapy, sicca cell therapy, embryonic cell therapy, and organotherapy—refers to various procedures in which processed tissue from animal embryos, fetuses or organs, is injected or taken orally. Products are obtained from specific organs or tissues said to correspond with the unhealthy organs or tissues of the recipient. Proponents claim that the recipient's body automatically transports the injected cells to the target organs, where they supposedly strengthen them and regenerate their structure. The organs and glands used in cell treatment include brain, pituitary, thyroid, adrenals, thymus, liver, kidney, pancreas, spleen, heart, ovary, testis, and parotid. Several different types of cell or cell extract can be given simultaneously—some practitioners routinely give up to 20 or more at once.

Chromotherapy or Color Therapy

The use of color (usually in the form of colored light) to produce beneficial or healing effects.

Colon Therapy

The therapeutic goals of colon therapy are to balance body chemistry, eliminate waste, and restore proper tissue and organ function. Colon therapy releases toxins, cleans the blood, stimulates the immune system, and aids in restoring the pH balance in the body. Colon therapy, also known as colonics, is believed to relieve a wide range of symptoms related to colon dysfunction.

Chelation Therapy

Chelation therapy is a series of intravenous injections of the synthetic amino acid EDTA, designed to detoxify the body. It is also often used to treat arteriosclerosis. Most frequently, this is administered in an osteopathic or medical doctor's office.

Chinese (Oriental) Medicine

Oriental medical practitioners are trained to use a variety of ancient and modern therapeutic methods—including acupuncture, herbal medicine, massage, heat therapy, and nutritional and lifestyle counseling—to treat a broad range of both chronic and acute illnesses.

Chiropractic

The chiropractic views, the spine as the backbone of human health: misalignments of the vertebrae caused by poor posture or trauma cause pressure on the spinal nerve roots, leading to diminished function and illness. Through manipulation or adjustment of the spine, treatment seeks to analyze and correct these misalignments.

Colonics

A colonic is a colon irrigation, the irrigation of the large intestine with sanitized, filtered water under gentle pressure to wash out or detoxify it of stagnated fecal material; it is a full intestinal enema.

Counseling/Psychotherapy

This broad category covers a range of practitioners, from career counselors to psychotherapies who treat depression, stress, addiction, and emotional issues. Formats can vary from individual counseling to group therapy. Some therapists may also incorporate bodywork, ritual, energy healing, and other alternative modalities as part of their practice.

Cupping

It is a traditional Chinese medical technique which applies suction to diseased parts of the body using ceramic glass or bamboo cups in order to increase the regional circulation and thereby promote healing. In very ancient times, the horns of animals were used for this purpose.

Craniosacral Therapy

This is a manual therapeutic procedure for remedying distortions in the structure and function of the craniosacral mechanism—the brain and spinal cord, the bones of the skull, the sacrum, and interconnected membranes. It is used to treat chronic pain, migraine headaches, TMJ, and a range of other conditions.

Dance/Movement Therapies

Dance and/or movement therapy uses expressive movement as a therapeutic tool for both personal expression and psychological or emotional healing. Practitioners work with people with physical disabilities, addition issues, sexual abuse histories, eating disorders, and other concerns.

Holistic Dentistry

Holistic dentists are licensed dentists who bring an interdisciplinary approach to their practice. They may incorporate such methods as homeopathy, nutrition and acupuncture into their treatment plans. Most holistic dentists emphasize wellness and preventive care while avoiding silver-mercury fillings.

Dowsing

Dowsing is an ancient art of searching for hidden things (water, precious metals, etc.) using one of the senses that many of us are not even aware of possessing; reportedly 80% of people have this special gift—an ability to sense things not perceptible to others. Some of these people do not need any extratools to do that—they just KNOW where is the best place to dig a well or where the gold treasure is hidden.

Ear Candling

Primarily used for wax build-up and related hearing problems, ear candling is also used for ear infections and sinus infections. Treatment involves placing the narrow end of a specially designed hollow candle at the entry of the ear canal, while the opposite end is lit.

Electropathy

Electropathy is a specialized system of therapeutics which involves the use of various forms of electric currents for medicinal purposes.

Fasting Therapy

Therapeutic fasting or fasting for health is a purifying and rejuvenating process by which toxic waste matters of the body are eliminated and regeneration of diseased tissues occurs.

Feng Shui

Ancient Chinese practice of arranging the home or work environment to promote health, happiness, and prosperity. Consultants may recommend changes in the surroundings—from color selection to furniture placement—in order to promote a health flow of chi, or vital energy.

Feldenkrais Method

The Feldenkrais method is a systematic approach to neuromuscular relearning. The method is suited to healthy people who want to increase the flexibility of their bodies and thinking, people with neurological and movement disorders, and those who want to achieve excellence in the arts, sports, or any endeavor.

Flower Essences

A method of alleviating negative emotional states that may contribute to illness or hinder personal growth. Drops of a solution infused with the captured 'essence' of a flower are placed under the tongue or in a beverage. The practitioner helps the client choose appropriate essences, focusing on the client's emotional state rather than on a particular physical condition.

Gem Therapy

A relatively recent discovery in the field of alternative medicines, it involves the use of specific gems to treat specific ailments.

Herbalism

An ancient form of healing still widely used in much of the world, herbalism uses natural plants or plant-based substances to treat a range of illnesses and to enhance the functioning of the body's systems. Though herbalism is not a licensed professional modality in the United States, herbs are 'prescribed' by a range of practitioners.

Heliotherapy

Heliotherapy is the science conducted on the positive effects of the Sun and is an effective tool in boosting the body's immune system.

Holistic Medicine

A descriptive term for a healing philosophy that views a patient as a whole person, not as just a disease or a collection of symptoms. In the course of treatment, holistic medical practitioners may address a client's emotional and spiritual dimensions as well as the nutritional, environmental, and lifestyle factors that may contribute to an illness. Many holistic medical practitioners combine conventional forms of treatment with natural or alternative treatments.

Homeopathy

A medical system that uses infinitesimal doses of natural substances—called remedies— to stimulate a person's immune and defense system. A remedy is individually chosen for a sick person based on its capacity to cause, if given in overdose, physical and psychological symptoms similar to those a patient is experiencing. Common conditions homeopathy addresses are infant and childhood diseases, infections, fatigue, allergies, and chronic illnesses such as arthritis.

Hypnotherapy

A means of bypassing the conscious mind and accessing the subconscious, where suppressed memories, repressed emotions, and forgotten events may remain recorded. Hypnosis may facilitate behavioral, emotional, or attitudinal change such as weight loss, or smoking cessation. It is also used to treat phobias, stress, and as an adjunct in the treatment of illness.

Hydrotherapy

It is defined as the scientific application of water for therapeutic purposes. Water may be used at various temperatures, in different modes and in different forms.

Iridology

The diagnostic system based on the premise that every organ has a corresponding location within the iris of the eye, which can serve as an indicator of the individual organ's health or disease. Iridology is used by naturopaths and other practitioners, particularly when diagnosis achieved through standard methods is unclear.

Kinesiology

Kinesiology is the study of the human body during movement. There are many disciplines within Kinesiology including anatomy, biomechanics, exercise physiology, motor control, motor learning, neuromuscular physiology, sports psychology, and philosophy. Kinesiology graduates enter a variety of careers and graduate programs related to the understanding of how the body works including medical school, physical and occupational therapy schools, athletic training, and other health professions, public school teaching, sport and exercise related fields, the military, business, and law.

Lymph Drainage Therapy

Therapy to drain and improve the lymphatic vessels, a system of tubes or canals through which lymph is carried from different parts of the body.

Massage Therapeutic

A general term for a range of therapeutic approaches with roots in both Eastern and Western cultures. It involves the practice of manipulating a person's muscles and other soft tissue with the intent of improving a person's well-being or health, and may include, but not be limited to, effleurage, deep tissue, percussion, vibration, and joint movement.

Magnetotherapy

The art of healing by the application of natural and artificial magnets to the diseased parts of the human body. It is a clinical system by which human ailments are treated and cured through the application of magnets to the body of the patients.

Midwifery/Childbirth Support

Midwives provide education and support during pregnancy, assist the mother during labor and delivery, and provide follow-up care. Practitioners of childbirth support include childbirth educators, assistants, and doulas (women labor coaches who also provide postpartum home care).

Native American Herbology

Native American healers and spiritual leaders seldom travel far from their homes and even more infrequently publicize their work—it is not the way. However, there is a body of knowledge about the herbal treatments used by various Native People. Much of the information has been tested and incorporated into our present herbal therapies.

Natural Products

Products composed of organically grown plants and containing no chemicals. These products may be used cosmetically as well as for health and nutrition.

Naturopathic Medicine

Naturopathic physicians work to restore and support the body's own healing abilities using a variety of modalities including nutrition, herbal medicine, homeopathic medicine, and orient medicine. A primary healthcare system which emphasizes the curative power of nature, treating both acute and chronic illnesses in all age groups.

Network Chiropractic

This refers to a network of independent chiropractic offices that use Network Spinal Analysis, a method characterized by the sequential application of a number of gentle, specific adjusting techniques. Care progresses through a series of levels that parallel spinal and quality-of-life changes.

Ohashiatsu

A system of physical techniques, exercise and meditation used to relieve tension and fatigue and induce a state of harmony and peace. The practitioner first assesses a person's state by feeling the hara, the area below the navel. Then, using continuous and flowing movements, the practitioner presses and stretches the body's energy channels, working in unison with the person's breathing.

Oriental Diagnosis

It is a diagnostic procedure by which the patient's pulse is examined to detect disease according to traditional Chinese medicine.

Osteopathic Medicine

Osteopathic physicians provide comprehensive medical care, including preventive medicine, diagnosis, surgery, prescription medications, and hospital referrals. In diagnosis and treatment, they pay particular attention to the joints, bones, muscles, and nerves and are specially trained in osteopathic manipulative treatment—using their hands to diagnose, treat, and prevent illness.

Physiotherapy

It is a wonderful manipulative technique by which the deformities of an individual are modified in order to notify the body and the vital organs in accordance with the principles of naturopathy.

Pyramid Healing

A potential healing method using pyramidal structures.

Radiesthesia

The use of dowsing or divining to diagnose disease and select remedies. It can be used to diagnose any condition according to leading practitioners. Basically, it is simply a method of arriving at a diagnosis and treatment using the human being as the diagnostic instrument.

Radionics

A therapy that has grown-up around the ability of the human being to use radiesthesia together with simple instruments to help in the diagnosis of disease in animals, plants and humans and then to treat this disease at a distance without the presence of the patient.

Reconstructive Therapy/Prolotherapy

Reconstructive therapy uses injections of natural substances such as dextrose, glycerin, and phenol in order to stimulate the growth of connective tissue and this strengthens weak or damaged joints, cartilage, ligaments, and tendons. This therapy is used to treat degenerative arthritis, lower back pain, torn ligaments and cartilage, carpal tunnel syndrome, and other conditions.

Reflexology

This modality is based on the idea that specific points on the feet and hands correspond with organs and tissues throughout the body. With fingers and thumbs, the practitioner applies pressure to these points to treat a wide range of stress-related illnesses.

Reiki

Practitioners of this ancient Tibetan healing system use light hand placements to channel healing energies to the recipient. While practitioners may vary widely in technique and philosophy, Reiki is commonly used to treat emotional and mental distress as well as chronic and acute physical problems, and to assist the recipient in achieving spiritual focus and clarity.

Rolfing

A massage technique using deep manipulation of the fascia (connective tissue) to restore the body's natural alignment, which may have become rigid through injury, emotional trauma, and inefficient movement habits. The process involves ten sessions, each focusing on a different part of the body.

Shiatsu

The most widely known form of acupressure, shiatsu has been used in Japan for more than 1,000 years to treat pain and illness and for general health maintenance. Using a series of techniques, practitioners apply rhythmic finger pressure at specific points on the body in order to stimulate chi, or the vital energy.

Sound Therapy

The use of sound waves to heal.

Tibetan Medicine

Evolved as a synsthesis of Tibetan, Chinese and Persian Medicine, and even Ayurveda. These remedies include indigenous herbs, fruits, flowers, metallic powders and minerals given in tablets, and are especially effected in treating rheumatism, asthma, gastritis, diabetes and many neurological disorders.

Unani

Involves the use of plants and herbs, these remedies are known to provide cures for diseases such as sinusitus , leukoderma, rheumatism, jaundice and elephantiasis.

Vision Therapies

Through exercise and relaxation techniques, vision may actually be improved to the point that glasses may no longer be needed. Therapies are typically offered by licensed optometrists and ophthalmologists.

Vitamin Therapy

A complementary therapy of vitamin usage combined with other treatments to address a range of illnesses and to enhance the functioning of the body's systems. Assists the immune system in combating diseases such as chronic fatigue syndrome and HIV/AIDS.

Wellness Restoration

A comprehensive program designed to increase muscle mass by using adequate nutrition, supplementation, anabolic steroid therapy and resistance weight training to prevent/reverse wasting in HIV disease.

Yoga Therapy

The use of yoga to address mental and physical problems while integrating body and mind.

PREVALENCE OF USE OF SPECIFIC THERAPIES

The most common CAM therapies used in the US in 2002 were prayer (45.2%), herbalism (18.9%), breathing meditation (11.6%), meditation (7.6%), chiropractic medicine (7.5%), yoga (5.1–6.1%), body work (5.0%), diet-based therapy (3.5%), progressive relaxation (3.0%), mega-vitamin therapy (2.8%) and visualization (2.1%).

In Britain, the most often used alternative therapies were Alexander technique, Aromatherapy, Bach and other flower remedies, Body work therapies including massage, Counseling stress therapies, hypnotherapy, Meditation, Reflexology, Shiatsu, Ayurvedic medicine, Nutritional medicine, and Yoga. Ayurvedic medicine remedies are mainly plant based with some use of animal materials. Safety concerns include the use of herbs containing toxic compounds and the lack of quality control in Ayurvedic facilities.

According to the National Health Service (England), the most commonly used complementary and alternative medicines (CAM) supported by the NHS in the UK are: acupuncture, aromatherapy, chiropractic, homeopathy, massage, osteopathy and clinical hypnotherapy.

Complementary medicine treatments used for pain include: acupuncture, low-level laser therapy, meditation, aroma therapy, Chinese medicine, dance therapy, music therapy, massage, herbalism, therapeutic touch, yoga, osteopathy, chiropractic, naturopathy, and homeopathy.

Many CAM approaches are used by a large percentage of people in the general public and cancer patients.

The 2007 National Health Interview Survey reported about 4 out of 10 adults used CAM therapy in the past 12 months, with the most commonly used treatments being natural products and deep breathing exercises.

One meta-analysis compared CAM use in various countries. On average, over half of all cancer patients use CAM therapies.

One large survey of cancer survivors reported on the use of complementary therapies. The therapies used most often were prayer and spiritual practice (61%), relaxation (44%), faith and spiritual healing (42%), and nutritional supplements and vitamins (40%). CAM therapies are used by 31–84% of children with cancer, both in and outside of clinical trials. CAM therapies have been used in the management of side effects caused by cancer or cancer treatment.

IN PALLIATIVE CARE

Complementary therapies are often used in palliative care or by practitioners attempting to manage chronic pain in patients. Integrative medicine is considered more acceptable in the interdisciplinary approach used in palliative care than in other areas of medicine. "From its early experiences of care for the dying, palliative care took for granted the necessity of placing patient values and lifestyle habits at the core of any design and delivery of quality care at the end of life. If the patient desired complementary therapies, and as long as such treatments provided additional support and did not endanger the patient, they were considered acceptable. The non-pharmacologic interventions of complementary medicine can employ mind-body interventions designed to" reduce pain and concomitant mood disturbance and increase quality-of-life.

POTENTIAL SIDE EFFECTS

Conventional treatments are subjected to testing for undesired side effects, whereas alternative treatments, in general, are not subjected to such testing at all. Any treatment—whether conventional or alternative—that has a biological or psychological effect on a patient may also have potential to possess dangerous biological or psychological sideeffects. Attempts to refute this fact with regard to alternative treatments sometimes use the appeal to nature fallacy, i.e. "that which is natural cannot be harmful".

An exception to the normal thinking regarding sideeffects is Homeopathy. Since 1938, the US Food and Drug Administration (FDA) has regulated homeopathic products in "several significantly different ways from other drugs." Homeopathic preparations, termed 'remedies,' are extremely dilute, often far beyond the point where a single molecule of the original active (and possibly toxic) ingredient is likely to remain. They are, thus, considered safe on that count, but "their products are exempt from good manufacturing practice requirements related to expiration dating and from finished product testing for identity and strength," and their alcohol concentration may be much higher than allowed in conventional drugs.

INSTRUCTIONS TO PATIENTS

Cancer patients using or considering complementary or alternative therapy should discuss this decision with their doctor or nurse, as they would any therapeutic approach. Some complementary and alternative therapies may interfere with standard treatment or may be harmful when used with conventional treatment. It is also a good idea to become informed about the therapy, including whether the results of scientific studies support the claims that are made for it. When considering complementary and alternative therapies, following questions should patients ask their health-care providers:

- What benefits can be expected from this therapy?
- What are the risks associated with this therapy?
- Do the known benefits outweigh the risks?
- What side effects can be expected?
- Will the therapy interfere with conventional treatment?
- Is this therapy part of a clinical trial? If so, who is sponsoring the trial?
- Will the therapy be covered by health insurance?

Further information on evaluating CAM therapies and practitioners is available from NCCAM.

CONCLUSION

Alternative therapies are an alternative to Western medicine. Some practitioners of alternative therapies will recommend against using Western evidence-based medicine. You should always discuss alternative therapies with your healthcare professional to ensure you understand the potential risks involved in stopping current treatment.

Many alternative therapies are only marginally regulated, if at all, by federal drug and medical regulation agencies and so the buyer should beware of the possible risks of these therapies. Even if there are scientific studies showing pain relief from alternative or complementary therapies, few use children as study participants. Often, there is no knowledge of whether an alternate therapy is safe for children, even if it has been shown to be safe or effective for adults.

Chapter 23

Entrepreneurship in Healthcare

The fundamental law of entrepreneurship is—What is good for the business is good for me? The entrepreneur think differently. They have historically been known as "Risk Takers". You should go out and reach for the stars.

SETTING GOALS

Good management is the key to success and good management starts with setting goals. Set goals for yourself for the accomplishment of the many tasks necessary in starting and managing your business successfully. Be specific. Write down the goals in measurable terms of performance. Break major goals down into sub-goals, showing what you expect to achieve in the next two to three months, the next six months, the next year, and the next five years. Beside each goal and sub-goal place a specific date showing when it is to be achieved.

Plan the action you must take to attain the goals. While the effort required to reach each sub-goal should be great enough to challenge you, it should not be so great or unreasonable as to discourage you. Do not plan to reach too many goals all at one time. Establish priorities.

Plan in advance how to measure results so you can know exactly how well you are doing. This is what is meant by "measurable" goals. If you cannot keep score as you go along you are likely to lose motivation. Re-work your plan of action to allow for obstacles which may stand in your way. Try to foresee obstacles and plan ways to avert or minimize them.

- *Getting started:*
  Before starting out, list your reasons for wanting to go into business. Some of the most common reasons for starting a business are:
  - You want to be your own boss
  - You want financial independence
  - You want creative freedom
  - You want to fully use your skills and knowledge

- Next you need to determine what business is 'right for you.' Ask yourself these questions:
  - What do I like to do with my time?
  - What technical skills have I learned or developed?
  - What do others say I am good at?
  - Will I have the support of my family?
  - How much time do I have to run a successful business?
  - Do I have any hobbies or interests that are marketable?
- Then you should identify the niche your business will fill. Conduct the necessary research to answer these questions:
  - What business am I interested in starting?
  - What services or products will I sell?
  - Is my idea practical, and will it fill a need?
  - What is my competition?
  - What is my business's advantage over existing firms?
  - Can I deliver a better quality service?
  - Can I create a demand for my business?
- The final step before developing your plan is the pre-business checklist. You should answer these questions:
  - What skills and experience do I bring to the business?
  - What will be my legal structure?
  - How will my company's business records be maintained?
  - What insurance coverage will be needed?
  - What equipment or supplies will I need?
  - How will I compensate myself?
  - What are my resources?
  - What financing will I need?
  - Where will my business be located?
  - What will I name my business?

  Your answers will help you create a focused, well-researched business plan, that should serve as a blueprint. It should detail how the business will be operated, managed and capitalized.

One of the most important cornerstones of starting a business is the business plan. Once you have completed your business plan, review it with a friend or business associate. When you feel comfortable with the content and structure, make an appointment to review and discuss it with your banker. The business plan is a flexible document that should change as your business grows.

"I'm sailing away, set an open course for the virgin sea
I've got to be free, free to face the life that's ahead of me
On board, I'm the captain, so climb aboard
We'll search for tomorrow on every shore
And I'll try, oh Lord, I'll try to carry on"

–"Come Sail Away", Dr. Pradeep Bhardwaj

A consultant is a knowledge worker. Therefore the first thing you need to ensure is that you have a sound *educational background* in your area of practice. In many areas of consultancy practice you also need to acquire a professional *certification* in your field. Each profession would have its own requirement for certification. The national nodal professional body for your profession will provide the necessary information in this regard.

A consultant is a person who works by selling their specialist knowledge. So you need to make sure you have this knowledge and have the propensity and appetite to develop it as the industry it serves changes. You may also need to acquire a professional qualification or certification. So make sure you have the requisite bits of paper. As soon as you do quit your job you will need to figure out your own balance between the time you spend marketing and the time you spend delivering. If you are delivering a lot then you will have little time for marketing. Do not neglect this or else when you run out of work to deliver there will be nothing in the future.

HOW IMPORTANT IS HANDS ON EXPERIENCE FOR A START-UP?

Can you Learn to Drive a Car by Reading the Instruction Manual?

While it is possible to think the big things through by going to a research stint, it gives little experience with the tactical skills and in dealing with ground realities. It is possible from a research perspective to come up with sound strategies and business ideas; but you may get severely hampered when it comes to actually implementing them. There is no denying that fact that you need a few years of hands on experience where you hone not only your technical skills, but also the people issues within the organization and outside.

Mentoring

Any business, including consultancy practice, is fraught with uncertainties. You may need to take decisions regarding issues beyond your immediate area of expertise. You will be buffeted by changing business realities due to myriad reasons, such as, competition, obsolescence, business cycles, regional and global geo-politics, and many more. To guide you through this jungle it is prudent to adopt a seasoned *mentor*. Ideally, he is a person whose professional background and expertise is from your area of consultancy practice, he has hands on experience in running a company and has a wide network of professional contacts. Adopt him, use him as a sounding board, treat him as your friend, philosopher and guide.

Entrepreneurial Thought Processes

Entrepreneurs think differently. The life of an entrepreneur is one of seeking and seizing opportunity. They have historically been known as risk takers. Learning to think in an entrepreneurial way could allow you to stay one step ahead of the competition, whether it be in your business or with other aspects of your life.

You should go out and reach for the stars. While you may not be successful in plucking one, you would not come up with a handful of mud either. It is a painful thing to start on your own. A 9–5 job gives a sense of security alright. But that security is given to you by those who take risks. And when you give that kind of security to others, the feeling is hard to describe. Makes you a humble and a fuller being.

Business Development

Once you are through with the initial phase of the start-up, you need to focus on the business development aspect of your consultancy practice.

A very important part of starting or growing a business is making contacts and creating a web of resources for your company. Creating both personal and professional bonds with other people is critical and could open doors for a budding consultant. To do this one could try to find common ground with new acquaintances and make some sort of connection with them. Always having business cards on hand and using them as a way to casually exchange phone numbers. One should try to go to as many social and business functions as possible. Making contacts is crucial to the future success of your business.

Some suggestions for doing this are: Make a list of individuals that you would like to meet. Then determine your common interests. Think of every possible connection you could have with these people. Are your children at the same middle school? Do you belong to the same religious/social organization? Are you both members of a certain club? Will they be attending an upcoming industry conference? Try to find the common link that will create a casual and relaxed first meeting. Once you do have the opportunity to meet, make a note of the place you met and the discussion you had. Pay attention to their interests and things that are important to them, whether they are business oriented or personal. It is appropriate to touch base with them or extend an invitation to some sort of gathering once every six months, just to keep the lines of communication open. To help you in your effort it could be useful to use a contact management program such as MS Outlook or Act! that allows you to keep updated information on contacts. These programs will also allow you to create notes on each individual and record your discussions. Creating a personal relationship with these individuals is the way to gain their trust and business. Keeping in touch with people is the way to maintain professional and personal relationships and the best way to promote your practice.

You never know how helpful the web of relationships could be to you in the future.

Conclusion

While you are contemplating at starting a consultancy practice, you may use these ideas to help you develop your thoughts. However, you must remember that each business is unique and there is no predefined roadmap for success. Ultimately, your convictions based on your unique experience, training, background and opportunities are the best guide. Best of luck!.

It is a great idea for a business start-up in these economically challenging times to sell your own knowledge and expertise as a consultant. Independent consulting is one of the fastest growing and most profitable business models around. More and more people are enjoying the independence and extra money it brings as well as the change in the quality of life through being in control of what you do and with whom you work.

So, what is a Consultant?

A consultant is someone who offers help to someone or a business trying to solve a problem. Consultants work in a specific field of knowledge and provide expert knowledge to help solve problems. This will be a field that you are most familiar with.

In theory almost anyone can be a consultant—as long as you have what a client wants. This usually means skill and knowledge to solve a problem. It is not necessary to be the world's leading expert in a particular field. Nor do you need to have been in the same line of business yourself, nor any other kind.

Among other things you will need to be able to '*sell yourself*', and have a very good appreciation and understanding of how to solve the problem that needs to be solved. This is normally good knowledge combined with experience and good communication skills.

Select something which you know about and something which you like. Can you communicate the benefits of your skills to a lay person? Can you write about what you know in a way that is easy for a person to understand? Can you explain how your knowledge and skill could solve a problem. These are all essential talents you will need to have in addition to the basic knowledge of the area in which you are offering expertise.

Save up as much Money as Possible before Starting

All too often, people go into business without any savings, exclusively using loan money from friends, banks, or the SBA. They except to be able to start paying the loans back right away with their profits. What these business owners do not realize is that it can take months or years to make a profit. And once a lender discovers a business is not as profitable as expected, the lender is likely to call in the loan or refuse to renew it for another year. Often new business owners then have to take out home equity loans or use credit cards to pay off their loans (which puts their home and credit rating at risk) [For more information, see Business Financing FAQ].

A better plan is to save up as much of the needed investment money as possible, including your living expenses for the first year, or even two. Odds are that your business would not be profitable for one to two years. Even if you get plenty of business coming your way—and your customers pay you on time, which is not always a sure thing—you will want to be able to invest most of that money back in the business for space, equipment, advertising, and insurance needs.

STEPS

Here are some steps that you will need to take to set-up your consultancy. Define your market before you do anything else. Who is it you are selling your consultancy and knowledge to and what do they want? Everything else rests on this. There is no point in doing anything until you can answer these questions. Where are the people you will be selling to and how do you know what it is they want. My point is this: however clever or knowledgeable you are about something is no guarantee that someone will pay you for it. So find out what they want first (related to your area of expertise of course) then go from there. This goes whether you are setting up as a sole trader or with others to create accompany. A mistake that many make is that they feel they are good at something and that the world owes them a living. Lots of businesses of all kinds go down the tubes for this reason. They invent or create a product and then look for someone to buy it. No! Look for something that people want then go away and create it!

Plan once you have answered the above question, prepare your business plan. A business plan will help you work through your vision and strategy for keeping the business working. What is the rationale that your business can succeed? Provide evidence! What exactly are your products and services (you may have a main one but develop other back end products too). What is it that you want to achieve by when. How much do you want to make be when. Be realistic and bold. What is your evidence that this figure can be reached. How are you going to market? What is your financial plan? Do you need to borrow? How will you convince lenders? There are lots more things that should be in a plan and each of these needs to be unpacked and detailed. Brainstorm these, then start putting them to a timeline.

Make a space to work, where are you going to work from? Many sole traders start from home. This is a good idea as it keeps overheads down. But if you do this make sure you inform the insurers of your house as turning your home into a workplace without telling them will render your insurance null and void. Choose a space in your home that is comfortable and warm. Obviously, you will need phone access, internet access, a place for your computer, files and books (consultants always have lots of books).

What about Marketing?

If you do not have clients or customers then you do not have a business. Usually, it pays to ensure that you have some before you leave your paid employment. The next thing to do is to inform them that you are ready and available for work.

Your marketing should narrow in on you being the expert that people need to solve their problems. A good way to do this is publish a few articles on the internet with links to your site (you must have a site!) which answers a question related to your field (you could go to *Answers.Yahoo.com* and look for a question to answer. Show your practical value to your potential customers. People need to get the idea that you are an expert, the expert. There are tons of ways you can market yourself and get your name out there. Here are 7 things you need to be thinking about:

1. *Networking*: Going to events where your target market congregates is one of the most effective. You will need business cards if you go to these. Also be prepared to speak to a wide range of people with a wide range of potential issues they may be looking for answers to. Start with the people you already know—your former colleagues and bosses, your friends and existing industry contacts. If there are name badges make sure you have the right information on yours. Talk to as many people as you can and collect business cards. Online networks are also important. These are

known as forums. Join the ones that form you target market. But do not abuse these through blatant marketing or you will just get banned. Use these to build relationships.

2. *Ask for referrals*: If you get work and it is successful ask your client for a referral or two. Normally people will be happy to recommend you. Ask for a quote you can put on your website. Even if the person to whom you are referred does not have any work for you at the present time ask if they too could refer you to other potential clients.
3. *Public presentations*: Consultants are usually good at communicating. You need to be able to talk about your area of expertise to all sorts of people. Speaking at events offers a great opportunity to get your message out there. This can terrify some. But fear not. Practice with a friend what you want to say. Use visual aids to detract attention from yourself. Keep what you want to say short and to the point and ask the audience questions frequently to maintain attention and interest and interaction. Volunteer to offer them free information. Contact you chamber of commerce, organizations and forums in your locality. See what possibilities there are at local colleges, universities and libraries.
4. *Adds and articles*: Try to get a short article in a publication or trade journal that your target market reads. This is good for your reputation and gets your message out there among potential purchasers. Make it interesting and engaging—not just an in-your-face advert. Approach a journalist or editor to write something for you. They are usually happy to have new information to provide. Put together a short e-book and put it on your website to sell.
5. *Direct mail*: You can distribute direct mail as sales letters, ad mailings, or brochures. The thing is to create a document that attracts the attention or your recipient, engages their interest, provokes their curiosity ultimately compels them to take action. It is absolutely imperative that you emphasize the benefits that your client will receive as a result of buying your services. Concentrate less on everything else.
6. *Cold calling*: Yes, I know—it sounds a pain and few people like it but do not neglect it. Practice cold techniques. Learn the first names of the people you want to speak to so that it sounds to the gatekeepers—of which there will be plenty—that you know them. Understand that the person you assume is the decision maker may not be. It could be the person above or below them or even along from them! Make your aim of a call to get an appointment. Keep it short, keep it clear and do it early in the morning—sometimes the person you want to speak to will be in before the secretary and may well answer the phone instead.

7. *Your website*: It is true that much of your business will be generated from face-to-face relationships. Some think that this means you do not really need a website. Think again! Your website is your presence on the web. A place for all those who do not know a person who can solve their problem personally—so they look online. It is a place where all those internet articles you are going to write can be stored so that people can see at a glance your expertise. It is a place where you offer back-end products and services, related business products and so on in addition to your consultancy service. Your site has the potential to send your income through the roof. Apart from having your contact details on there you absolutely must have lots of great copy (Yes, '*salescopy*'), and for goodness sake have an opt-in section so that you can collect all the email addresses of people who are interested in what you do.

Starting a consulting business or selling your knowledge takes not only your specialist expertise but also business knowledge and wisdom, tactics and patience. It relies on good communication and marketing, the ability to build rapport and to understand the needs of your potential clients.

Being a Consultant is Being in Business

The days of spending large sums of money on advertising have gone. That was last century's way of building business. These days, the focus is on building contacts, creating a reputation by helping people and solving their problems. All of this can be done at very low cost.

One of the biggest mistakes that new consultants make is to focus too much on being the expert and not enough on marketing themselves. You can be the most knowledgeable person in your field, but without marketing yourself, you are unlikely to win a consistent pipeline of clients that are ready to pay you for your consulting services.

Below is a list of key points that you should keep in mind each and every day. All of these simple statements can be put into practice with little or no money, yet together they can help you build a successful consulting business.

- Select a niche and remain focused
- Commit to yourself to being the undisputed expert in your niche
- Agree with yourself that you are in this business for the long-haul
- Be sure you have guts, determination and the ability to succeed
- Move away from negative people
- Listen and learn from those successful consultants who have trod before you
- Preserve your time and money

- Help people and give away an abundance of free advice
- Accept help from smart people when they offer it
- Never forget that you will need to consistently market yourself
- Do not make the mistake of selling. Instead, help people solve their problems.

Out of all the above, you might still be asking the question; "are you sure I do not need a large budget to market my consulting business?" I can fully appreciate that concern, especially when there is so much advertising in newspapers, magazines and TV these days.

I can assure you that plenty of very successful consultants all over the world have attained their success without a large advertising budget. In fact some of the principles of advertising are so simple, they are overlooked by most.

Knowing these simple marketing principles can make the difference between a successful consultant and a failed consultant who has to go back to working for someone else, all because they neglected the importance of marketing. Knowing your subject might be sufficient to 'get a job', but it is very insufficient if you want to be a successful independent consultant.

There are some very good resources on the internet and books on the subject of consulting. Some spend more time discussing business cards, premises and tax than on the more critical success factors such as marketing. However, there are some excellent resources available that will show you how to market yourself as an independent consultant using a small budget.

If you are committed to succeeding and are prepared to listen to the right people, there is no reason why you cannot become a successful consultant.

TIPS FOR INTERNAL CONSULTANCY

From our considerable experience of internal consultancy work, we have listed below a few of what we feel are the key tips for anyone working in this field. We hope that you find them helpful.

—Fred Sherwin

- *Success in consultancy is as much about managing relationships as content*: Of course, for some 'expert' assignments the content is crucial. However, for most, it is the building and maintaining of relationships—particularly between consultant and client—that leads to successful assignments.
- *What all clients want*: Each client is different—in the way they see your role, in the level of involvement they wish, and in the sort of results they seek. With experience, one learns to read the situation, adapt, and

establish an agreed working relationship. However, the following are common to virtually all clients:

- *No unexpected surprises*: More anything else, this needs to be the touchstone that governs any consultancy assignment. If anything is going amiss, clients want to know in case it impacts on something else they or others are doing.
- *A success*: It is easy to forget this at times, but almost all clients want a success—it reflects on them just as much as it reflects on you. But how does your client define success?
- *Clarity and flexibility*: They want to be clear what your role is and what you are planning to do, but also expect you to be flexible and able to adapt to changed circumstances. Thus, work to define your role and then stay in it, but be prepared to flex and adapt when needed.
- *Your interest*: They expect you to be interested in their work, their ideas, their people, and the issues they face.

- *Have a consultancy process*: You need to have in mind a consultancy process that you expect to progress through, as a game-plan for both yourself and the client. Not just because it is tidy but because it helps you to manage the client relationship. The one that we use envisages an assignment as progressing through five broad stages:
  - *Entry*: Where one builds the initial relationship with the client and carries out an initial survey or scoping to establish what the assignment is about, what it should aim to achieve, the likely time and effort required, and possible risks and difficulties.
  - *Contracting*: Where one agrees with the client what the task is, what the consultant's role is, and how it should be tackled.
  - *Diagnosis*: Gathering information and ideas to arrive at options and a plan of action.
  - *Intervention*: Taking actions to deliver the results, be it a report or organizing the changes.
  - *Withdrawal*: Ensuring that the client organization can carry on without you and leaving the ground clear for your future involvement.

    This is a general model and you may find it best to amend it to something that suits your own particular work and style. You may need to customise a process for a particular assignment.
- *On the practice of consulting:*
  - *The golden rule—Start with an initial survey or scoping*: The initial meeting between client and consultant is crucial. If the client is in a rush or under pressure, there is a danger that you might be agreeing to a brief, resources and timescales without knowing

very much at all about the issues and difficulties. An initial survey followed by a brief proposal and a further meeting, gives both you and the client a much better basis for moving forward.
- *If you are unsure or wish to change the brief—go back to the client*: During the assignment, if you become at all unsure about the brief or feel that it needs to be changed, go back to the client and discuss it. If you feel that way, then the likelihood is that the client feels the same. If things are deviating from what the client expects—tell them. What they want most of all is no unexpected surprises.
- *Be organized*: If you are acting as a consultant, the client expects that you will be professional. To maintain that image, you do need to be well organized. If you start to make errors or miss meetings, then that image will be eroded. Plan and project manage your assignment well.
- *Managing expectations is key*: When assignments do start to flounder, in most cases, it is because a mismatch develops between the clients expectations and the consultants plans and activities. This is why in many assignments, regular stock-takes, perhaps by note or phone, are needed.
- *Get connected and stay connected*: If you want to get and retain the client's confidence and respect, you need to convince them that you are connected—that you understand their world. Some key pointers are:
  - Get to know the client's business so that you understand their pressures, concerns and priorities.
  - Be aware of other projects going on so that you have a similar context to them.
  - Try to keep connected with the daily happenings in the team, e.g. concerns and priorities.
- *Consciously build your own reputation with the client*: The more respect that the client has for you and your work, the more impact you will have and the more they will ask you to input. It also means that at the end you can withdraw to return.

• *Learning to read situations*: If managing relationships is the key to success in consulting, then it is the behavior and interpersonal skills of the consultant that make that happen. All really skilled consultants have excellent interpersonal skills. They need them in order to:
  - Read situations
  - Build empathy with clients and others
  - Gain the trust and respect of those they are working with
  - Facilitate meetings
  - Influence others

- Tailor communications to suit the audience
- Predict peoples' reactions
- Avoid or get out of difficult situations.

These skills—listening, observing, questioning, challenging, influencing, negotiating—are fundamental to good consulting and can all be developed through training and experience. They form a key element of our consultancy skills training.

- *About you as a consultant*:
  - *Where is your consulting 'comfort zone'?*: Your comfort zone is the style that you are personally most comfortable with. For some it is "process consulting", for others "facilitation", for yet others it is "expert advice". We can all flex and operate outside of this comfort zone—but only within limits. What is your comfort zone and what are the limits?
  - *What are your strengths and weaknesses?*: Planning, organizing, interpersonal skills, creativity? Identify them and then major on your strengths and start to develop to remedy your weaknesses.
  - *What is your organizational role?*: Internal consultants often have a dual role. They consult but they are part of a group with functional responsibilities which carry a monitoring accountability, e.g. internal audit. Such dual roles can make uneasy bedfellows and confuse both you and the client.
- *Consultancy ethics*: And finally—consultancy can be a seductive role. One can be in a situation of having influence and knowledge far beyond what people in the client's team have. Some consultants can be tempted to misuse this. But as a consultant you do need a set of ethics to work to.

  If a client invites you into their operation to help them, they have the right to expect that you:
  - Respect the client's knowledge
  - Be careful not to be over-prescriptive or judgemental
  - Respect confidentiality
  - Avoid becoming involved in the internal politics
  - Remain in the role that the client expects you to fulfill.

INTERNAL CONSULTANCY SKILLS CASE STUDY

For four years, we supported a Central Government Department with the introduction of their '*professionalism through quality*' initiative to their thirty local operating sites located all over the UK.

After an initial survey, we developed a proposal to run training workshops for members of change teams based at their 30 local operating sites.

- The teams were to start and lead local initiatives
- The workshop covered both process and service improvement techniques and consultancy skills for change agents
- The teams would be guided by a national steering group which also sponsored UK-wide improvements.

The whole program was highly successful. We ran workshops across the UK covering one hundred and fifty members of PTQ teams who then 'kick-started' and led local initiatives.

Thereafter, we advised senior managers and the steering group, developed a self-assessment 'health-check' to help to steer progress at each operating site, and introduced further training as required. The momentum and interest grew and by the end of that period every site in the UK had an active team working on identifying local customer improvements.

Outcome

All the PTQ teams were able to return to their sites and develop a local initiative. These led to numerous improvements in working practices and procedures to improve customer service.

Consulting Skills

A workshop to train participants in the consultancy skills needed to successfully work with clients. It covers:

- *Operating as a consultant:*
  - The consultancy phases
  - What clients want and building a relationship
- *Entry and contracting:*
  - Managing initial contacts
  - Key skills and behaviors
  - Client and consultant roles
- *Diagnosis:*
  - Research and analysis
  - Stakeholder and clients needs
  - Establishing the issues
- *Intervention:*
  - Different intervention styles
  - Scoping the project
  - Developing proposals
- Withdrawal and the future role
  - It includes key interpersonal skills of listening, questioning, and influencing.

Facilitation Skills

A workshop to train participants in the key interpersonal skills of facilitation. It covers:

- The facilitation process and role.
- Establishing and building the relationship.
- Facilitating meetings—how groups develop and behave
- Intervention strategies—what to use; when and how?
- *Key interpersonal skills:*
  - Observing
  - Listening and questioning
  - Challenging and influencing.

A self-assessment helps participants to identify their own strengths and weaknesses.

Research, Analysis and Problem Solving

Aimed at all who wish to become better acquainted with the approaches, tools, and techniques of structured problem solving. It covers:

- Scoping the problem
- Collecting the information required—hard and soft information
- Establishing the 'real' problem—the root causes
- *Tools and techniques:*
  - Brainstorming, mindmaps
  - Fishbone analysis, process mapping and beyond
- *Finding solutions:*
  - Tools for creativity
- *Implementing:*
  - Roadblocks and how to remove them.
  - Plans, pilots and implementation.

We have taken that framework as the structure of this consultancy skills toolkit. The toolkit is in four parts, each accessed by the buttons at the top of the page or by the links here:

TOOLKIT

Overview	The key aspects of the consultancy role and approach.
Working with clients	The skills to work with and manage clients and their expectations.
Delivering projects	The skills to manage consultancy projects to the clients requirements.
Dealing with people	The interpersonal skills to work with and deal with people.

THE CONSULTANCY PROCESS

You need to have in mind a consultancy process that you intend to progress through. You need it as a game-plan both for yourself and the client. Not just because it is tidy, but because it helps you to manage the client relationship. The one that we use envisages an assignment as progressing through five broad stages:

Five consultancy stages

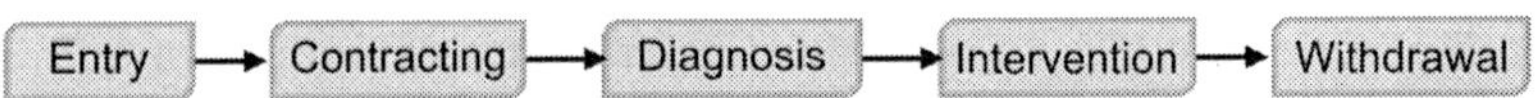

- *Entry*: Where one builds the initial relationship with the client and carries out a survey or scoping to establish what the assignment is about, what it should aim to achieve, the likely time and effort required, and possible risks and difficulties.
- *Contracting*: Where one agrees with the client what the task is, what the consultant's role is, what the client's role is, and how the work should be tackled.
- *Diagnosis*: Gathering information and ideas to arrive at options and a plan of action.
- *Intervention*: Taking actions to deliver the results, be it a report or organizing the changes.
- *Withdrawal*: Ensuring that the client organization can carry on without you and leaving the ground clear for your future involvement.

This is a general model and you may find it best to amend it to something that suits your own particular work and style or for a particular assignment.

WHAT ALL CLIENTS WANT?

Each client is different—in the way they see your role, in the level of involvement they wish, and in the sort of results they seek. With experience, one learns to read the situation, adapt, and establish an agreed working relationship. However, the following are common to virtually all clients:

- *No unexpected surprises*: More anything else, this needs to be the touchstone that governs any consultancy assignment. If anything is going amiss, clients need to know. In particular in case, it impacts on something else they or others are doing.
- *Success*: You want success but so do your clients—it reflects on them just as much as it reflects on you. But how does your client define success? Spend some time in the early days establishing just that.
- *Clarity and flexibility*: They want to be clear what your role is and what you are planning to do, but also expect you to be flexible and able to

adapt to changed circumstances. Thus, work to define your role and then stay in it, but be prepared to flex and adapt when needed.
- *Your interest in them*: They expect you to be interested in their work, their ideas, their people, and the issues they face. Try to exhibit that.

On the Practice of Consulting

These are simply seven key points on the practice of consulting—tips and guidelines.

1. *The "Golden Rule" always start with an initial survey*: The initial meeting between client and consultant is crucial. If the client is in a rush or under pressure, there is a danger that you might be agreeing to a brief, resources and timescales without knowing very much at all about the issues and difficulties.

   Always aim to leave that initial meeting with an agreement to you carrying out an initial survey so that you can assess the task, issues and difficulties. This together with a short proposal and a further meeting, gives both you and the client a much better basis for moving forward.
2. *If you are unsure or wish to change the brief—go back to the client*: During the assignment things change. If you become at all unsure about the brief or feel that it needs to be changed, go back to the client and discuss it. If *you* feel that way then the likelihood is that the client feels the same. If things are deviating from what the client expects—tell them. What they want most of all is no unexpected surprises.
3. *Be organized*: If you are acting as a consultant, the client expects that you will be professional. To maintain that image, you do need to be well organized. If you start to make errors or miss meetings, then that image will be eroded. Plan and project manage your assignment well.
4. *Managing expectations key*: When assignments do start to flounder, in most cases it is because a mismatch develops between the clients expectations and what the consultant is doing. This is why in many assignments, regular stock-takes, perhaps by note or phone, are needed.
5. *Get connected to their world*: If you want to get and retain the client's confidence and respect, you need to convince them that you are connected—that you understand their world. Some key pointers are:
   - Get to know the client's business so that you understand their pressures, concerns and priorities.
   - Be aware of other projects going on so that you have a similar context to them.
   - Try to keep connected with the daily happenings in the team, e.g. concerns and priorities.

6. *Consciously build your own reputation with the client*: The more respect that the client has for you and your work, the more impact you will have and the more they will ask you to input. It also means that at the end you can withdraw to return.
7. *Learn to read situations*: If managing relationships is the key to success in consulting, then it is the behavior and interpersonal skills of the consultant that make that happen. All really skilled consultants have excellent interpersonal skills. They need them in order to read situations, build empathy with clients, and gain the trust and respect of those they are working with. The skills of listening, observing, questioning, challenging, influencing, negotiating—are fundamental to good consulting.

About You as a Consultant

Consultancy Styles (Fig. 23.1)

There are a variety of consultancy styles—each suited to different people and different situations. For example:

- Some consultants adopt the *expert style*—they see themselves as bringing a knowledgeable, independent approach to the client—a depth of knowledge and expertise that the client lacks. A style often employed by medical practitioners, technical/IT consultants, and business strategy analysts. Extremely useful in some situations but absolutely inappropriate in others.
- Others see their prime contribution as working on and helping with the *process*. Sometimes working with the client to help them to decide what is to be done and how it is to be achieved, sometimes working

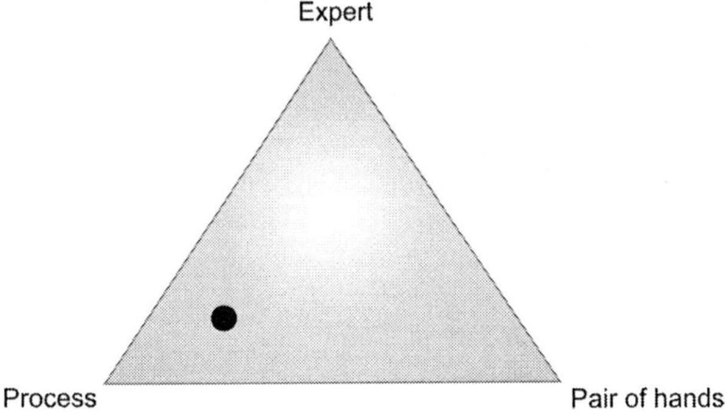

Fig. 23.1 Consultancy styles

with a manager to help them review their management style, or at other times working with a team to help them work together more effectively. Coaching, counseling, and organizational development all fall under this heading.

- Yet others see themselves as essentially a *pair of hands*. Their task is to help the client to implement the clients strategies, plans, and decisions. A style often employed by some of the larger consultancy bureaus.

So, which style is the best one? Clearly, it depends on what the situation and the client requires. In some situations, the expert style may be most effective, whereas in others the process style would be best employed.

In practice, consultants rarely work within one single style—their position is somewhere within the triangle above. The dot in the triangle depicts someone who has a strong preference for process working but who can flex into other styles as the situation requires.

For practicing consultants the message from this is quite simple:

1. Try to establish your own preferred style of consultancy—essentially where you lie within the triangle—and then develop your ability to flex and operate in your less preferred styles. (*Note: Process consulting is covered best in books by Edgar Schein who pioneered the field.*)
2. When starting an assignment, consciously assess what style of consultancy the situation and the client require and what you can provide. Attempt to avoid a style mismatch, e.g. working in a process mode with a situation and client that requires an expert mode.
3. In your contracting, ensure that you agree this with the client—so that they are clear about the style you will be adopting.

Consultancy Development—Key Points

- *Where is your consulting 'comfort zone'?*: Your comfort zone is the style that you are personally most comfortable with. For some, it is 'process consulting', for others 'facilitation', for yet others it is 'expert advice'. We can all flex and operate outside of this comfort zone—but only within limits. What is your comfort zone and what are the limits?
- *What are your strengths and weaknesses?*: Planning, organizing, interpersonal skills, creativity? Identify them and then major on your strengths and start to develop to remedy your weaknesses.
- *What is your organizational role?*: Internal consultants often have a dual role. They consult but they are part of a group with functional responsibilities which carry a monitoring accountability, e.g. internal audit. Such dual roles can make uneasy bedfellows and confuse both you and the client.

Consultancy Ethics

Finally, consultancy can be a seductive role. One can be in a situation of having influence and knowledge far beyond what people in the client's team have. Some consultants can be tempted to misuse this. But as a consultant you do need a set of ethics to work to.

If a client invites you into their operation to help them, they have the right to expect that you:

- Respect the client's knowledge
- Be careful not to be over-prescriptive or judgmental
- Respect confidentiality
- Avoid becoming involved in the internal politics
- Remain in the role that the client expects you to fulfill.

WORKING WITH CLIENTS

If there is anything that distinguishes the excellent consultant from the average it is the way that they relate to and work with (and in fact manage) their clients.

This does not simply happen automatically and without effort. To really work effectively with a client the consultant has to invest time and effort in:

- Understanding the clients world—their business and organization, and the pressures they face
- Understanding how it feels to be the client dependant on the consultants efforts
- Keeping in touch with the dynamics of the clients situation
- Keeping the client in touch with how the consultant is progressing
- Sorting out those things that need to be brought to the clients attention from those which would only confuse and distract.

This section contains some models and analyses from the field of customer service that our own clients have found valuable. Use them to think through what you feel your clients requirements are.

Professional Versus Mass Services

Clearly, good customer service is vital in any consultancy assignment. However, when thinking about customer service in consultancy, it is vital to distinguish between:

- A *mass service* as provided by a fast food restaurant or a shop
- A *professional service* as provided by a solicitor, architect, or doctor.

Most customer service ideas are based on providing a mass service. Although there are elements in common, there are also significant differences, summarized in the Table 23.1.

Table 23.1 Differences between mass and professional services

Mass services	Professional services
• Has customers	• Has clients
• Usually a one-off contact	• Regular or repeating contact
• Brief contact—a transaction	• Extended client contact—a project
• Customers with similar needs	• Clients with varying needs
• Pre-prepared service	• Service created/customized for particular client
• Customer often knows exactly what they want	• Clients often does not have the technical expertise to know what they want—they just want a solution to their problem

KEY CONCLUSION

Serving clients is different to serving customers.

Each client is unique with particular needs and all consultants need to invest time and effort in building and maintaining the relationship. In particular:

- In understanding their clients situation
- In building trust and a relationship with them
- In ensuring that their client is up-to-date with progress
- In ensuring their client keeps them up-to-date on relevant developments
- In ensuring that their client understands sufficiently the professional or technical options available—even at times coaching or training their client in this.

Key Point

Clients and professionals, by nature, tend to have different views as to what the service is. Professionals tend to emphasize the core specialist elements, clients value the softer 'helpful' peripheral elements.

Successful professionals recognize this and adapt their style to suit. In particular, they invest time and effort in ensuring that they have a good grasp of the clients world and perspective, and attempt to accommodate to that.

Its all about perceptions and expectations. A survey was carried out of accountancy practices in three countries—UK, Sweden, and Canada. The researchers identified eight elements of service provided by such practices:

1. Technical expertise
2. Taxation advice
3. Statutory
4. Peace of mind/confidence
5. Problem solving

6. Ideas testing
7. Financial advice
8. Prestige.

Each practice and their clients were asked to score these for importance. The results can be seen by clicking on the picture here.

The key points were as follows:

- In all cases the professionals providing the service rated the core technical elements as being the features that the client valued most (financial advice, technical expertise).
- Whereas the actual clients placed much more emphasis on the softer peripheral elements (peace of mind, confidence, statuary, tax advice).

Surveys of solicitors gave similar results, with clients rating approachability highest.

WHAT IT FEELS LIKE TO BE A BUYER (FIG. 23.2)?

The following was taken from a slide presentation about buyers reviewing competitive tender proposals. It summarizes some of the thoughts that go through a buyer's head when making such decisions and choices.

It is particularly relevant to consultants when an assignment is being established, but also some of the feelings described continue during the progress of the assignment.

Clients and Professionals Working Together

Clients and professionals do not always have comfortable relationships.

For example, some typical comments clients make about professionals are:

- Know their subject but are not always easy to work with
- Can be inflexible—wants to provide Rolls Royce next year when Mini today would do
- They do not understand my situation, nor do they want to. They just want to design computer systems (or accounts/layouts/reports, etc.)
- Too many unexpected surprises

Also, some typical comments professionals make about clients might include:

- Just too political.
- Only does what their boss wants them to do
- Just wants to protect their own back
- Would not make decisions—always wants to wait to see what others think
- Does not really understand the technical issues involved.

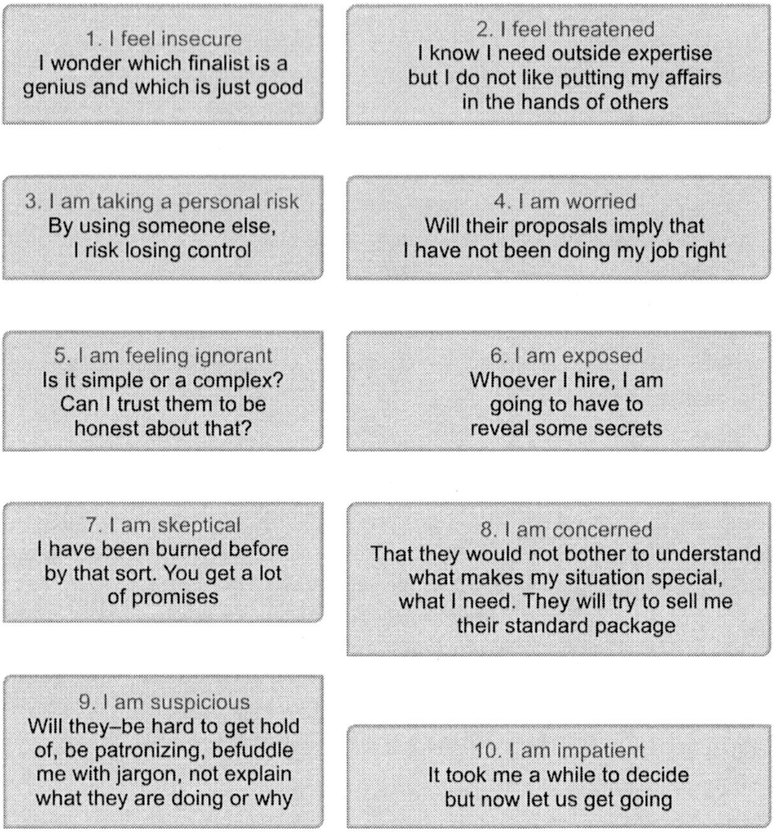

1. I feel insecure
I wonder which finalist is a genius and which is just good

2. I feel threatened
I know I need outside expertise but I do not like putting my affairs in the hands of others

3. I am taking a personal risk
By using someone else, I risk losing control

4. I am worried
Will their proposals imply that I have not been doing my job right

5. I am feeling ignorant
Is it simple or a complex? Can I trust them to be honest about that?

6. I am exposed
Whoever I hire, I am going to have to reveal some secrets

7. I am skeptical
I have been burned before by that sort. You get a lot of promises

8. I am concerned
That they would not bother to understand what makes my situation special, what I need. They will try to sell me their standard package

9. I am suspicious
Will they–be hard to get hold of, be patronizing, befuddle me with jargon, not explain what they are doing or why

10. I am impatient
It took me a while to decide but now let us get going

Fig. 23.2 Feelings of a buyer

The Clients World

They are buying your service, and almost by definition they are buying a service the details of which they do not understand and probably do not want to understand. How ideally should one handle them?

The key is to working successfully with clients is to really understand them and the world they operate in, and ensure that your actions as a consultant help rather than hinder the client-without compromising your professional standards. Three points about the clients world:

1. *They are representatives of others*: Often, a representative for others in the customers organization, nominated or appointed to represent them in terms of what they want and expect from you.

Clients have to respond to and manage the pressures and wishes of these others—perhaps why they often change their minds frequently. They may need the professionals help in doing so.

2. *The project to them is "Just another brick in the wall"*: To the professional the project is very important, vital. It is their main if not sole task. To the client it is only a small part of a larger scheme.

   When professionals get angry at clients for changing (for example) the wording in the booklet, they forget that to the client it is not just another booklet but a Government White Paper committing the country to a new tax. Delays or weaknesses in the service provided often have a ricochet effect on the larger scheme and then on the clients career.

3. *Their future career depends on your performance*: For many clients the project is only a part of their working world. They have bosses, colleagues, peers, and perhaps aspirations of a career. Yet their performance in that world often depends upon the professional.

   So what they invariably want from their consultant is:
   - Understand my world, my problems
   - Treat me as an individual
   - No unpleasant surprises
   - Help me look good with my bosses and my colleagues.

It is this perspective of the client that explains the value they place on the softer peripheral aspects of the service.

The Professionals World

The main point about professionals is their specialism and expertise. They enjoy practising their craft and get a lot of pleasure and satisfaction from practising it *well*, as judged by their colleagues, fellow professionals at large, and of course their clients; often in that order.

They often belong to a group of similar such professionals with whom they discuss their craft, even at lunch or after hours. People outside the group often do not understand the finer nuances of their craft.

To them it is the *core technical elements* that are important. It is where they practice their craft, it is what that their colleagues respect, and it is often where they see as their future. And it is through this that they themselves define *quality of service*.

CASE

Clients and professionals, by nature, tend to have different views as to what the service is. Professionals tend to emphasize the core specialist elements, clients value the softer "helpful" peripheral elements. Of course, there are always other issues which affect that quality (managing resources, staff appraisals, internal conflicts, etc.), but this difference in perceptions is the key one.

This short case illustrates a number of the issues often found in organizations providing professional services, be they computer consultancies as above, or advertising, designers, solicitors, accountants, etc.

BACKGROUND

The Division was meeting for a one-day workshop to review the results of its recent customer survey. About 30 people strong, a mixture of professionals and administrative support, it specialized in designing and providing tailor-made computer systems. Because of recent outside pressures the managers had been trying to improve the performance and image of the Division over the last two years through a mixture of restructuring, teambuilding, and quality improvement initiatives. The customer survey was the latest step in this.

DIVISION

The Division had a fairly high *esprit de corps*. People were interested and committed to their field and viewed themselves as very professional. They worked hard on their projects and saw themselves as the equal or better of any of their competitors. Working on projects as they did, they rarely had a chance to meet as a whole team and people generally enjoyed these occasions, although some did get on their hobby-horses rather.

Nobody, aside from the managers, knew the results of the customer survey, but people were not too worried. They knew that some customers were rather particular and grumbled a little, but they were confident that the group was respected and their work valued. After all, the customers did seem to come back, usually.

The Clients' View

The group broke into small teams to review the results and a quiet hush descended on the room, to be broken after some ten minutes or so by a growing buzz with occasional loud expletives. The survey results were not at all what they had expected. It was not that they were disastrous but they were different and a far cry from the Divisions own perception of itself. The customers surveyed were not critical of what the Division saw as its core service, the systems it delivered; in fact there were not many comments about that. What most customers criticized were what the people in the Division saw a peripheral and incidental aspects. Typical comments included:

- They know their subject but are not always easy to work with.
- They can come over as rather arrogant. They seem to always think that they know best.
- They can be rather inflexible. A feeling that they always want to provide a Rolls Royce next year when a Mini now would do.
- Sometimes I feel that they do not understand my situation, nor do they want to. They just want to design computer systems.
- The final system was good but there were too many unexpected surprises on the way. I only heard about problems at the last moment.

The Response

The team discussions became heated and rather angry. "But this is not fair" was a common cry. The customers were ignoring the quality of the systems and that surely was the main thing. They also ignored all the hard work, often done after hours, that people put into the projects. All the criticisms seemed to be about incidental aspects. Perhaps we should all be trained to say "Have a nice day" was one comment. "Perhaps we should get McDonalds or Disneyland to run a training course" was another? Some people queried the way in which the survey was done, perhaps the wrong questions had been asked. Others questioned whether the client sponsors were the right ones, perhaps all projects should be sponsored by the top managers.

They all returned to the main room and in the general discussion that followed, it was agreed that the Division clearly had an image problem and a working party was set-up to create a new promotional brochure. After lunch, the Division had a fascinating speaker on "ISDN and the latest developments" and then everyone returned to their desks and offices to resume their projects.

Ingredients of a Service

From the Clients viewpoint, any service has three ingredients, illustrated in Figure 23.3.

1. Does the core package provide the elements that I want?
2. The performance—Is it OK for quality, delivery reliability, reaction times, etc.?
3. The experience—Are they easy to work with?—Was the journey good?

From the clients perspective, professionals often tend to overvalue the first, the core, and underestimate the value that clients place on the other two, softer peripheral items. Success comes from delivering on all three.

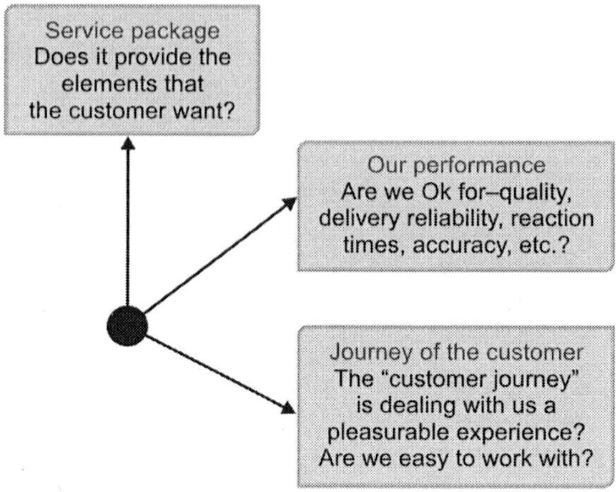

Fig. 23.3 Three dimensions of service

JOURNEY OF THE CUSTOMER: ANALYSIS (FIG. 23.4)

Background

This analysis is based on one of the iconic "customer strategy" tales of the 1980s.

In the early 1980s Jan Carlzon, the then president of Scandinavian Airlines (SAS), took an airline that was failing and turned it around to be one of the most respected airlines in the industry. His strategy for achieving this was as along the following lines:

1. The SAS business depended on repeat business on ensuring that its customers were so impressed with their trip that they booked on SAS the next time they flew. In Jan Carlzon's words, from this viewpoint, the real assets of SAS were not the planes and equipment, but satisfied customers—customers who would return to SAS.
2. In the eyes of those customers, SAS really existed only as a whole series of moments of truth—*Anytime a customer comes into contact with any aspect of a business, however remote, is an opportunity to form an impression.*

   These moments of truth cumulatively create the image—good or bad—of SAS.

   Some examples of moments of truth for SAS were:
   - When you call to make a reservation to take a flight
   - When you arrive at the airport and check your bags curbside
   - When you go inside and pick up your ticket at the ticket counter

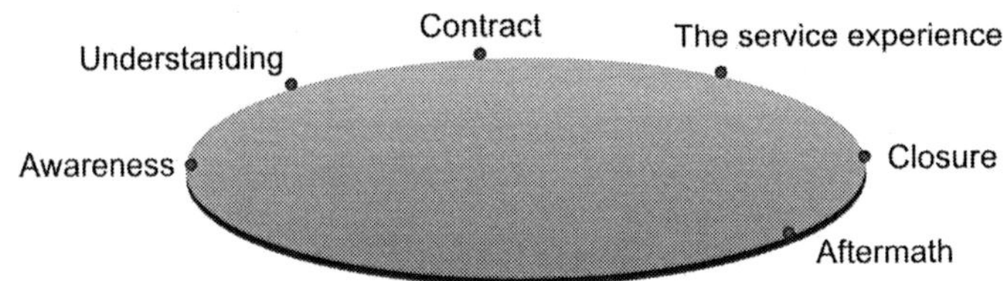

Fig. 23.4 Journey of customer: analysis

- When you are greeted at the gate
- When you are taken care of by the flight attendants onboard the aircraft
- When you are greeted at your destination.

3. In order to build up that image of SAS in the customers eyes and thus ensure repeat business he set about to get the whole organization to focus on these Moments of Truth and ensure that SAS managed them better. The impact was not just upon training and procedures, but extended even to the design of the aircraft and the scheduling of flights. Gradually, over a few years, this focus led to a major turnaround in SAS's fortunes and enabled it to survive and prosper when so many others failed to do so. In 1986, he summarized his experiences in his book called *Moments of Truth*-still worth reading.

JOURNEY OF THE CUSTOMER: DIAGNOSIS

The following diagnosis is based on those ideas—mapping the journey of the customers and the moments of truth that they face. It has been used with considerable success in a wide variety of improvement projects.

Step 1: Map out your Journey of the Customer

Figure 23.5 provides a good starting point for many services

- *Awareness*: How the customer becomes aware of the service you provide?
- *Understanding*: How the customer learns about the service and what it can do for them?
- *Contract*: How the customer contracts to take the service?
- *Service experience*: How the customer progresses through the service? It may help to make a detailed process map like the one below.
- *Closure*: How the service is completed and how the customer experiences that?
- *Aftermath*: How things are handled afterwards—in particular, how post-service difficulties are handled?

Step 2: Identify the Moments of Truth and the Hot-Spots

There are two main approaches to this:

1. *Internally*: As a team, go through the map step-by-step and brainstorm the Hot-Spots—those places where the customers may find the journey uncomfortable. In most cases this identifies the main hot-spots.
2. *Externally*: Use the map to develop a survey questionnaire for customers to complete or to be interviewed about. This can be very powerful for identifying hot-spots that your own people are blind to.

Step 3: Tackle the Hot-Spots

List the hot-spots, prioritise them, and then set-up teams to resolve them.

DELIVERING PROJECTS

In recent years the formal use of projects as a style of working has escalated in all organizations, both private and public sector.

In consultancy work, it is crucial that the consultants are all capable of designing and delivering projects to client requirements—it is fundamental.

However, unless projects are tackled with thought and care, they can go amiss. Typically, in terms of either not delivering what was required, delivering late, delivering at a higher cost in money or resources than was envisaged, or simply by causing too much disruption in the process.

Project management approaches were developed to tackle this situation. This section summarizes the key features which impact on consultancy skills. Those who wish more detailed information on the project management approaches and tools should visit our companion toolkit *Project Management Guide.*

SUMMARY OF THE PROJECT APPROACH (FIG. 23.5)

All organizations that manage projects on a regular basis develop a set of "ground rules" that summarize the way projects are managed in their organization. The following are our ground rules. They will apply to all projects, but will need to be tailored to suit a particular project.

1. *Projects are best managed through a broad structure of stages:*
   - Projects progress through the five broad stages—proposal, scoping and planning, start-up, implementation, and closure.
2. *Project organization:*
   - All projects to have a formal Project Manager and Project Sponsor.
   - The *Project Manager* is responsible for delivery of the project. To be chosen on the basis of skills, capability and knowledge of the project task, and their ability to get things done.

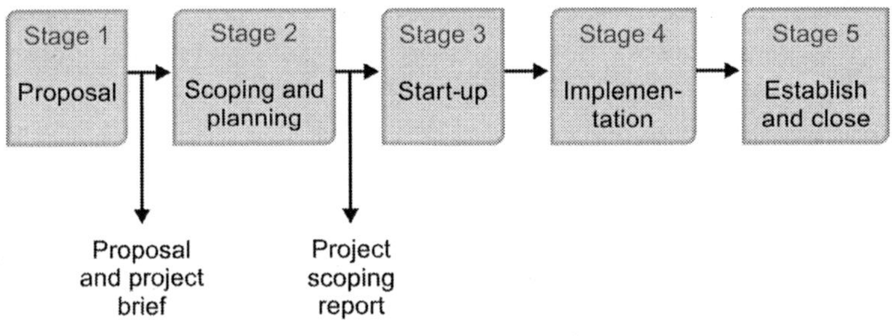

Fig. 23.5 Project approach

- The *Project's Sponsor* is responsible for looking after the project and the outcomes on behalf of the organization, and supporting the project manager. The sponsor may be an individual or a group.

3. *Projects are always scoped:*
   - The project proposal stage establishes what the project is to deliver. The project scoping stage is to plan and organize that delivery.
   - All projects to have a Project Scoping Stage where the Project Manager has the opportunity to scope the project.
   - This stage will normally last a few days (or weeks for larger projects).
   - It will focus on clarifying:
     - What the project objectives and terms of reference are?
     - What the issues are?
     - How the project should be organized and tackled—what tasks, what resources needed, what the schedule should be?
   - The conclusions should be summarized in a brief (typically two to five pages) Project Scoping Report (sometimes called project initiation document or project plan).
4. *Project scoping report:*
   - A brief two-to-five page document which describes what the project is to achieve and how it will be organized and tackled. It should cover the following:
     - Project terms of reference and objectives.
     - Benefits to be realized and costs and disruption to be contained.
     - Top level plan showing planned progress in terms of stages, milestones and activities.
     - Project organization showing who is involved and the key responsibilities—project manager, project sponsor, team and contributors.
     - Risks and implementation issues which may occur.

5. *Project control*: Project progress needs to be monitored and controlled. Progress control needs to be established to suit the particular project. This is normally achieved via discussion, meetings, and project reports.
6. *Project reporting*: There are four main project reports used in project management—project brief, project plan, progress report, postproject review.
7. *Key company procedures*: As well as project specific procedures, the project manager will need to follow particular organization-wide procedures, such as Contracts, Finance, IT, and human resources.
8. *Projects are often coordinated within programs*: Many organizations coordinate individual projects via a number of strategic programs. Each programe is built from a portfolio of inter-related projects, all contributing to a common outcome.

PROJECT PLANNING

No plan survives the first contact with the enemy

—Sun Tzu in the Art of War

Planning is one of the main secrets to successful project implementation.

- In the first place, during the planning stage a good plan enables the Project Manager to analyze how the work needs to be carried out and identify the options.
- In the second place, during the implementation stage, it provides a "baseline" to enable the Project Manager to judge whether the project is on course or not and thus control it.

To do this in practice, you need to focus on the project and draw up a complete list of the activities and tasks to be carried out showing the people or sections that would need to do them. Then chart these activities using a Critical Path analysis network, a Gantt chart, or milestone plan.

With this chart, talk to the people who would need to be involved about their contribution and to get their ideas, their estimates of time involved, and their availability. Continue this until, you have a fairly complete map of the project. During this process, you will start to identify possible difficulties and blockages and should become clear as to which activities are the critical ones—those, which could delay the whole project.

Having done that, simply get the team and other contributors to talk and think about what needs to be done, and then use charts to communicate that to others.

Planning Sheets, Milestone Plans and Gantt Charts

You will almost certainly need to use one of the following planning techniques to plan your project.

- *Stages plan* lays out the progress in a series of stages.
- *Critical path analysis* links the activities together to form a network. To use this technique, you will most likely need to have received training in it.
- *Milestone plans* focus mainly on the end-dates by which something needs to be complete or by which certain objectives need to be achieved.
- *Bar or Gantt Charts* focus more on the activities to be carried out to complete the project.

Each technique has its strengths and weaknesses and you need to select the technique most suited to your particular project. Each is illustrated in Table 23.2.

Table 23.2 Planning sheet

Activity	Date activity can start	Date activity must finish by	Estimated duration	People and resources involved	Estimated cost in time or resources

Critical Path Analysis

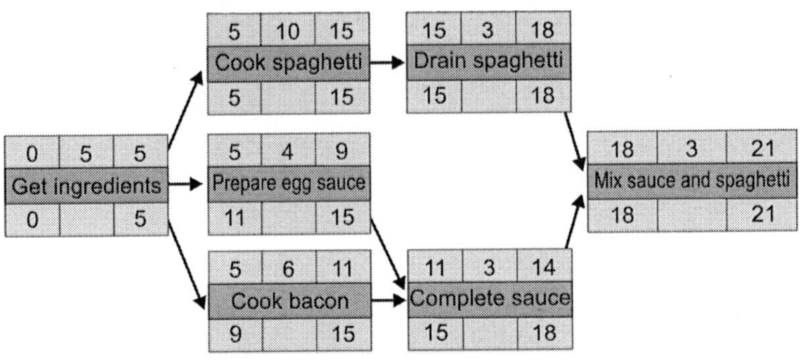

Stages Plan

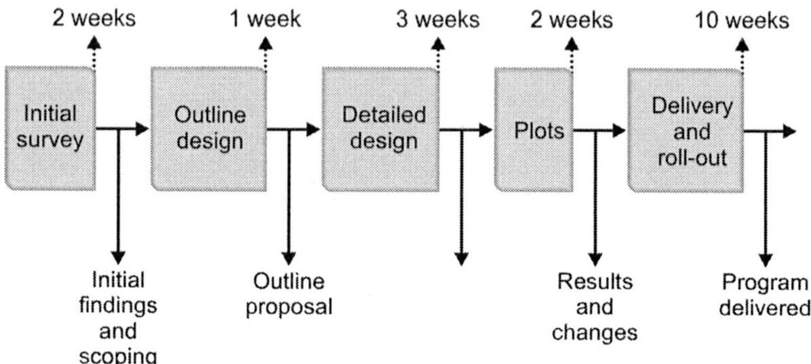

Gantt Chart

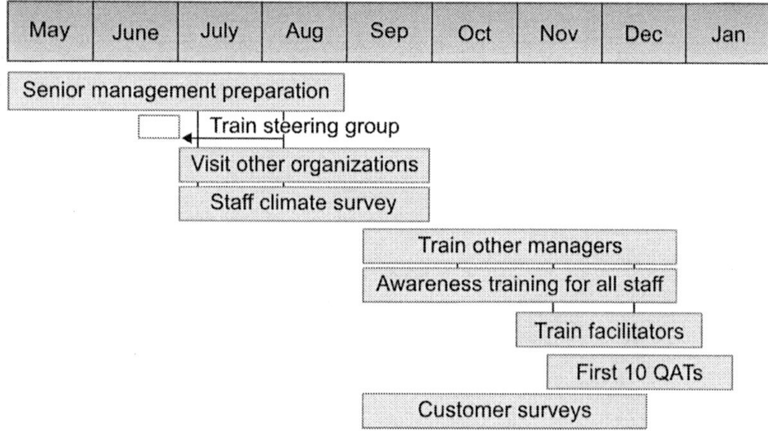

Milestone (End-Date) Plan

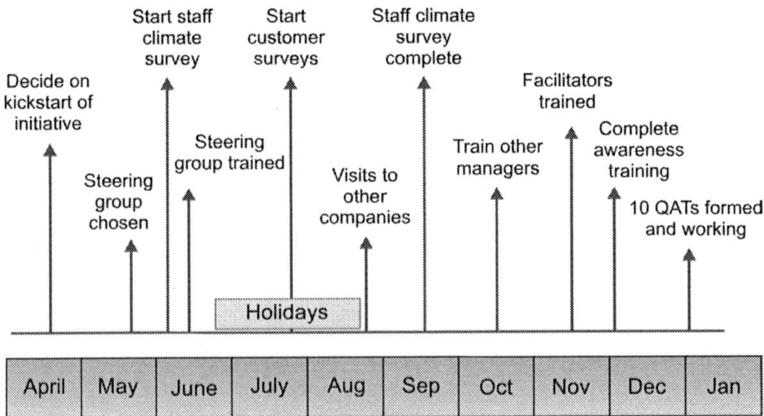

Project Reports

This section introduces the five main reports commonly used for project control and reporting. The sequence of reports is represented in the Flow chart 23.1.

KEY POINTS

- Some reports are more specific than others. The structure for the Project Scoping Report Plan is the most specific as this document will be used for central coordination of the organizations projects. Others are less specific in that their content may need to vary from project to project. For these the content should be agreed between project manager and project sponsor.
- The reports are progressive, for example, information in the Project Brief provides the basis for similar information in the Project Scoping Report.
- The Project Brief and Project Scoping Report templates are based on scoping a project.
- Regarding timing of the reports, it is generally best practice to produce them at a natural end-of-stage rather than at regular intervals.

MANAGING PROJECTS

In recent years, the formal use of projects as a style of working has escalated in all organizations, both private and public sector. All team leaders manage projects at some point in their work.

Flow chart 23.1 Sequence of reports

Project brief	The *Project Brief* is generally the first document. It is produced when the project is initiated by the Project Sponsor following a Project Proposal stage. It should establish for the project manager: • What the project is to achieve, by when, and within what resources?
Project scoping report	The *Project Scoping Report* (sometimes called project initiation document or project plan) is the second document. It is produced by the Project Manager following a brief *Scoping Project Study.* It should build on the Project Brief developing it to establish: • What the project is to achieve? • A detailed time schedule for carrying out the project • Details of the resources required—people, money, sections • Who is to be involved in the project? • What the risks and implementation issues are?
Project progress report	The *Project Progress Report* is produced by the Project Manager in agreement with the Project Sponsor. It should establish: • What progress has been made, what work is left remaining, and what the issues are?
Past project evaluation	The *Post Project Evaluation* is not produced for all projects. When it is produced by the Project Manager at the request of the Project Sponsor. It should establish: • How did the project progress and what were the issues we should be aware of for future projects?

However, unless projects are tackled with thought and care, they can go amiss. Typically, in terms of either not delivering what was required, delivering late, delivering at a higher cost in money or resources than was envisaged, or simply by causing too much disruption in the process.

Project management approaches were developed to tackle this situation. This section is a brief summary of the main features and contains two articles:

- Five key to success
- A success checklist for projects.

More detailed information on the project management approaches and tools can by found on our companion "Project Management Guide".

Five Keys to Success

So, what is a project? In practice, the distinction between what is "normal work" and "project work" can be quite gray. Many activities that we classify as just normal work can be called projects. Typically, the characteristics of a project are as follows:

1. A start and a finish
2. A time frame for completion
3. A unique event
4. An involvement of several people on an adhoc basis
5. A limited set of resources
6. A sequencing of activities and phases.

Over the past 50 years or so, project management has evolved as a pragmatic and structured approach to bringing some order to such situations. It can partially succeed in this but no one would claim that it is a universal panacea. It depends on the managers and staff applying the approaches—poor managers plus project management approaches only delivers poor project management.

It is a pragmatic approach, developed over time by drawing together a variety of approaches and methods from other areas—the point at which these started to form into a discipline was probably during the project for the development of Polaris missiles in the 1960s.

The essence is best summarized in the following five main features—five keys to success:

1. Objectives
2. Stages
3. Organization
4. Planning and Control
5. Leadership and Management.

Objectives

It is the project objectives which perhaps more than anything else "define" a project and make it concrete—what is the project there to achieve and by when?

The difficulty is often that everyone involved or affected by the project has their own ideas and interpretation of what those objectives should be, and even when agreement has been reached, as time moves on the ideas and interpretations diverge again.

Establishing and maintaining clarity and agreement on this, and then communicating it well—that is the first of the keys to success in projects.

Stages

All projects progress naturally through phases, e.g. a research and exploration phase, a decision phase, a planning and organizing phase, an implementation phase, and then a closure phase (This also applies to many of our personal projects—buying a car or a house, arranging a holiday).

The second key to successful project management is to not try to tackle the project as one great whole, but to "chunk" it down in appropriate stages (chunks), making each stage a "mini-project", and each end-of-stage a milestone. The stages that we use in this guidance are project proposal, scoping and planning, set-up, implementation, and establish and close.

Organization

Because projects often operate outside of the normal hierarchy, often also crossing boundaries, the Project Manager needs to establish organizational foundations for it. Typically, there are two issues:

- Who in the organization is sponsoring the project—who does the Project Manager report to for that project?
- Who needs to be organized to work on the project—the project team and how to do it?

Planning and Control

All projects, be they a new building or a cultural change project, are always moving into uncharted territory. The project manager has a choice—to cross fingers and hope, or to plan and replan to try to chart that territory and then adjust to suit, and communicate the changes. Project management opts for the latter. In it planning is done throughout the whole project on three levels:

- *Top-level planning*: To establish the viability and sense of the project and to structure (chunk) it into stages.
- *Implementation strategies*: To identify likely implementation issues and devise strategies to handle them; and finally.
- *Activity scheduling*: To plan in detail, what actions need to take place when, and who should be carrying them out.

Leadership and Management

The four items covered so far all create the foundations for managing the project but are not of themselves sufficient. You can have done all that but the project still goes amiss. They still need the fifth and most important key of all—the management and leadership of the Project Manager to make them work.

In almost, all projects these are simply the normal management skills that managers employ in their normal work—team development, negotiating, influencing, etc. applied to three strands:

1. Progressing the project.
2. Gaining and maintaining the support of "others".
3. Keeping the "team" connected, committed, and energised.

Where the "team" may be a formal team or simply a group of people providing occasional support, and "others" covers both the formal and informal "stakeholders" of the project.

In conclusion, a focus on these five does not guarantee success—no one can promise that—but it will lead to fewer crises, errors and time wasted on unnecessary remedial actions.

SUCCESS IN PROJECT MANAGEMENT

There is no "magic formula" to success in project management. In practice, it is simply a matter of introducing definition, focus and clarity into the project and then managing people and tasks actively to ensure progress. Experience of projects has shown that the successful ones have the following in common:

1. *The project is clearly relevant*: When the project is seen to be sensible, valuable and useful, and linked to the key tasks and objectives of the organization.
2. *There is a single project focus*: When there is a clear, named single Project Manager for the project.
3. *The sponsorship is sound*: When the project is well sponsored in the sense that there is a person or group who are clearly named as responsible for sponsoring the project on behalf of the organization, and who fulfill their duties well.

   In particular, this involves agreeing and approving the project and project plans with the Project Manager, linking and positioning the project in relation to others, and providing support to the Project Manager when required (enabling resources and support).
4. *There is a skilled and capable project manager*: When the project manager is competent and has the appropriate skills and knowledge for the work, and also has experience and expertise in project management approaches.

5. *There is a clear project management framework*: When the project is managed within a clear project management framework that is well understood and accepted within the organization.
6. *The project is well-scoped and planned*: When the project manager invests sufficient time and energy in the early days of the project in scoping it and planning it in detail.
7. *Empowerment and delegation are sufficient*: When the project manager is sufficiently empowered—in the sense that they can gain access to the resources needed to carry out the project and has the necessary delegated authorities to take decisions and act on their own authority when needed.
8. *The organizational climate is conducive*: When the project is carried out within an organizational climate where there is a high degree of cooperation, openness, and responsibility in terms of people doing what they have agreed to do.

In essence, it is through these eight factors that one reduces project risk. None of the above guarantee success on their own, but all contribute to reducing the risk of failure. Having them in place on your project does not guarantee success, but it will increase your chances considerably.

How Teams Develop?

The researchers were studying groups and in particular how groups developed.

They identified that generally groups have a fairly clearly defined growth cycle. Groups develop and mature, and in doing so they progress to maturity through four stages: Form, Storm, Norm, and Perform (Fig. 23.6).

1. *Stage 1—Forming*: The group is not yet a group but a set of individuals. This stage is characterized by talk about the purpose of the group, the definition and the title of the group, its composition, leadership, pattern, and life-span. At this stage, too, each individual tends to want to establish their personal identity within the group, make some individual impression.
2. *Stage 2—Storming*: Most groups go through a conflict stage when the initial, often false, consensus on purposes, on leadership and other roles, on norms of work and behavior, is challenged and re-established. At this stage a lot of personal agendas are revealed and a certain amount of interpersonal hostility is generated. If successfully handled, this period of storming leads to a new and more realistic setting of objectives, procedures and norms. This stage is particularly important for testing the norms of trust in the group.

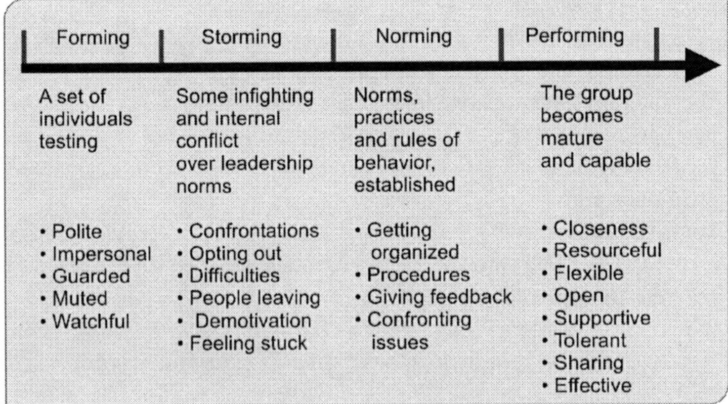

Fig. 23.6 Four stages of group development

3. *Stage 3—Norming*: The group needs to establish norms and practices. When and how it should work, how it should take decisions. What type of behavior, what level of work, what degree of openness, trust and confidence is appropriate. At this stage there will be a lot of tentative experimentation by individuals to test the temperature of the group and to measure the appropriate level of commitment.
4. *Stage 4—Performing*: Only when the three previous stages have been successfully completed will the group be at full maturity and are able to be fully and sensibly productive. Some kind of performance will be achieved at all stages of development but it is likely to be impeded by the other processes of growth and by individual agendas. In many committees the leadership issue, or the objective and purpose of the group, are recurring topics that crop up in every meeting in some form or other, seriously hindering the true work of the group.

TEAM FOCUS

1. Teams always go through the stages although some develop very rapidly, some slowly. Some teams stick in any of the early phases, and in fact never reach their maturity and their performing stage.
2. The team must pass through the stages, but they are able to influence and manage their progress so they pass through the stages quicker so that they become mature and effective more quickly. This is essentially what teambuilding does.
3. This model also links with the Adair model. The group will 'grow up,' will mature very rapidly when:

- the task is very important.
- the individuals are highly committed to the group.
- individual and group objectives are identical.

4. The different stages need to be managed differently. What is appropriate in a performing stage is not appropriate in the forming stage and vice-versa. There is alike here with the *Tannenbaum and Schmidt* Leadership Style Continuum.
5. Some of the disruptive behavior seen in groups (bickering, etc.) is not so much "bad behavior" as the natural development of the group, the working-through of the team issues.
   Experienced leaders recognize it as that and resist the temptation to "stamp down" on it, knowing that it will pass of its own accord.

TEAM ROLES

Everyone, by nature of their background and personality, has one or two preferred roles in a team—roles in which they feel most comfortable and are also most effective. Some people bring creativity to a team by introducing new ideas, others are good at planning and scheduling, others are good at chairing, and so on. The key point is that people have preferred team roles and that often, the key to success lies in getting the right mix of team roles.

In the 1960s, Meridith Belbin carried out research into this, showing that teams with a good balance of team roles performed better than teams with a poor balance, *even when the latter had more capable and brighter individual team members* (Fig. 23.7).

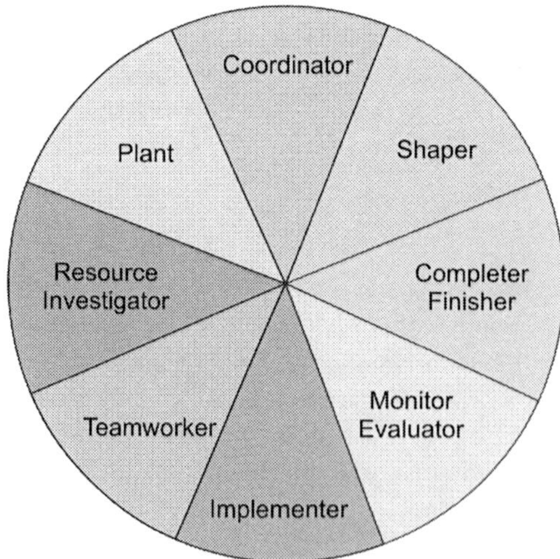

Fig. 23.7 Belbin team roles

His research laid the foundations for these ideas and he developed his Team Role Analysis described in more detail in his book *Management Teams—why they succeed or fail, R Meredith Belbin.* This also contains a self assessment to help you identify your own preferred team roles.

The ideas have been taken forward and many organizations (particularly in the USA) now always use team role analysis for project teams, either for selecting the team or as a means of team-building (Table 23.3).

Table 23.3 Belbin team roles with examples

	Plant: Often creative, imaginative and unorthodox, solves difficult problems. Not always good at communicating with and managing ordinary people
	Resource investigator: Often extrovert, enthusiastic, and communicative. Explores opportunities and develops contacts. Has been known to lose interest once initial enthusiasm has passed.
	Coordinator: Mature, confident, and trusting. A good Chairman. Clarifies goals, promotes decision making. Not necessarily, not the most clever or creative member of a group
	Shaper: Tends to be dynamic, outgoing, highly strong. Challenges, pressurizes, and finds ways round obstacles. May be prone to impatience and short-lived bursts of temper
	Monitor/Evaluator: Sober, strategic and discerning. Sees all options. Judges accurately. Sometimes appears to lack drive and ability to inspire others
	Teamworker: Usually social, perceptive and accommodating. Listens, builds, and averts friction. Sometimes not sufficiently decisive in crunch situations
	Implementer: Disciplined, reliable, conservative and efficient. Turns ideas into practical actions. Can sometimes appear to be a little inflexible and unwilling to adjust
	Completer/Finisher: Painstaking, conscientious, and anxious. Searches out errors and omissions. Delivers on-time. May appear to be inclined to worry unduly and be reluctant to delegate.

The Belbin self assessment is often used by teams as part of a team-building session—it helps team members to understand better where others are "coming from". People who complete it are often amazed at some of the aspects of their personality that it can highlight.

Even without that, an experience team leader can use the ideas behind Belbin together with the descriptions to make their own estimate of people's preferred team roles and allocate tasks within the team on that basis.

Dealing with People: Interpersonal Skills

If managing relationships is the key to success in consulting, then it is the behavior and interpersonal skills of the consultant that make that happen. All really skilled consultants have excellent interpersonal skills. They need them in order to:

- Read situations
- Build empathy with clients and others
- Gain the trust and respect of those they are working with
- Facilitate meetings
- Influence others
- Tailor communications to suit the audience
- Predict peoples' reactions
- Avoid or get out of difficult situations.

These skills—listening, observing, questioning, challenging, influencing and negotiating—are fundamental to good consulting and can all be developed through training and experience. They form a key element of our consultancy skills training.

Active Listening

But do not we all listen? Yes, certainly but there are different types of listening, in particular:

- *Normal listening*: Here, the listener is just listening to enjoy the story or argument being told—almost coasting. This is the listening, we might use in a restaurant, bar, or meeting. The listener is joining in the conversation whilst sometimes half-listening, sometimes thinking about other topics, sometimes thinking about their own next comment.
- *Competitive listening*: Where the listener is more interested in promoting his or her point of view instead of considering the speaker's thoughts. The listener listens, but also looks for breaks in the conversation to deliver their own point of view, perhaps even attacking any points they may not agree with.

- *Active listening*: Here the listener moves onto another level. Not just enjoying the story but actively working with the speaker to understand the speaker's story, how the speaker feels, what they think, and actively showing their interest and understanding through their body language, questions, responses, etc.

Active listening style is a very effective way to gain a deep understanding of the speaker's knowledge, beliefs, thoughts and feelings. It is used widely by counselors, psychologists and psychiatrists in their daily work, and in consultancy work, it is an invaluable skill. It focuses on two elements:

1. *Creating an atmosphere that makes it easy for the speaker to talk about the topic and the issues concerned.*

   The best atmosphere in terms of physical location/environment and lack of distractions, but in particular in the behavior of you as the listener—a behavior of listening that:
   - Encourages them to talk
   - Shows that you are paying attention
   - Ensures that they realize that you are listening noting what they are saying
   - Helps them to say what they want to say.
2. *Using communication skills to steer and guide the conversation in the direction that you wish it to go, and providing the context and detail you need.*

   This is achieved mainly through the following communication skills:
   - *Questions*—obtaining information by the use of questions.
     - Open questions—What should we do to ...?
     - Specific questions—How much are we talking about?
     - Closed questions—Was she late?
     - By asking closed questions to check assumptions—yours and theirs.
   - Summarizing—in order to check your understanding of what they have said.
   - Supporting—encouraging communication by using supporting statements: I see. And then?
   - Listen and paraphrase—use their words to demonstrate that you were listening (Perhaps using their words to form questions).
   - Main Points—identifying the main points they make and how they differ from yours.
   - Facts versus Opinion—distinguishing fact from opinion in the other person's statements.

Tips for Active Listening

It really is all about self-discipline and the use of some very simple tactics. The following summarize the key points.

1. *First and foremost, stop talking!*: It is difficult to listen and speak at the same time.
2. *Put the other person at ease*: Give them space and time and "permission" to speak their piece. How we look at them, how we stand or sit, makes a huge difference. Relax, and let them relax as well. (see Body Listening below)
3. *Show the other person that you want to hear them*: Look at them. Nod when you can agree, ask them to explain further if you do not understand. Listen to understand them and their words, rather than just for your turn.
4. *Remove distractions*: Good listening means being willing to turn-off the TV, close a door, stop returning emails or reading your mail. Give the speaker your full attention, and let them know, they are getting your full attention (See Control Distractions below).
5. *Empathize with the other person*: Especially, if they are telling you something personal or painful, or something you intensely disagree with, take a moment to stand in their shoes, to look at the situation from their point of view (See Build Rapport below).
6. *Be patient*: Some people take longer to find the right word, to make a point or clarify an issue. Give the speaker time to get it all out before you jump in with your reply.
7. *Watch your own emotions*: If what they are saying creates an emotional response in you, be extra careful to listen carefully, with attention to the intent and full meaning of their words. When we are angry, frightened or upset, we often miss critical parts of what is being said to us (See Control your Emotional Hot Buttons below).
8. *Be very slow to disagree, criticize or argue*: Even if you disagree, let them have their point of view. If you respond in a way that makes the other person defensive, even if you "win" the argument, you may lose something far more valuable.
9. *Ask lots of questions*: Ask the speaker to clarify, to say more, give an example, or explain further. It will help them speak more precisely, and it will help you hear and understand them more accurately (See Questioning on next page).
10. *Stop talking!*: This is both the first and the last point, because all other tools depend on it. Nature gave us two ears and only one tongue, which is a gentle hint that we should listen twice as much as we talk.

Become a 'Whole Body' Listener

To be effective listeners, we must involve our whole body. Not only are our ears tuned in, but so are our eyes, our mind (the intellect), our bodies and hearts. Good listeners give both non-verbal and verbal signals that they are listening. A 'whole body' listener listens actively by:

- Conveying a positive, encouraging attitude
- Sitting in an attentive posture (facing the speaker)
- Remaining alert, but comfortable
- Nodding in acknowledgement of the speaker's words
- Making good eye contact
- Ignoring or eliminating distractions
- Tuning in to the speaker's feelings
- Looking like a listener.

If you are in total rapport you will naturally match the speaker's physical movements, tone of voice, vocabulary and breathing patterns. Good listeners are in sensory balance with the speaker. According to Albert Mehrabian, an expert in human behavior, our communication is:

- 55% nonverbal.
- 38% inflection and tone.
- And only 7% words.

If Mehrabian is correct, then most of the messages are seen and sensed, and the words are far less important than the non-verbal cues and tone of voice.

Finally, think about your personal mannerisms and behavior. Do you have any of the following habits that would distract or confuse a speaker? Fidgeting, blinking, biting your lip, frowning deeply, playing with your hair, tie or jewelry, looking at your watch. Stop for a moment and think about these habits. Would they distract you, if you were the one speaking? If your answer is yes, you need to find a way to modify your behavior.

CONTROL DISTRACTIONS

A telephone is one of the biggest distractions to listening in a business environment, because unseen, others choose when the phone will ring. If the phone were the only distraction, we could probably learn to tolerate it. Everyday, we must deal with many internal, external, visual and auditory distractions.

To be good listeners, we must control our responses to distractions or they will control us. Distractions affect our ability to listen well because of their variety, novelty or intensity. External distractions include the telephone, background noise, unfamiliarity with vocabulary, seating, lighting, etc. Internal distractions can be things such as headaches, hunger, fatigue, or a current emotional state, such as anxiety.

Build Rapport by Pacing the Speaker

Pacing is a method listeners use to build rapport with a speaker by imitating or mirroring his or her behavior. This involves gestures, breathing, voice rate, vocabulary, favorite phrases and facial expressions.

When pacing, a good listener focuses on who the speaker is and what he or she is saying. The listener then makes a conscious effort to overcome the differences between them. The sooner the speaker and listener find common ground, the sooner they can communicate at a comfortable level. From that point, their opportunity for mutual understanding will be greater. As a listener, you can pace a speaker in any of the following ways:

- Match your voice rate to theirs
- Change your voice volume to match theirs
- Notice and use some of the same words and phrases as the speaker
- Approximate the speaker's gestures
- Breathe at about the same rate, without being very obvious.

Control Your Emotional 'Hot Buttons'

Words, issues, situations, and/or personalities trigger us emotionally. When these issues trigger our emotional 'hot buttons' a verbal message will become distorted (either positively or negatively). Because issues are emotional, they create barriers to effective listening.

Emotional 'hot buttons' are intense, complex feelings that affect everyone. Each may initiate a different emotional reaction, but our physical responses are similar. If you cannot eliminate your emotional 'hot buttons', the best alternative is to develop acceptable responses. The triggers warn you that emotions are taking over. When emotional levels go up, objectively comes down. Problems are never satisfactorily resolved at an emotional level.

The following is a list of coping skills for preventive maintenance when your hot button is activated by someone's anger or frustration.

1. Listen attentively without interrupting
2. Make a conscious choice about your response—get angry, try to solve the problem, or ignore it
3. Acknowledge the other person's feelings.

4. Ask objective questions for clarification—open-ended questions are useful
5. Try to see the other person's point of view
6. Stick to the subject
7. Be patient
8. Express your point of view and evidence—without backing them into a corner
9. Explain why
10. Work out a 'win-win' plan—fair and workable for both.

How Well do you Listen?

Discovering your attitude about listening is an important first step towards successful listening. Attitudes determine our behavior (Table 23.4).

Table 23.4 Listening attitudes and behavior

		YES	*NO*
1.	I am interested in many subjects and do not knowingly tune out dry-sounding information		
2.	I listen carefully for a speaker's main ideas and supporting points		
3.	I take notes during meetings to record key points		
4.	I am not easily distracted		
5.	I keep my emotions under control		
6.	I concentrate carefully and do not fake attention		
7.	I wait for the speaker to finish before finally evaluating the message		
8.	I respond appropriately with a smile, a nod, or a word of acknowledgment, as a speaker is talking		
9.	I am aware of mannerisms that may distract a speaker and keep mine under control		
10.	I understand my biases and control them when I am listening		
11.	I refrain from constant interruption		
12.	I value eye contact and maintain it most of the time		
13.	I often restate or paraphrase what the speaker said to make sure I have the correct meaning		
14.	I listen for the speaker's emotional meaning as well as subject matter content		
15.	I ask questions for clarification		
16.	I do not finish other people's sentences unless asked to do so		
17.	When listening on the telephone one hand is kept free to take notes		
18.	I attempt to set aside my ego and focus on the speaker rather than on myself		
19.	I am careful to judge the message rather than the speaker		
20.	I am a patient listener most of the time		
	Total Scores		

To discover your listening attitudes. complete the following exercises. If a statement describes your listening attitude or behavior accurately, tick 'Yes.' if not, tick 'No.' Be hard on yourself.

The following scale will help you to interpret your present listening skill level based on your current attitudes and behavior patterns:

- *1—5 'No' answers* You are an excellent listener. Keep it up!
- *6—10 'No' answers* You are a good listener, but can improve.
- *11—15 'No' answers* Through practice you can become a much more effective listener in your business and personal relationships.
- *16—20 'No' answers* Listen harder!

Communication Skills—Asking Questions

Listening alone will not, always give you all the information you require. You will need to guide and direct the conversation using questions. There are two important considerations: type of questions and level. The type of question, we habitually use can determine the sort of response, we get. The level at which we probe will determine the insight, we gain into the other person.

There are five types of question:

1. *Closed questions* usually get one word ("Yes", "No") answers. Useful for checking facts but do not give much information.
2. *Open questions* give the other person a chance to express their opinion. The other person has more control over the discussion. Open questions usually begin with "how", "where". An easy way to make sure your questions are open is to put "Tell me about ..... before the topic.
3. *Probing questions* push the other person to develop their thinking. They can be more difficult to ask because we may become more inhibited about pushing the point. Probing questions can be translated as "Tell me more about ......"
4. *Leading questions* produce no information at all. They tell the person what the answer is in the question. They can be very irritating and give the impression you are not interested in what the other person has to say.
5. *Multiple questions* often start out as good probing questions. Sometimes, we find it difficult to tolerate the silence so we fill in with supplementary questions. This ends with confusing the other person as well as ourselves.

If we can discover what is important to the individual, we are well on our way to understanding their behavior, and their priorities. We can do this by focusing our questions on what they want, what they value. This information is often less accessible and can be said to be on a deeper level than, for instance, conversation. It may be necessary to build an atmosphere of trust before someone is prepared to disclose at this level. This can take some time.

Effective Team Communication Behavior

The researchers were carrying out studies into what it was that made some groups successful whereas others were not. They looked in detail at the way people in the groups behaved and identified the following particular behaviors (Table 23.5).

In the Successful Groups:

- Members contributed in roughly equal amounts
- Over 25% of all proposals were built-on
- Far more positive supportive behavior than negative
- 10% of the time was spent on "Testing Understanding and Summarizing"
- Significant time was spent on discussing how a problem should be tackled, rather than leaping straight into it.
- *Typical behavior profile of a group*:
  - 16%—Initiating (proposing 12%, building 4%)
  - 14%—Reacting (supporting 8%, disagreeing 6%)
  - 70%—Clarifying (seeking information 17%, giving information 43% Summarizing and testing understanding 10%).

CRITICAL EXAMINATION

Introduction

Critical examination technique as a tried and tested method of analyzing an organization or system.

Table 23.5 Effective team communication behaviors

Seeking Ideas	Asking other people for their ideas
Proposing	Putting forward ideas as statements (i.e. we should do this!)
Suggesting	Putting forward ideas as questions (i.e. how about doing so and so?)
Supporting	Agreeing with something someone else has said
Seeking clarification/ information	Asking other people for further clarifications or information
Clarifying/explaining/informing	Giving information, opinions and explanations
Disagreeing	Explicitly disagreeing with something someone has said
Difficulty stating	Point out the snags or difficulties with something someone else has said

It is the systematic analysis of information about a problem, procedure or activity by which it is subjected to exhaustive challenge, with regard to need, simplification, combination, sequence and alternatives. Its aim is to determine the valid reasons for each activity, and to draw up systematically a list of alternatives which can be developed into a new and improved method.

Critical examination of policies, objectives and activities helps the team leader to challenge what is happening now, accepted policies and objectives, how work is carried out, the timing and sequence of activities and so on. It has long been part of the 'tool kit' of the management consultant.

Technique

In order to ensure that critical examination of all appropriate functions is carried out, a structured approach in applying the technique can be used. This requires the consultant to ask a series of specific questions of relevant activities, objectives and policies depending on the level at which the investigation is being conducted. The questions are as follows:

- What is being done?
- How is it being done?
- Where is it being done? I Why?
- When is it being done?
- Who is doing it?

As this suggests, the question "why?" is asked of the responses to the other questions; this is the validation of the answers.

The first question is always "what?". It is crucial when answering this question that care is taken to state exactly what is achieved and not be confused by describing how something is done. This appears an obvious statement but is very easy to fall into this trap. The reason for first asking what is achieved is that if the activity is not validated—by the response to the subsequent question 'why?'—then the indications are that the activity need not be carried out at all. In such circumstances, the subsequent questions are unnecessary.

Assuming the activity is satisfactorily validated, the remaining primary questions are asked—each response being challenged by the question 'why?' and validated or otherwise by the answers. If all responses to the question 'why?' are satisfactory, this does not necessarily mean that the situation should remain unchanged. It simply means that some activity is necessary and that it should be carried out somehow, at some dine, in some place and by someone.

In adopting the structured approach to critical examination, further searching questions are then posed:

Table 23.6 Critical examination sheet

Purpose	What is achieved? Why?	Is it necessary?	What else could be done?	What should be done?
Place	Where is it done?	Why there?	Where else could it be done?	Where should it be done?
Sequence	When is it done?	Why then?	When else could it be done?	When should it be done?
Person	Who does it?	Why that person?	Who else could do it?	Who should do it?
Means	How is it done?	Why that way?	How else could it be done?	How should it be done?

- What else could be done?
- How else might it be done?
- Where else might it be done?
- When else might it be done?
- Who else might do it?

Alternatives are being consistently sought. In doing so, the consultant must guard against assuming that a better, alternative situation must in some way conform to what is happening now. In attempting to generate alternatives by answering the questions above, the consultant is not necessarily challenging the correctness of the present situation; what is being challenged is its uniqueness.

Below is a Critical Examination sheet (Table 23.6) which sets out the questions in tabular form for easy reference and analysis.

STYLES OF INFLUENCING

Here, we introduce two models on influencing style:

1. Tough Battler, Friendly Helper, Logical Thinker
2. Push-Pull Influencing with self assessment questionnaire.

Tough Battler, Friendly Helper, Logical Thinker

This model is based on work by RW Wallen in which he identified three types of executive personality. Charles Handy summarized it in his book *Understanding Organizations* 1986.

The model describes three types of executive personality, each of which employs quite different styles of influencing others, and each of which needs to be influenced in particular ways (Fig. 23.8 and Table 23.7).

This is a nice simple little model with the advantage that in many cases one can "spot" quite quickly the preferred style of someone else, and then adjust ones own influencing style to suit.

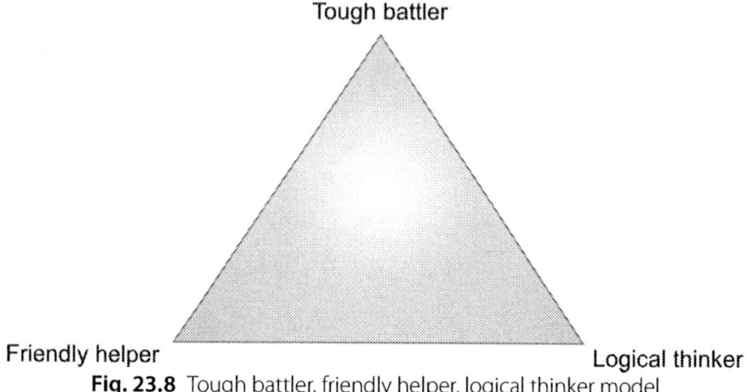

Fig. 23.8 Tough battler, friendly helper, logical thinker model

Table 23.7 Ways of influences in model

Tough battler • Has drive, energy, commitment • Self-assertion using power, leverage points • Concerned with winning/doing it my way • Has a "Distributive" world view—a world of conflict, fight, power and assertiveness	**Influences through** • Giving orders • Offering challenge • Threatening • Asserting • Broken record
Friendly helper • Friendliness, openness • Cooperation include others • Appeal to emotions, trusting • Concerned with "positive" relationships • Has an "Integrative" world view—a world of helpfulness, cooperation, love and sympathy	**Influences through** • Appeasing • Appealing to pity • Trading favors • Making friends • Lateral appeal
Logical thinker • Calm, logical, thoughtful, organized • Use logical argument/debate • Appeal to commonsense, precedence • Concerned with facts and information • Has a "Rationality" world view—a world of understanding, logic, systems and knowledge	**Influences through** • Appealing to logic • Presenting 'facts' • Swamping with detail • Quoting rules and regulations • Using the hierarchy

Push-Pull Influencing Styles

Research over several years into the behavior of effective influencers has revealed two basic types of influencing called Push and Pull.

Push Style

The Push style is characterized by extensive use of three types of behavior. The influencer spends 70% or more of their time in these activities:

- Proposing
- Giving Information
- Blocking/shutting out

The rationale of the Push style is that people are influenced by convincing proposals which are well supported. The keys to successful use of the push style are: the quality of the proposals; the information given; the ability to get those proposals heard by shutting others out.

The Push style tends to be most effective under one or more of these conditions:

- The recipient has little experience or understanding of the issue and recognizes the need for help or guidance.
- There is no vested interest in the status quo and the recipient does not feel threatened by accepting the proposal.
- The recipient recognizes the legitimacy of the influencer's power base (e.g. expert, position, physical).
- The recipient trusts the influencer's motives.

Pull Style

The Pull style is characterized by concentration upon three different behaviors. The influencer spends 35% or more of their time in these activities:

- Testing understanding
- Seeking information
- Building.

The rationale of the Pull style is that people are influenced more readily by uncovering their needs, motives, aspirations and concerns. The keys to effective use of the Pull style are: the quality of questions used to test understanding and to seek information, and the ability to build upon ideas and proposals.

The Pull style tends to be effective in most situations, but is particularly useful under these conditions:

- The recipient of the influence attempt has strong opinions and views
- The recipient has a vested interest in the status quo and could have difficulty in accepting the influencer's proposals
- It is unknown what the recipient will find acceptable
- The influencer has no recognized power base, or wishes not to use an established power base

- It is important that the influence attempt has a long-lasting effect, i.e. the influencer wishes to obtain more than compliance from the recipient
- The relationship between the two parties is new, or there is a history of mistrust
- Previous attempts using a Push style have failed.

Research evidence suggests that when Push and Pull styles are mixed during an influence attempt, the result is a decrease in effectiveness. The two styles appear to cancel each other out. It is therefore important to consciously choose a particular style before attempting to influence another and to stick to that style throughout the meeting.

It is, of course, possible for an influencer to use a different style with the same recipient on another occasion or after an adjournment. Sometimes, the two styles can be used together, if a pair of influencers, acting as a team, each employs one of the styles.

Self-assessment Questionnaire

Please read each of the following statements carefully and decide the extent to which they describe your behavior in situations where you need to influence others. Base your answers on typical day-to-day activities which occur in your job.

Please be as frank as possible. The questionnaire will be of little value, unless you provide an accurate and objective description of your behavior.

Against each statement, enter in the appropriate box the score which corresponds to your choice from the five possible responses given here.

Enter the Score

1. 4, if you definite agree, that is, if the statement accurately describes your actions
2. 3, if you are inclined to agree, that is, if the statement describes your actions with reasonable accuracy
3. 2, if you are undecided, that is, you are genuinely unsure whether or not the statement describes your actions accurately
4. 1, if you are inclined to disagree, that is, if you think the statement probably does not describe your actions accurately.
5. 0, if you definitely disagree, that is, if the statement definitely does not describe your actions.

Please answer the questionnaire as quickly as possible and do not hesitate to use the extreme score where appropriate (Table 23.8).

Table 23.8 Influencing style questionnaire

	Influencing style questionnaire	A	B
1.	I often delegate important tasks to others even when there is a risk that I will be personally criticized, if they are not done well		
2.	I put forward lots of ideas and plans		
3.	I am willing to be persuaded by others		
4.	I usually put together good logical arguments		
5.	I encourage people to come up with their own solutions to problems		
6.	When opposed, I am usually quick to come forward with a counter argument		
7.	I am usually receptive to the ideas and suggestions of others		
8.	I often provide detailed plans to show how a task should be done		
9.	I am quick to admit my own mistakes		
10.	I often suggest alternatives to the proposals which others have made		
11.	I show sympathy towards others when they have difficulties		
12.	I push my ideas vigorously		
13.	I listen carefully to the ideas of others and try to put them to use		
14.	It is not unusual for me to stick my neck out with ideas and suggestions		
15.	If others become angry or upset, I try to listen with understanding		
16.	I express my own ideas very clearly		
17.	I readily admit my lack of knowledge or expertise in some situations		
18.	I defend my own ideas energetically		
19.	I often put as much effort into developing the ideas of others as I do my own		
20.	I often anticipate objections to my point of view so as to be ready with an answer		
21.	I often help others to get a hearing		
22.	I frequently disregard the ideas of others in favor of my own proposals		
23.	I often listen sympathetically to people who do not share my own views		
24.	When other people disagree with my ideas I do not give up: instead I try to find another argument to persuade them		
25.	I am quite open about my hopes, fears and aspirations and my personal difficulties in achieving them		
26.	I am imaginative in producing evidence to support my own proposals		
27.	I usually show tolerance and acceptance of other people's feelings		
28.	I usually talk about my own ideas more than I listen to those of others		

Contd...

Contd...

	Influencing style questionnaire	A	B
29.	I usually accept criticism without becoming defensive		
30.	I present my ideas in a very organized way		
31.	I often help others to express their views		
32.	I frequently draw attention to inconsistencies in the ideas of others		
33.	I go out of my way to show understanding of the needs and wants of others		
34.	It is not unusual for me to interrupt others while they are talking		
35.	I do not pretend to be confident when in fact I feel uncertain		
36.	I often put a lot of energy into arguing about what I do		
	Now calculate your overall scores in boxes A and B and see below for how to interpret your scores		
	Total All Pages		

INTERPRETATION OF SCORES

The questionnaire gives an indication of the extent to which you use two different styles of influence in your job.

1. Box A gives your overall score for the *Pull* influence style.
2. Box B gives your overall score for the *Push* influence style.

Your overall score for each style can be interpreted as follows:

- *54–72*: Definite use of the style
- *42–53*: Tendency to use the style
- *30–41*: Neither use nor avoidance of the style
- *18–29*: Tendency to avoid use of the style
- *0–17*: Definite avoidance of the style.

POLITICAL RESOURCES: INVENTORY

The following questions are designed to help you think about the political resources you have. They are divided between the four types of power-base:

1. *Authority*—the power and authority that goes with the position or office that you hold.
2. *Expertise*—the power that goes with the particular skills that you possess that others need to access.
3. *Resource*—the power that goes with the resources that you control.
4. *Interpersonal*—the power and influence that derives from you and your personal skills, in particular skills in influencing, and leadership.

The questions help to identify whether you have the particular type of power in each section, but there is space for you to add additional indicators of your own. The more positive indicators you have, the greater your power.

1. *Do you have formal authority?*

		Yes	No
a.	Do you have the formal right (say, in your job description) to make decisions, other than trivial ones?		
b.	Do other people need your approval before they take action?		
c.	Do you supervise someone else's work?		
d.	Do your decisions significantly affect important aspects of the organization's work long-term?		
e.	Does your manager typically support your decisions and not over-rule them?		
f.	Do you encounter any resistance to your right to make decisions, supervise others, give approval, from subordinates, peers, more senior managers?		

- *Yes* answers to any of (a)–(e) indicate your possession of authority.
- *Yes* to (d) indicates a high level of power based on authority.
- *Yes* to (f) suggests a reduction of your political resources which you may need to do something about.

2. *Do you have the power of expertise?*

		Yes	No
a.	Does it take a year or longer to do your job adequately?		
b.	Do you need a qualification to do your job?		
c.	What is the highest qualification in your field — do you have it?		
d.	Are you the only person in your organization who can do your job?		
e.	If you were to leave your organization would they have difficulty in replacing you?		
f.	Does your knowledge and skills relate to a major aspect of the organization's work?		
g.	Do people frequently consult you and follow your advice?		
h.	Do more senior managers clearly show that they value your contribution?		

- *Yes* to any of (a)–(h) indicates your possession of expert power.
- But *No* to (g) and (h) suggests a lack of perception of your expertise by others, and you may need to do something about this, if this political resource is to be fully used.

3. *Do you control resources?*

		Yes	No
a.	Can you give or withhold access to the following resources of your organization: • Money • Information (non-trivial) • Promotion • Training • Senior managers and other powerful people • Computers and other operational or administrative facilities • Perks		
b.	Are others aware that you can give or withhold access to these things, perhaps because you have on occasion refused them?		
c.	Do others have alternative sources to these resources?		

- *Yes* to any of the items in (a) indicates that you have power based on resource control.
- *No* to (b) suggests that you may need to do something about this in order to fully use this political resource.
- But *Yes* to (c) in reference to any resource indicates a low level of power in relation to that resource, to which you may not wish to draw attention.

4. *Do you have interpersonal power?*

		Yes	No
a.	Are you on good terms with a number of people in the organization across different departments and hierarchical levels?		
b.	Do you know who the powerful people are, and are you on good terms with them?		
c.	Do people confide in you?		
d.	Do you usually speak at meetings?		
e.	Are you an "active listener"—you make sure you have understood the other person's point of view?		
f.	Do you make sure that other people take your views seriously when it matters to you?		
g.	Do you avoid being either passive or aggressive in formal or informal discussion with others in the organization?		
h	Can you hold the attention of a group or larger audience?		

- *Yes* to any of these questions indicates your power based on interpersonal skills.
- *No* to any of (d)–(h) suggests that training would help you develop your political potential.

Looking back over your answers to the question in this paper, you will probably have found that you have in some degree each of the types of power-base. If you give yourself a rating for each of the four types on the chart here, you will have a profile of your political resources.

You may wish to take action to alter the profile which emerges. Two questions which are useful to ask when deciding what to do are:

1. Do the people who have got to the top of your organization have any characteristics in common?
2. Are there any trends which might demand different characteristics for success in future?

Profile of political resources					
High	**5**				
	4				
Medium	**3**				
	2				
Low	**1**				
		Authority	Expertise	Resource control	Interpersonal skill

NEGOTIATING OVERVIEW

What makes a good negotiator? There have been a number of studies in this area, two important ones being carried out by Professor Gerald R Williams who specialized in legal negotiating and Neil Rackham of the Huthwaite Research Group who focused on sales negotiating.

Table 23.9 summarizes their main findings, more details of which are included here and also under Negotiating—Planning and Negotiating—Behaviors.

Williams—Cooperative Problem-solvers Versus Competitive Adversarials

In the early eighties, Professor Gerald R Williams asked negotiators, after a negotiation, to rank the other, their goals and their attributes. The other being those they were in negotiation with.

Table 23.9 Negotiating overview

Summary
Negotiating styles • There are two broad negotiating styles which Williams labeled as Cooperative problem-solvers versus Competitive adversarials. • The key conclusion of his study was clear. A cooperative problem solving approach is generally far more effective than a competitive adversarial approach. Cooperative problem-solvers were more likely to be rated as "effective" or even as "average". • 97% of cooperative problem-solvers got positive reviews as opposed to the 67% of the competitive adversarial negotiators.
Neil Rackham Neil Rackham studied effective and non-effective negotiators from two aspects: (1) Planning and Preparation (see Negotiating—Planning) and (2) Negotiating Behavior (see Negotiating—Behaviors).
Effective negotiators use stages Six typical negotiation stages are: • *Stage 1*: Preparation • *Stage 2*: Relationship building • *Stage 3*: Exchanging task-related information • *Stage 4*: Persuading • *Stage 5*: Making concessions • *Stage 6*: Reaching agreement
Effective negotiators prepare and plan well Not just the basics such as location, timing, and attendance; but particularly looking at the issues, options, common grounds, differences, settlement ranges, and best approaches. See Preparation.
Effective negotiators use ranges • Each side has a range of positions in mind—sometimes called the settlement zone, sometimes described as Fallback–Realistic–Ideal). • One other indicator of expert flexibility is that expert negotiators approach the negotiation table with these ranges in mind. Average negotiators do not. They have a fixed figure in their head, and if they do not get that figure they have, by definition, failed. • Expert negotiators come to the negotiation table prepared to craft a wise outcome that meets the long- and short-term interests of the parties, an agreement that will last the tests of time. They know that standing in cement will not help them move.
Effective negotiators face negotiation as a problem solving event Unlike many an ineffective negotiator who views the other as either a friend to be won over or as an adversary to be beaten, effective cooperative negotiators focus their energies first and foremost on solving the problem that got their clients to the negotiation table in the first place. Hence, the effective cooperative asks at all times, How will what I am proposing solve the problem? Sometimes called principled negotiation.

Contd...

Contd...

Effective negotiators focus first on building common ground

- Average negotiators, even when they focus on the problem that brings them to the negotiation table, address their differences first. Expert negotiators do not, choosing instead to identify common ground. They recognize human realities.
- This is the approach that senator George Mitchell reportedly took when facilitating the negotiation in Northern Ireland. Well aware that all parties were deeply entrenched in their positions, the senator spent the first year of the negotiations helping each party recognize the humanity of the other. People ate dinner together, went to each other's children's sporting events, saw movies and discussed them, and through this process they learned how very much all parties had in common. This permitted them to reframe their argument from one of sheer power politics to one of shared economic interdependency, embedding their future across-the-table negotiations deeply in common ground.

Effective negotiators do not fear differences

Experts do not pretend common ground exists when there is not any and they do not hide show-stoppers when there is one.

Effective negotiators behave effectively in negotiations

They employ the sort of interpersonal behaviors that lead to successful outcomes. Some behaviors help the negotiating process, others inhibit it. Those adopting "pulling" behaviors were more effective than those using "pushing" behaviors. Rackham covered this fully and the results are summarized in Skilled Negotiators 2.

Effective negotiators manage the need for both assertiveness and empathy

One of the hardest things for law students to learn is that, if they want to be effective cooperative negotiators, they need to be both assertive about the interests of their client and empathetic to the interests of the other. Failure at either makes reaching a negotiated agreement all the harder.

- Without assertiveness, the other can never fully appreciate the needs of your client.
- Without empathy, you can never fully understand the needs of the other, and without that knowledge you will always be unsure what to concede, what to propose, and what to shy away from.

- *65% of the negotiators were reported to be cooperative problem-solvers*: Of these, 38% were rated "effective", 59% were rated as "average", and only 3% were rated "ineffective".
- *24% competitive adversarials*: Of these, 25% were rated as "effective", 42% were rated as "average", but 33% were judged as "ineffective".
- An 11% could not be readily classified.

The key conclusion is clear. Cooperative problem-solvers were more likely to be perceived as "effective" or even as "average" with 97% of them getting positive reviews as opposed to the 67% of the competitive adversarial negotiators.

Rackham

For this insight, we have to turn to one of the first studies where trained observers actually sat in on negotiations and measured what the negotiators were doing, before and during the negotiation, to reach settlements that would stand the tests of time. These researchers, led by Neil Rackham, found that expert negotiators plan and communicate differently than average negotiators—the difference is measurable; it can be learned.

Rackham defined experts as negotiators who:

- Routinely came to agreement
- Shaped agreements that were routinely implemented successfully
- Who left the negotiation table with the other willing to negotiate with them again.

Average negotiators lacked one or more of the three measures. For example, some could come to agreement, but their agreements were not always successfully implemented. Others could come to agreement, but their other did not want to negotiate again.

The detailed results are tabulated in *Skilled Negotiators 1* and *Skilled Negotiators 2*.

PREPARATION

All research into this field indicates that:

1. A Cooperative problem solving approach is generally far more effective than a competitive adversarial approach.
2. *Preparation works*: Effective problem-solving cooperatives enter the negotiation with a whole lot of strategic and tactical thinking already done, so they can react flexibly and concentrate on listening with the goal of understanding. They know what they very much need and what concessions they can readily make. They even recognize what can do them in and they have thought of clever and credible ways to undermine those weaknesses in the eyes of the other, maybe even turning them into strengths in the process. They have even thought through settlement options just as thoroughly.

Why so much emphasis on preparation? Because as Rackham's findings proved, they who prepare best, most deeply and most broadly, usually "win." They get their clients' interests met. Solid preparation provides the problem-solving negotiator with:

- A better understanding of the problem facing them.
- They know the strengths and weaknesses of their perspective as well as those of the other.
- It also gives them a game plan that permits them to set their perspective aside and listen understandingly, especially for new information, and respond empathetically to the other.

The Range: The Settlement Zone

Experts base their starting, target, and reservation points and their concessions on a solid grasp of the strengths and weaknesses of their case and that of the Other, as well as on a broad and deep mastery of the contours of the market and a nuanced appreciation of the short and long-term value their client brings to the table. And they do not do it alone. They do it with their client, as legal ethics make clear the shape of any settlement is for the client to determine.

Before they involve their client in their estimations though, experts repeat the same thinking, this time from the vantage of the Other. They know that the Other is going through the same exercise in an effort to set their settlement box. So the expert stands in their shoes, trying to figure out with whatever information they have what the Other's starting point, target point, and resistance point may be, for armed with that knowledge, the expert can knowingly advise their client what a good settlement may look like.

How do they do that? They take the information they have collected and tested to the extent that any information unilaterally devised can be tested—and lay it out as follows (Fig. 23.9):

Note: Alternative descriptions of the three positions are:

1. Ideal outcome for starting point.
2. Realistic outcome for target point.
3. Fall-back position for resistance point.

It is the area that lies between the two resistance points (or fall-back positions) that is of most interest to them, for within this area both parties can find room to settle.

- Are the resistance points close to each other and the settlement zone tight? Could be problematic if both parties hold on to their guns; everyone will get shot. However, if counsel can maintain their heads,

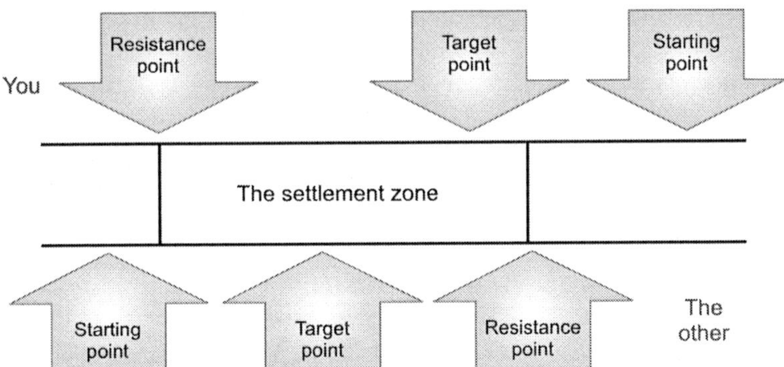

Fig. 23.9 The range between the settlement zone of you and the other

they can point out that the costs of walking away probably exceed the costs of getting closer.

- Are the resistance points spread? Now is the time to start thinking creatively with the goal of not just closing the gap, but of creating value in the process.

Behavior, Particularly Communications

Experts communicate specially, transmitting information in a way that will allow it to be received.

When Rackham sat in on negotiations, he measured discrete communication behaviors that fell into three primary categories:

1. *Initiating:*
   - Making a proposal
   - Building on the proposals of another
2. *Reacting:*
   - Supporting
   - Disagreeing
   - Defending/attacking
3. *Clarifying:*
   - Testing for understanding
   - Summarizing
   - Seeking information
   - Giving information

Also noted were two additional behaviors observed mostly in group interactions: bringing in, that is soliciting input; and shutting out, that is interrupting, cutting off and the like.

Some negotiators relied primarily on proposing, giving information, and shutting out to get across their ideas. Others used those three behaviors in part, but relied mostly on building on the proposal of another, testing for understanding, and seeking information to persuade.

The difference was so measurable that Rackham could classify the two respectively as "Pushers" and "Pullers." Both types of persuaders enjoyed successes, but the expert negotiators most often fell into the Puller category. These negotiators used communication behaviors to help the Other persuade themselves. In other words, if there were any persuading to be done of the Other, the Other was the one who was helped to do it.

Unconvinced about the value of Pulling? Let us return to the data. Research shows that 20% of an expert negotiators' behavior revolves around using questions; they seek information from the Other nearly three times more often than the average negotiator. 10% of their behavior has them testing for understanding more than twice as often as the average negotiator. That means at least fully a third of their behaviors involve pulling. When they do make statements, some 8% of their behavior involves summarizing what they heard the other say. And they use this summarizing, a clarifying technique, nearly twice as often as the average negotiator. Putting those percentages ages all together, some 40% of expert negotiators' behavior involves clarifying the other's thinking twice as much as average negotiators' behavior.

Why do expert negotiators rely so heavily on questions and other clarifying behaviors? For many reasons. Perhaps the most compelling is that questions help you persuade the other. Test it out in the quiet of your home. Try to alter your significant other's behavior by telling him (or her) what to do.

Skilled Versus Average Negotiators

Planning

The Huthwaite Research Group conducted a study in the United Kingdom on the behavior of successful negotiators. The researchers interviewed and observed 49 successful negotiators in a total of 102 negotiations. The 49 comprised 17 union representatives, 12 management representatives, 11 contract negotiators and 9 others.

The negotiators were not considered successful unless they were rated as effective by both sides, had a track record of significant success and had a low incidence of implementation failure. Successful negotiators planning behavior differed from that of their less skilled colleagues (Table 23.10).

1. *Planning time*: Both skilled and average negotiators used about the same amount of time for planning, however, the time was used differently.
2. *Exploration of options*: Skilled negotiators considered twice as wide a range of options and outcomes. This is essentially a creative process. The greater the range of options, the greater the likelihood of finding a mutually beneficial option.
3. *Common ground*: All negotiators focus more on areas of conflict than of agreement, but skilled negotiators spent over three times as much time talking about areas of commonality.

Table 23.10 Summary of planning behavior differences between the skilled negotiators and the average negotiators

Summary of planning behavior differences	Skilled negotiators	Average negotiators
Overall time spent planning	No significant difference	No significant difference
Number of options and outcomes considered per issue	5.1	2.6
Percentage of comments about areas of anticipated common ground	8%	11%
Percentage of comments about long-term considerations of issues	8.5%	4%
Planned order	Issues	Sequences
Average use of sequences during planning per session	2.1	4.9
Setting limits	Range	Fixed-point

4. *Long-term versus short-term*: All negotiators spend most of their time on immediate issues. However, skilled negotiators spent more than twice as much time on long-term issues.
5. *Setting limits*: Average negotiators set single point objectives, like not paying a penny more than £90,000. Skilled negotiators set a range, e.g. £85,000–£95,000. This gives more flexibility and also allows for exploration of the interests underlying the position.
6. *Sequence versus issue planning*: Average negotiators use sequence planning, e.g. point A must be agreed before being able to move on to negotiate on point B and so on.

   Skilled negotiators in contrast use issue planning. Each issue is negotiated on its merits unlinked to other issues and time sequencing is therefore less important. This does not mean that issues cannot be linked only that there is no predetermined order.

Source: Neil Rackham, "The Behavior of Successful Negotiators, 1982.

Skilled Versus Average Negotiators 2

Negotiating Behavior

The Huthwaite Research Group conducted a study in the United Kingdom on the behavior of successful negotiators. The researchers interviewed and observed 49 successful negotiators in a total of 102 negotiations. The 49 comprised 17 union representatives, 12 management representatives, 11 contract negotiators and 9 others.

The negotiators were not considered successful unless they were rated as effective by both sides, had a track record of significant success and had a low incidence of implementation failure. Successful negotiators planning behavior differed from that of their less skilled colleagues (Table 23.11).

Table 23.11 The negotiating behavior differences between the skilled negotiators and the average negotiators

Negotiating behavior	Skilled negotiators	Average negotiators
Use of irritators per hour of face-to-face negotiating time	2.3	10.8
Frequency of counterproposals per hour of face-to-face negotiating time	1.7	3.1
Percent of negotiator's time classified as a defence/attack/spiral	1.9%	6.3%
Disagreeing	0.4%	1.5%
Testing for understanding	9.7%	4.1%
Summarizing	7.5%	4.2%
Questions, as a percent of all negotiating behavior	21.3%	9.6%
Feelings commentary, giving internal information as a percent of all negotiating behavior	12.1%	7.8%
Argument dilution, average number of reasons given by negotiator to back each argument or case that s/he advances	1.8	3.0

1. *Irritators* are words that, while having negligible value in persuading opponents, cause annoyance. Irritators include such phrases as "generous offer," "fair price," and "reasonable arrangement." Average negotiators use over four times as many irritators as do skilled negotiators.
2. *Counterproposals* involve negotiators responding to their opponents' proposals by simply offering their own proposal. Average negotiators use counterproposals twice as frequently as skilled negotiators. Skilled negotiators clarify their understanding of opponent's suggestions before responding with their own proposals.
3. *Defend/attack spiral*: Negotiating, by definition, involves conflict. That conflict often leads to heated, value-laden accusations and defensive statements. Average negotiators frequently respond defensively and often attack, first gently and then harder and harder. Skilled negotiators, by contrast, rarely respond defensively. Although, they also rarely attack, when they do so, they hit hard and without warning. Average negotiators attack more than three times as frequently as do skilled negotiators.
4. *Behavioral labeling* refers to describing what you plan to say before you say it. For example, "Can I ask a question?" and "Can I make a suggestion?" are behavioral labels for a question and a suggestion. Behavioral labels forewarn opponents. For all behavior except disagreement, skilled negotiators use labelling over five times as often as their colleagues. Average negotiators label disagreement three times as often as do skilled negotiators.
5. *Active listening* involves demonstrating to oneself and to one's opponent that the previous statement has been understood. Active listening does not convey agreement or approval—it strictly reflects understanding. Skilled negotiators use two powerful active listening techniques—testing

for understanding and summarizing—more than twice as often as their average colleagues.

6. *Questions* are a primary source of gathering information. Skilled negotiators use more than twice as many questions as do average negotiators.
7. *Feelings commentary* involves describing what a person feels about a situation. A negotiator might say, "I am uncertain how to react to what you have just said. If the information you have given me is true, then I would like to accept it; yet I have some doubts about its accuracy. So part of me feels happy and part feels suspicious. Can you help me to resolve this?" Skilled negotiators give almost twice as much feelings commentary as do average negotiators.
8. *Argument dilution*: Weak arguments generally dilute strong arguments. Skilled negotiators know that the fewer arguments, the better. Average negotiators use almost twice as many reasons to back up of their positions as do skilled negotiators.

PRESENTATIONS: PREPARATION

This page is in three parts:

1. Outstanding presenting skills—what research shows.
2. Preparation for presentations—what to cover and how to do that.
3. The presentation proper—the start, handling questions, and the closure.

Outstanding Presenting Skills

The five skills most frequently used by people rated by their colleagues as outstanding presenters.

1. *Fine tuning*: Materials refined to audience, before and during the presentation.
2. *Focused on outcomes*: What do I want to achieve? How will they respond to this?
3. *Chunking*: Chunking the information down to manageable segments.
4. *Viewpoint*: Seeing their presentation from the others viewpoint.
5. *Unshakeable belief*: In the success of the presentation.

They achieve this because they make use of three pieces of knowledge when they design their presentation.

Media is the Message

Many studies in this all indicate a very simple and important conclusion—that we tend to base our judgment of others on three main characteristics:

1. Verbal content = 7%.
2. Vocal interest = 38%.
3. Body language = 55%.

Thus, at least 90% of your public image depends on how you look and sound rather than what you actually say. In terms of impact, the best speech you write will depend for its success on your presentation style and not on the contents of the speech itself.

Attention Span

Other studies have shown that most people have an attention span of between 25 and 40 minutes, and can only process 5 to 9 new chunks of information at any given time. We can maintain attention span longer by the way that we structure and "chunk" the presentation into smaller sections.

On Recall

Further studies carried out on recall of information indicate that we can effectively recall.

- 20% of what we *hear.*
- 30% of what we *see.*
- 50% of what we *hear* and *see.*
- 70% of what we *do.*

The implication for your presentation is simply: *Tell* it to them; *Show* it to them; Get them to *use or interact* on it.

Preparation for Presentations

Nearly everyone approaches a presentation with some nervousness and sometimes panic. A certain degree of nervousness is quite normal and can actually help you to give a better performance. Preparation can help you manage that nervousness.

Setting Objectives

Spend some time thinking about and summarizing:

- My aims. What do I want to achieve with the presentation?
- The audience. What is the audience like—who are they, how many of them, how familiar are they with the topic?
- Venue. What is the venue likely to be like?
- The subject. What is the best structure—what sections should I have?
- Timing. How long have I got—what timing for each section?
- Visuals, etc. What equipment shall I need?

Chunking the Presentation into Sections

Break the subject down into separate sections with a list of points you wish to make under each and any information, including examples, statistics, etc., which you may need to support the points.

Often best done in a "storyboard" approach—using a sheet of A4 for each section. For each section, think about the use of audio-visuals and handouts, and about what audience participation you would such as—exercises, questions, comments.

Draw up your final plan with the selected sections and points laid out in sequence. Then go through the storyboard and decide how you are going to:

- Introduce the presentation. *Tell your audience*:
  - What you are going to say and how long it will take
  - What audio/visuals you are going to use
  - What part you want them to play and when (e.g. questions during or at end).
- Link each part to the next.
- Link the audio/visuals to your text.
- Control people's reading of any handouts, e.g. when and how much tine.
- Sum up your conclusions and relate them to your objective.

Finally, check your plan for:

- Content
- Sequence
- Timing
- Balance (the right weight for each section, balance between spoken word and audio/visuals).

Preparing Your Audio/Visuals

Audio/visuals are there to convey information, to reinforce the spoken word, and to provide background information and atmosphere.

The best advice is to keep it as simple as possible. Too many audio visuals can be difficult to coordinate, and may well distract the audience.

Preparing Your Notes or Script

Unless you can memorize an entire speech and still seem spontaneous on the day some form of notes or script is essential.

Generally, cards are best for notes as they can be easily held in the hand— write on one side only. For simple headings, notes should include:

- The sequence of headings and sub-headings.
- Opening remarks, link phrases and summaries, and your carefully worked out conclusions.

- The points where audio/visuals will be used.
- The points where audience participation is required, with, perhaps, leading questions or prepared discussion topics.
- The timing.

Rehearsal and Practice

For some presentations, a rehearsal is valuable/essential. The main reasons are:

- To make sure you can set the stage and arrange the equipment so that everyone will be able to see and hear.
- To make sure that your words and visual aids do what you have planned.
- To check the timing.
- To gain confidence from the experience.

Whenever possible, rehearse your presentation in the actual venue, using the equipment you will use on the day. If this is not feasible, talk through the whole presentation, if possible in similar accommodation and using similar equipment.

The Presentation Proper

Make sure that you arrive in good time, not least to check that all your equipment, materials and props are where they should be. Thank the chairman, greet the audience with a smile and start at once on your introduction. Be as natural and relaxed as you can. Keep an eye on the time. The most common mistake is not facing the audience when you are talking to them, especially when you are using visual aids.

If anything goes wrong, treat it humorously—do not get irritated or embarrassed. Answer questions briefly and clearly. Make sure you are answering what has been asked and repeat the question for the benefit of anybody in the audience who may not have heard the question. After the presentation assess your performance and decide what improvements you can make to your next one.

The Presentation Start

To be able to give your session the attention it deserves, your audience needs to:

- Settle down.
- Understand where you are going—what your roadmap for the session is.
- Become hooked—give you their attention and stop thinking about other things.

To achieve this, you need to manage your own nerves and appear confident and comfortable, prove that you and the session are worth listening to, and get the audience's attention and show them you care about them. Thus:

- Get yourself comfortable and prepared in terms of equipment, stage, and the presentation.
- When starting, start formal—you can move to informality later.
- Check the audience for—comfort, sight and hearing.
- Do not rush—take your time.
- Give them the information they need:
  - *What your session is about*: what the topic is and how it links to the conference.
  - *Where your presentation is leading*: in broad terms—what your conclusions will be.
  - *What your planned roadmap*: .. for the session is.
  - *Your behavior Ground Rules*: Questions, pauses, etc.

Handling Questions (5 Key Points)

1. At the outset, make sure they know what your groundrules for questions are	For example: "I will be delighted to take any questions of clarification at any time, but any others will be dealt with at the end of the session."
2. Wait and listen one hundred% to the question	We often start working out the answer to a question while the questioner is still speaking. Try to avoid this and while a questioner is speaking-listen. Only start thinking about the answer when the question is complete.
3. Rephrase the question	Too often, only the presenter, the questioner and the first few rows of the audience know what question the presenter is answering. A useful tactic is to rephrase the question and then repeat it to the whole audience before you answer it. The benefits are:
	• Everyone in the audience knows what is going on • It confirms your understanding with the questioner • It gives you time to think about your answer.
4. After answering, move your gaze on elsewhere	Looking at someone as you finish speaking is an implied cue for a reply. Only do so if you actually want the dialog to continue. Perhaps reinforce the message by asking something like "Does that answer your question?". To avoid a follow-on question, simply direct your gaze to some other part of the room as you finish speaking and indicate that you are ready to take a new questioner.
5. When you don't know the answer—be honest	Perhaps say "I don't know; or better still; "I don't know but I will find out", or even "I don't know, but I'll find out by the end of the lunch break". Then make sure that you do so.

Closure: When you Come to the End-stop

The two parts of your presentation that will be remembered most clearly are the introduction and the conclusion especially the conclusion. Try to finish a presentation on a positive note—make the audience feel that you and they have shared a worthwhile experience. As they say in show business, "Always leave them wanting more".

Know When to Stop

Do not be afraid to finish early. Speakers often fall into "endless maze" or "more the merrier" mode when they find that they have finished ahead of time and thereby snatch defeat from the very jaws of success.

To put it bluntly, few presentations fail by ending early unless the premature ending is due to lack of adequate preparation. Do not spoil the effect by trying to pad your speech up to the official length.

What was it All About?—Summarize it for Them

The closing section of a presentation is the vital part of that structure and must be something more than just the end of the event. It must summarize all that has gone on before and create a bridge to whatever happens after the presentation is all over. What your audience will really need to know is:

- *What* (Are we supposed to do)?
- *When* (Do we do it)?
- *How* (Will we know when we have done it satisfactorily)?
- *Closing comments.*

Some Common Errors

- *The emergency stop*: Without a hint of warning the speaker pulls up—*Well, I think that is all I have to say, so I'll stop there.*
- *The endless maze*: Where the speaker clearly ends up as lost and confused as his audience, *And so I will finish on that point and remind you of the comment I made earlier about ...*
- *The more the merrier*: Often due to lack of order and structure—*And in addition ... I had also like to say/point out/remind you.*

CHAIRING MEETINGS

As a Chair your task is to utilize the talents of the group and move them towards the meeting's objectives. This can be difficult to achieve. Looking back at your own experiences of chairing meetings, or through your observation of meetings, what elements of leading meetings can go wrong?

In this section, we look at some key pointers that will help you to lead meetings more effectively.

- *Setting up the meeting:*
  - Type of meeting
  - Size of meeting
  - Membership
  - Developing the aims and agenda.
- *Chairing the meeting:*
  - Opening the meeting
  - Keeping control
  - Discussing each item
  - Encouraging participation
  - Summarizing and closure
  - Actions after the meeting.
- Consensus building

Setting Up the Meeting

Type of Meeting

Different types of meeting need to be chaired or led differently. Clarify what type of meeting, it is that you are chairing. Is it for information gathering, information giving, negotiating, problem solving, decision making, or some other type of meeting?

Size of the Meeting

Meeting tend to fall into two size categories:

1. *Small groups, as around 3–7 people*: Small groups can be highly productive and focused. generally all participants are visible, there is a low drop out rate, and there is less possibility of cliques forming. However, they may have a narrow range of skills, have limited discussion, be a little too informal, and result in less reliable decisions.
2. *Large groups, say over 10 people*: In such groups there are often a range of view points and this can lead to sound decisions. Because of the size, there is more group pressure on saboteurs to fall in line. However the size also means that it can be hard to achieve consensus, people may be intimidated into silence, and the chair may have exert visible control. Sometimes there can be a high drop out rate, and side meetings with the danger of cliques forming. The larger the group (say exceeding 15-20), then the more these difficulties are compounded.

Membership

- The decision about who is to attend depends on what you want to accomplish in the meeting. This may seem too obvious to state, but it's surprising how many meetings occur without the right people there. Try not to ensure that those who attend can contribute rather than being simply "representatives" of their sections.
- Rather than relying solely on your own judgment about who should come, ask others for their opinion as well.
- Think about the size of room and layout that would suit the meeting—horseshoe, round table, cabaret, conference style, theater.
- Prepare the ground. Depending on the type of meeting, you may wish to prepare the ground more along the following lines:
  - Talk to each person to tell them about the meeting, it is overall purpose and why their attendance is important.
  - Follow-up with a meeting notice, including the purpose of the meeting, where it will be held and when, how long it will last, the list of participants and whom to contact if they have questions.
  - Send out a copy of the proposed agenda along with the meeting notice.
  - Have someone designated to record important actions, assignments and due dates during the meeting. This person should ensure that this information is distributed to all participants shortly after the meeting.

Developing the Aims and Agenda

- Think of what overall outcome you want from the meeting and what activities need to occur to reach that outcome. The agenda should be organized so that these activities are conducted during the meeting. In the agenda, state the overall outcome that you want from the meeting.
- For some meetings, it is best to develop the agenda together with key participants, or simply solicit agenda items in advance.
- Design the agenda so that participants get involved early by having something for them to do right away and so they come on time.
- Next to each major topic, include the type of action needed, the type of output expected (decision, vote, action assigned to someone), and time estimates for addressing each topic.
- Do not overly design meetings; be willing to adapt the meeting agenda if members are making progress in the planning process.
- Think about how you label an event, so people come in with the right frame of mind.

Chairing the Meeting

Opening the Meeting

A good start to the meeting will make a great deal of difference. It is your chance to assert your authority and lay down the ground rules.

It is worth giving thought to how you are going to open the meeting. If nothing else, it will help you to steady your own nerves. Some things to take into account are:

- Start on time.
- State the purpose and objectives of meeting.
- Make appropriate introductions, check that everyone knows each other, try and put everyone at ease.
- Announce the timetable of the meeting (finish and break times).
- If leading a new group, give information on all participants attending, their expertise and relevance to the task.

KEEPING CONTROL

Possible weaknesses of the Chair are their lack of ability to keep control of the meeting, or their tendency to be too domineering or autocratic.

You may need to exert more control at the *beginning of a meeting,* when a group is newly formed, or when the *meeting is particularly* large. Being over-controlling, however, will inhibit debate and may reduce participants' sense of ownership of the tasks.

The trick is to strike a balance between control and participation:

- Stick to the agenda and keep to time.
- Bring discussion back to the point by summarizing and asking questions.
- Deal with emotional outbursts by referring to the task, whilst acknowledging the feeling being conveyed, e.g. *"I can see you feel very strongly about this point, but time is pressing upon us and we need to try and reach a conclusion".*
- Try to avoid leading with your opinion. Give your own opinions as a member, e.g. *"if I may leave the Chair for a moment..."*
- *Control the talkative*: If a speaker gets long-winded, watch for an opportunity to break in and ask someone else about their view.

DISCUSSING EACH ITEM

An effective meeting will have a well thought out agenda with clear items. The meeting leader needs to present each item positively, and must deal with them separately.

- Refer to the agenda.
- Introduce the item briefly, so all present are clear about its nature and purpose.
- Remind participants about how much time is allocated.
- Vary your approach to introducing items, e.g. invite someone to open the discussion to the whole group.

ENCOURAGING PARTICIPATION

One of the central elements of an effective meeting is the quality of participation and involvement of those present. The Chair plays a key role in encouraging and managing the contributions of participants.

Before looking at this more closely, give some thought to the range of feelings and attitudes that meeting attendees may have during a meeting.

As the Chair of the meeting, you need to manage all the people and personalities involved. We shall be spending time during the workshop looking more closely at this. For now, here are some general pointers.

- Always ask for a range of viewpoints. Use questions—open, general, direct and probing.
- Try to be unbiased.
- Make eye contact with all attendees.
- Observe—notice who is not contributing, bring them in by asking them if they have any views or ideas.
- Avoid putting down someone's suggestions or contribution.
- Thank people for their contributions.
- Make sure everyone understands what is being said.
- Allow debate, but do not allow hostility or conflict to develop.

SUMMARIZING AND CLOSURE

Summarizing is a particularly useful strategy to adopt when leading meetings. It can be used:

- When discussion is drying up or is degenerating into social *Chitchat*, e.g. *"Can I just recap on what has been said so far..."*
- To highlight and emphasize the mood of the group, *"I can see that there is a great deal of enthusiasm for this particular option."*
- When contributions become rambling or repetitive, *"I am picking up a consistent theme here, it seems that..."*
- To conclude a particular item before moving on to the next one, *"Points arising from this item are can I now suggest we move on."*

- To clarify what has been agreed. This is especially helpful for the person taking minutes, *"We have agreed that Jane is going to John will report back..."*
- At the end of the meeting—highlighting what has been achieved and re-emphasizing who is doing what helps to end the meeting positively, *"We have covered a lot of ground this morning. Just to quickly clarify, John you will be, and finally..."*

Close the meeting by thanking everyone for their attendance and their contributions. If there is to be a further meeting, aim to set the date and venue before closing the meeting. This will save a lot of time later on if venues or meetings have to be changed due to attendees' previous commitments.

Actions after Meetings

After the meeting, it is tempting to breath a sigh of relief and forget about it until the next scheduled meeting looms. However, there are several actions you need to take after the meeting has concluded.

The meeting is not an end in itself. An effective meeting can be measured by its results—the actions people take as a consequence of the meeting.

Consensus Building for Teams

One of the most important, yet poorly understood or applied, tools in a problem solving team is consensus. Consensus often is reduced to meaning "a vote," "what the most verbal agreed to," or some other dysfunctional process. But real consensus decisions can empower groups and produce superior solutions, definitions and results. Some guidelines for team members are given here.

TEAM CONSENSUS DECISION RULE

No judgement may be incorporated into the group decision until it meets at least with the tacit approval of every member.

(This is not a ground rule of unanimity, where each person is in total agreement; rather, it represents a feeling that one can "live with" the judgement or is at least willing to give it an experimental trying out.)

Guidelines for Team Member

- *Avoid arguing for you own position*: Present it as dearly and logically as possible, but be sensitive to and consider seriously the reactions of the group in any subsequent presentations of the same point.

- Avoid "win-lose" stalemates in the discussion of opinions. Discard the notion that someone must win and someone must lose in the discussion.
- Avoid changing your mind only in order to avoid conflict and to reach agreement and harmony. Withstand pressures to yield which have no objective or logical sound foundation.
- Avoid conflict-reducing techniques such as majority vote, averaging, bargaining, coin-flipping, trading out, and the like. Treat differences of opinion as indicative of incomplete sharing of relevant information on someone part.
- View differences of opinion as both natural and helpful rather than as a hindrance in decision making. Generally, the more ideas expressed, the greater the likelihood of conflict will be; but the richer the array of resources and creativity will be as well.
- View initial agreement as suspect. Explore the reasons underlying apparent agreement; make sure people have arrived at the same conclusions for either the same basic reasons or for complementary reasons before incorporating such opinions into the group decision.
- Avoid subtle forms of influence and decision modification, e.g. when a dissenting member finally agrees, do not feel that he must be "rewarded" by having his own way on some later issue or point.

When to Use a Consensus Process

Any complex issue requiring maximum input and agreement. Examples could include choosing a team problem to work on; defining your team's charter; creating a corrective action plan, etc.

When not to Use Consensus

Since consensus building is usually time consuming, routine or non-complex issues can often be resolved by other means. They might include. Team operating guidelines; lists of problems and barriers; and most other group decisions. Consensus is a powerful tool, but should not be overused!

Chapter 24

Postgraduate Medical Education Management

The availability of Doctors in India is far less than what the international average is – 0.6 per 1000 population against world average of 1.6 per 1000. The position is much more precarious when one considers the postgraduate scenarios and still worse when we consider the super specializations fields. For example India can turn out only 60 nephrologists per year.

It was, therefore necessary to come up with solutions which are cost effective, take the shortest possible time to set-up and yet produce post-graduate doctor specialists as per the norms of the Medical Council of India. The National Board of Examinations (NBE) was set-up to fill up these critical deficiencies by encouraging suitable Hospitals to get accredited for running the identified postgraduate courses which would be on par with the post-graduates coming out of Medical Colleges and would be so recognized by the Medical Council of India.

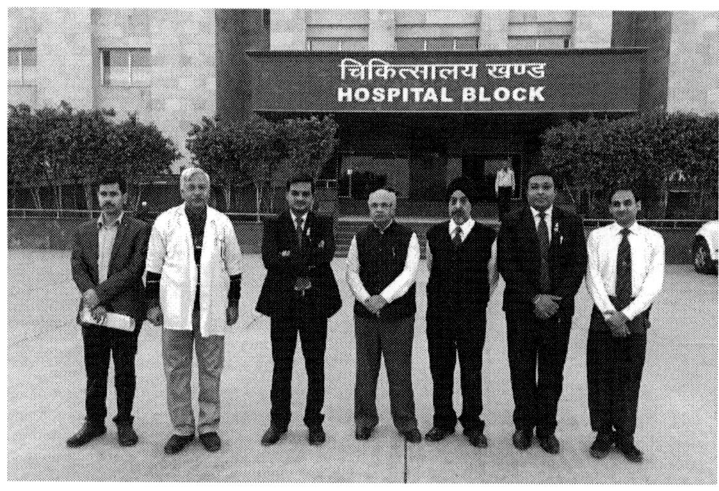

Medical College Establishment Team Member in a Hospital Visit

The NBE was to act as a facilitator for hospitals desirous of chipping in with facilities at their set-ups for this National cause. However, over the years, the Board has not been able to come up to the expectations reposed in it. It has, with passage of time, acquired a hegemonistic approach. This primarily appears not as much due to the over-zealous approach of those administering its functioning as due to their inexperience and misplaced priorities/facets of postgraduate medical education. The personal whims and fancies of those administering the Board also have been a significant contributory factor; or why should there have been drastic change of rules (with periodic changes of guard) for accreditation of hospitals willing to run postgraduate courses at their establishments. The medical fraternity feels that the National Board of Examinations has failed in its duties as with its wrong or unacceptable and wavering policies, the hospitals have been forced to withdraw from this route.

Some serious points worth considering for augmenting the availability of postgraduate doctors with the least additional costs (and without any burden on the exchequer) through the well meaning establishment of National Board of Examinations are enumerated below. These, if implemented, would certainly provide incentives to not only the doctors desirous of upgrading their qualifications but to the existing Hospitals to consider the same seriously.

- *Attitude of the accrediting agency*: The attitude of the National Board of Examinations is intimidating instead of being accommodating. The very fact that NBE wants the prospective hospitals applying for its accreditation to mention in its application form if it has engaged in any litigation/any case(s) in the court against NBE does not send a healthy message. It wants the applicant hospital to attach a list of all such cases with their application. It fails to understand that going to the court for redressal of one's grievances is the fundamental right of any individual/ institute and no one can intimidate the other from doing so. If the NBE is so concerned about anyone resorting to the legal route, it must search for the reasons within its methods of functioning and try to set them right.
- *Anarchic directives*: Medical education is an activity which is not the core-competence of the Hospitals. If they come forward to consider accreditations from NBE for conducting postgraduate courses, their intentions must be encouraged and efforts lauded. They should be permitted to consult or seek assistance from those experienced in this activity. Rather than do so, the NBE ordains that the Head of the Hospital shall declare on its official letterhead the following: "That I/We or this hospital has not sought/taken the help/assistance of an agency/agency

or part who is not employee of the applicant organization to prepare, submit and/or follow the accompany of application". In today's world it is unimaginable that someone cannot only harbor but issue such dictatorial directives—and that too for professional bodies like 200-bed hospitals. Why should a body like NBE be apprehensive of the hospital seeking help from a professional agency or an experienced consultant? The National Accreditation Board for Hospital and Health care Providers (NABH) which is a similar agency for quality accreditation of hospitals does not have any such stipulations. In fact it encourages those also who willingly come forward to help the hospitals acquire quality accreditations. The message which comes out is that NBE is dictatorial and issues anarchic guidelines.

- *No incentives to hospitals who offer their facilities as institutes of post-graduate medical education*: The Hospitals who come forward to conduct postgraduate courses at their establishments, if found fit, for the same by the NBE do not get any incentives or benefits. Many find it a losing proposition, financially. At today's cost, the hospital gets only ₹ 80,000/- per year as fees from each student. It pays back this amount through the mandated stipend(s) over the next three months. The remaining nine months it keeps paying these stipends thus incurring a significant financial loss. The cost of creating additional facilities (especially in today's scenario where the cost of space is phenomenally high) goes waste if not accredited by NBE. The facilities created become a financial burden to maintain. It can be argued that the student is providing services of a doctor to the Institute for which it needs to be paid for at par with similarly placed students in medical colleges. Yes, but then what is the incentive for the Institute/Hospital? The infrastructure, faculty and patients, etc. are provided by the Institute for the student to build himself. More than anything else the hospital is taking the risk liability of the student which in today's scenario can be enormous for a single botched up medicolegal case.

The hospital can be provided some incentives in the form of tax rebates, soft loans, and deferred repayments for the services it renders in the medical education field. The cost of creating extra infrastructure can be offset against the income to be taxed. The cost of expensive books can be similarly reimbursed or offset against the taxable income. Many more such small incentives, if granted to the hospitals, would encourage many of them to come forward to offer their existing set-ups for use by students for acquiring postgraduate medical education.

The NBE can have the publishers of reputed journals (both Indian and foreign) supply a fixed number of their journals free or at highly discounted prices for distribution to the hospitals running various postgraduate courses.

- *Not providing a 'level playing field'*: The Medical Colleges providing postgraduate education and hospitals accredited by NBE for the same purpose do not have 'level playing fields'. For example, a postgraduate teacher at Professor Grade can accept two postgraduate students under him in a medical college but in the NBE set-up he is allowed only one. Allowing each professor in the accredited hospitals to accept two candidates would immediately double the capacity of turning out postgraduate specialists per batch.

  It could be argued that for subjects/disciplines where there are secondary candidates, it automatically amounts to the same. The point is, provision of secondary candidates is permitted in only about 30% of the disciplines under NBE. Therefore, there is a need to have this stipulation for all courses, across the board, as a directive and not by implication.

  It would be a better idea if the NBE can run workshops for the inexperienced faculty (say, in thesis guidance) in such hospitals rather than downright reject the hospitals for lack of such trained or experienced faculty.

- *Unwarranted age stipulations for private hospitals/institutes make 'Over-qualification a disqualification'*: The age stipulations for faculty in hospitals accredited for postgraduate education are again without a sound logic. It is stipulated that a professor on the Faculty in a Hospital should be less than 65 years of age and a senior resident cannot be having more than 42 months of post-postgraduate (PG) degree experience. It defies logic. We all know that all well established hospitals wait for the Professors in medical colleges to superannuate to enable them seek their services for a better healthcare delivery. A professor has superannuated not because he ceases to be a good teacher/faculty after the midnight of his superannuating date, but because of the administrative necessity in the medical college (or in any government establishment) to ease him out so that those in the queue can also get a chance to occupy the seat of eminence. However, the NBE refuses to consider them as a good teaching faculty after that 'cut-off' date.

  We all are aware that a teacher, a lawyer and a doctor only 'grow' with experience and age. Rather than encourage such scarce talent and experience and utilize their services to the maximum possible, we dub them as unacceptable to teach/guide postgraduate students. Many a hospitals miss out on accreditations simply because they have highly experienced professors but over 65 years of age. This works a disincentive for the others.

In the case of senior residents, a postgraduate in the discipline was acceptable till sometime ago. This meant that even a diploma holder would have been eligible for this category of faculty. This itself was a big burden on majority of the hospitals as it would necessitate for them to have Four PG qualified members in each discipline (two degree holders as consultants and two diploma holders as junior faculty of senior residents). This stipulation has been further amended to having the senior residents also having postgraduate degrees. For a hospital to have four fulltime postgraduate degree holders for each disciplines would be a tremendous financial burden as it would require that high a patient load to merely sustain itself. Further, a post-PG experience of more than 42 months for this category of the faculty becomes a case of disqualification for NBE. It must be the only institution where over qualification becomes a disqualification. If this stipulation has been necessitated because of restricting mal practices, then it is for the NBE to 'sharpen its administrative teeth' rather than make a case of 'over qualification as a reason for disqualification'.

- *Stringent stipulations for technical publications are a damper*: The requirement of publications by the faculty is an important indicator of its involvement in educational activities—but then it is not the only indicator. It can be assessed by many other yardsticks other than those stipulated by NBE—presenting papers in professional gatherings of certain level being one.
- *Stiff penalty for rejection after paying an abnormally high application fee*: The hike of application fee from ₹ 70,000/- to ₹ 2,00,000/- per subject is rather too stiff. (This is in addition to ₹ 3,000/- charged for each application). What pinches the hospitals is the fact that their applications are summarily rejected and half of the application amount is forfeited—an unimaginably high penalty of ₹ 1,00,000/- for having one's application rejected after desk review. The penalty could be a fraction of the present one and add termed as secretarial charges. The term 'Penalty' is an indicator of the hegemony of NBE rather than their pious intention to be a facilitator for augmenting postgraduate medical education. The hospitals are not allowed a retrial if they do not come up to the accreditation standards in the first go and forfeit the entire amount of ₹ 2,00,000/-. What incentive is there for any right minded hospital administration to try for the accreditation from NBE if the penalty is stiff for a failure? The National Accreditation Board for Hospital and Healthcare Providers (NABH) is much more accommodating as it encourages a hospital to keep striving for improving its quality of service and be subjected to further inspections for accreditation. NABH approach does

not discourage the willing hospital from trying for their accreditation. But NBE accreditation means a totally different game for the applicant.

The irony is that many a time, the reason for the rejection is also not intimated. The hospitals have come to feel that it could be that the persons employed at NBE for reviewing the applications are not as well conversant as expected with the rules/norms and hospital infrastructure. Since many of them keep changing from batch to batch, it gives an impression that to cut on costs, the NBE may have employed them, as if, on contract basis for a specific duration or for a specific job.

- *Stipulation of bed strength for accreditation*: The new rule of a hospital having 200 beds for accreditation in broad specialities has brought about a tremendous reduction in the numbers of aspirants for the NBE accreditations. (It was 100 beds till about 2 years ago). If the NBE has to meet its intended function of getting more postgraduate doctors for the country, this move is certainly not in its interest. How many 200-bed hospitals can one find in our country especially in tier-II or tier-III cities? Hardly any. Yes, it would be appropriate if one limits the number of disciplines for accreditation in a hospital depending upon its bed-strength.

  More surprising is the stipulation for beds for exclusive set-up in specialities like ophthalmology, pediatrics, oncology, DVD, etc. where one should have a dedicated hospital with co-located bed strength of one hundred. The scope is drastically reduced with such stipulations.
- *Stand-alone diagnostic units not eligible for accreditation*: Making stand-alone units like diagnostic centers or laboratories ineligible for accreditation for the past 2–3 years is a retrograde step. When NBE permits stand-alone set-up of ophthalmology, dermatology and venereology, pediatrics, etc. for accreditation, the ban on stand-alone diagnostic units defies logic.

  It is well known that the work load in such centers for their areas of specializations is much more than what one expects in them when a part of a hospital. The faculty there is also much more experienced in the areas they handle. They also generally take the lead in introducing the latest technology for their areas of specialization. The concentration of highly qualified and experienced faculty in such facilities is waiting for one to exploit it for propagating postgraduating medical education. The sudden change of eligibility now by NBE making them ineligible for accreditation is therefore, not understood.

The intention of the Government in setting up the National Board of Examinations to overcome the shortage of postgraduate doctors in the shortest possible time was a very laudable effort. It intended to make use of the vast infrastructure available in our hospitals, the highly qualified and experienced doctors and the regular inflow of patients for teaching and training those aspiring to acquire postgraduate qualifications and making them available thereafter for services of our large population. But these lofty intentions have failed to fructify due to whimsical attitude and wavering guidelines of the National Board of Examinations.

To reduce the deficiency of postgraduate doctors in our country, the authorities concerned have to follow a pragmatic management approach to meet the urgent requirements of meeting the deficiencies of post-graduate doctors. To help it form policies, NBE should preferably involve managements of accredited hospitals in formulation of its policies and decision making so that their experience in running such postgraduate courses is also effectively made use of.

Chapter 25

Business Models in Clinical Research Management

MEANING OF BUSINESS MODEL

Business model is a buzzword that everybody uses (or overused) during the dotcom boom. It is the plan implemented by a company to generate revenue and make a profit from operations. The model includes the components and functions of the business, as well as the revenues it generates and the expenses it incurs. To extract value from an innovation, a start up needs an appropriate business model. Business models convert new technology to economic value.

A business model draws a multitude of business subjects, including economics, entrepreneurship, finance, marketing, operations and strategy. The business model itself is an important determinant of profits to be made from an innovation. A mediocre innovation with a great business model may be more profitable than a great innovation with a mediocre business model.

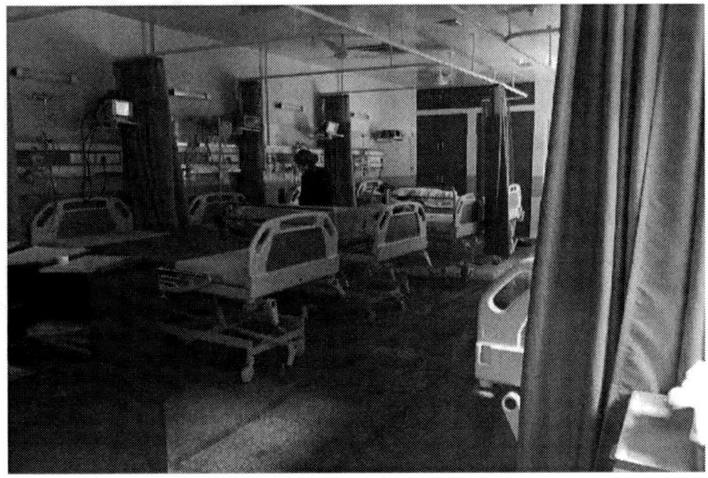

Clinical Research Ward

BUSINESS MODEL IN CLINICAL RESEARCH

Clinical Trials market in India has shown significant growth symptoms in the recent past. Clinical research experienced over 84% growth during 2006-2008 and it has its own merit in regards to further prospect considering global clinical market is growing at 12%. Clinical research industry in India touched US$258 million in 2008, up from US$140 million in 2006. An estimate shows that clinical research in India is expected to be US$320 million by 2009. The cost of conducting clinical trials in India, for instance, is 20–60% of the cost in developed countries. Not surprisingly, about 20–30% of the clinical development activity is now outsourced to developing countries such as India. Currently, there are more than 150 clinical research organizations (CROs) in India, out of which 20 comply with ICH-GCP guidelines. The leading players in India include Clinigene International, Vimta Labs Ltd, and Lotus Labs, besides multinationals like Quintiles Spectral, Pharmanet, SIRO Clinpharm and Clintec, etc.

Clinical testing of new medical therapies is an arduous process, which is difficult to plan, costly and habitually delayed. The industry spends over $30 billion a year on clinical trials, yet nearly 90% of trials fail to meet their timelines or budgets. The result has been longer delivery times and great disappointment among patients researchers and clinical trial sponsors. Clinical trials are the key interfaces of basic science findings, product development, rationalization of existing therapies, and their translation into effective clinical therapy. Thus, all translational research depends upon clinical trial data. However, clinical trial design is a specialty field in its own right and few basic scientists, clinician investigators, and clinicians have formal training in this field, particularly in neurosurgery and orthopedics. The performance of clinical trials and the outcomes of those trials form the most severe bottleneck of new therapy development, particularly in surgical fields and device development, where many alternative pathways for product introduction exist and no specific criteria are available for trial format. Thus, particularly in product development (unlike drug development), the manufacturer may omit clinical trials of efficacy determination altogether to focus only on safety issues, rather than risk a failed clinical trial that could doom FDA approval because alternative pathways to approval exist.

The primary motivations for considering and initiating clinical trials highlight the needs for well-designed clinical trial formats, for innovations at the FDA approval level, and in translational research as a whole.

Although they are important for surgical research, designs such as decision analysis, surveys, health economic, and qualitative studies will not be covered. A special attempt will be made to demystify some of the concepts inherited from classical "evidence-based medicine" without further judgment. In particular, the role of randomized controlled trials for evaluating treatment efficacy will be scrutinized—emphasizing differences between surgical and nonsurgical research while stressing the importance of making a surgical study both feasible and generalizable to a "real-world" patient population.

In the light of the developments, is there a need for the pharma industry to review its business models? The answer is an emphatic yes. The traditional Risk-Innovation-Reward model followed by the pharma industry has stopped fetching timely rewards, at least for now. Further to this, the concept of personalized medicine is slowly evolving in the pharma industry and is catching up fast in the healthcare industry. Decision-makers in the healthcare industry are seriously evaluating patient-centric strategies and in the not too distant future, these strategies will be implemented industry-wide. As a consequence, developing drugs customized to target populations and genetic traits will soon become the norm.

In such a scenario, the current "one-drug-fits-all" concept would be outdated and the traditional innovation-based business model will no longer hold good. Therefore, in enlightened self-interest, pharma majors will need to give serious thought to a variety of business models.

TYPES OF BUSINESS MODELS

The business models in clinical trials have certain unique aspects. One is the drawn out, highly structured value chain determined in large part by the regulatory process itself. Another is the high cost of product development, with associated high risks of failure. Offsetting these high costs and risks are the high returns for successful product development. A further defining characteristic is the focus on innovation. The pace of innovation both in terms of product innovation and in the process of drug discovery and development has intensified over at least the last decade. Some of the peculiar business models are listed and described here:

Individual Project Outsourcing Model

Outsourcing is a strategic management tool wherein business processes are transferred to another company. The concept is to let the third party service provider perform the management and/or day to day execution of one or more business functions. The third party service provider is insourcing those same processes. Outsourcing occurs when a company uses an outside firm to provide necessary business function that might otherwise be done inhouse. In its most advanced form, outsourcing makes it possible to build a large, entirely virtual company.

Outsourcing in clinical trial activities is a burgeoning industry, and it has seen exponential growth reminiscent of the boom in the IT industry. Among the clinical trial activities that can potentially be outsourced to India, the emergence of medical writing as a niche area for outsourcing is a recent phenomenon.

There are various models of outsourcing used in medical writing. The fractionated service outsourcing and full service outsourcing models are generally acknowledged to be the most successful models. The fractionated model allows a CRO to provide best in class services for individual operational functions. A client may choose, via this model, to outsource all its medical writing needs to a single CRO that offers services in this niche area. Numerous contracts are therefore managed across a given program (one per operational function) and the client has to ensure accountability of the various players in a multifaceted program.

Internal expertise of substantial depth is required to manage various players over long programs. This may be a resource challenge for the client especially in the case of specialized skills such as statistical analysis and medical writing. One may also encounter varying work cultures, standard operating procedures (SOPs) and incompatibility of data or operational systems such as the document management systems of the various providers. Unless managed with a great degree of discipline, this model is highly prone to unhealthy competition among the providers, which works to the detriment of the program.

Companies such as SIRO that have an operational base in data management in India and Europe are able to work on hybrid models that provide the advantage of the best expertise from Europe coupled with scale from India to provide high quality, optimal cost solutions. Big CROs offer their Indian counterparts to use their global server, software and other infrastructure with addition of user licenses to extend their data management business. Hence, they can save costs on some hardware and software to start the data management business.

Full-time Equivalent Model

The definition of full-time equivalent (FTE) is the number of working hours that represents one full-time employee during a fixed time period, such as one month or one year. FTE simplifies work measurement by converting work load hours into the number of people required to complete that work. FTE models assemble and relate workload data to job positions, processes, products, customer segments, and other performance drivers that an organization may use. FTE models are constructed with statistical tools and methods, and are organized as data models with data charts and graphs. Data models are used because they accurately measure workloads and required FTEs while also making scenario forecasting (what if analysis) easy and accurate.

In the FTE model, pharma companies outsource the job of developing the facility, offices and human resources (FTEs) to a service provider, who could be a CRO or an IT company with the understanding of the clinical trial data management and biostatistics business. The human resources in this case could be statistical programmers, statisticians, data viewers, DB designers and medical writers.

In this model, the client chooses to outsource all (or the bulk) of a given program or project to a single service provider. The service provider would be a full-service CRO that has expertise in each relevant functional area. Typically, the medical writing department of the CRO would be linked to the data management and statistics department(s) of the CRO with some level of integration in operations. This results, at best, in synchronized SOPs being used across functions and an umbrella project management. This allows the client and vendor to operate under a single contract and leads to efficiencies in contract processes. When this model works well, it often leads to a seamless integration between the client and vendor with each complementing the other's competency levels. The client derives the benefits of critical thinking and team work. However, the services provided may be a mixed bag as it would be difficult to find the perfect CRO with best-in-class services in each operational area.

FTE analysis models guarantee that you will:

- Reduce and optimize staffing costs
- Increase and optimize productivity
- Meet and exceed service quality levels
- Define and maintain the skills that your processes need
- Utilize all of your human resource capacity and skills in the most productive ways
- Provide rewarding work and careers to your employees
- Rationalize and optimize your organization with the right generalists and specialists.

This model offers client companies several advantages to:

- Have sufficient personnel at hand for their entire project related requirements and meet the peak time demand, without the need to recruit staff on permanent head count.

- Have access to experienced clinical research staff who are skilled in a variety of job functions which can eventually lead to reduced labor costs
- Reduce time spent in training the staff, and overall conduct of clinical trials
- Improve quality of research through quality staff and supervision
- Retain control over their existing projects without the need to outsource the entire project.
- Provide a solution for the high attrition rate in this Industry. This method allows the sponsor to work jointly with the CRO to provide innovative incentives and support for quality staff retention. This service also guarantees a timely replacement in the face of attrition.
- Minimize long-term risk
- FTEs/contract staffs are priced based on the cost of their salary, the overheads and the margin. It could be charged to the sponsor on monthly basis.

Functional Service Provider (FSP) Model

Many Life Sciences companies are moving towards specialized, niche providers with the experience and dedication in specific clinical service areas. These niche providers, often referred to as Functional Services Providers allow companies to focus on their core competencies and reduce costs while at the same time receiving high-quality solutions to their needs.

Initially, the functional outsourcing model was employed for just a few functions (e.g. monitoring or data management). Today, however, FSPs provide far more than just monitoring and data management. Rather than outsourcing a complete trial to a single CRO, a growing number of pharma and biotech companies are opting for this outsourcing strategy in regulatory document preparation, investigator contract negotiations, site identification and initiation, biostatistics, medical writing, and more.

Because project ownership remains in-house, companies that use functional outsourcing may experience higher levels of quality control yet have access to specific services at a lower overall cost. Sponsor companies benefit from being able to ramp up and draw down resources relative to their development activity levels without affecting their internal head count.

In some cases, companies have effectively collaborated with functional service providers by negotiating strategic staffing transfers (i.e. they have transferred some of their internal employees to the employ of the FSP team). This arrangement produces a provider team that is already steeped in the sponsor company's culture, processes, and systems. Most companies also find that by focusing on their core competencies and outsourcing other noncore functions, they can better allocate internal resources and operate more efficiently. Another advantage is that once companies are relieved of personnel worries, they can give greater attention to their clinical development strategies.

Cultural fit is a major factor in successful sponsor—FSP relationships. Be wary of the vendor with a knight on a white horse attitude. "We know what you want, we are the experts, now leave us alone to deliver," is not a philosophy that fosters collaboration. And collaboration is essential for a partnership to manage changes such as implementing new technologies. A successful partnership requires consideration and assessment of each party's interests; these are essential to addressing such issues as: What happens when the sponsor requires a quick ramp up by the FSP provider due to new development activities? What if there are lulls in the pipeline when the FSP may receive no work? These are issues that require advanced planning and mutual trust.

Functional service providers provide services function by function but have the added advantage of providing full service through IT+BPO+IS. India's service providers are on the leading edge of FSP services and are positioned for helping pharmaceutical companies transition to a single strategic partnership model for clinical trials. FSPs take up functions within the data-management process and provide flexible solutions. FSPs are especially effective in situations where the study size requires flexibility, start/stop/start prioritization, fast-tracking of certain studies, and more visibility to the study's progress.

The key strengths of FSPs lie in converting complex business processes into simpler activities with quality measurements; in turn, this helps the teams produce consistent, repeatable results every time. FSPs also bring in synergies with their IT background, which certainly brings about productivity improvements. In addition, FSPs use Six Sigma and Lean methodologies for process reengineering, which leads to significant cost savings. But the strategic value from a partnership—between a pharma company and a full-services provider requires many key relationship elements.

First, there must be a robust joint governance structure with leadership members from strategic, operational, and business transformation teams. Other imperatives include:

- Transparency in knowledge-sharing and best practices
- Baseline operational metrics and defined year-on-year productivity improvements with measurement systems, rewards, and recognitions
- Sharing of metrics and balanced scorecard to assess ongoing quality and health of the partnership
- Creating and leveraging cross-functional synergies within the partnership.

Example: Here is an example to illustrate the ramifications of advanced planning. A mid-size biotech deployed the FSP model for selecting a vendor for EDC. The sponsor was careful to evaluate potential FSPs months prior to implementing EDC on a specific program or study. They sent comprehensive RFPs six to nine months prior to final selection, scheduled capabilities demos, and selected a short list of preferred vendors on whom they performed complete vendor selection audits to ensure due diligence and appropriate fit within the organization. The sponsor requested pricing on a full program (four studies) in order to see if they would obtain cost reductions on subsequent studies due to the efficiencies gained. These efficiencies were seen in database development and programming, eCRF screen designs, and several other data management services where the EDC provider could provide reduced pricing by recycling the previous study material with minor modifications for the subsequent studies.

Once the right FSP vendor was identified, they negotiated the Master Service Agreement terms carefully to ensure that they established balanced obligations and a clear definition of all parties' roles and responsibilities, appropriate governance for issue resolution, and communication between the two organizations. This upfront evaluation process ensured that they selected the right vendor for the best price and that they wasted no time on vendor selection activities when they needed to begin work on the first EDC study.

A mid-sized pharma company used a similar approach. When our organization made the decision to use FSPs for data management, we did so in a structured and deliberate way. The head of the Data Management Group knew the capabilities, skills, and cultural profile that he needed in a provider for this approach to work effectively for his team and the company overall. He identified potential providers and carefully evaluated them from multiple perspectives. Face-to-face interactions were essential to the evaluation and final decision. The importance of understanding providers and how they work in their own environments cannot be overemphasized.

Build-Operate-Transfer (BOT) Model

Some companies reject outsourcing to third-party vendors and instead opt to start their own foreign subsidiaries, a process that frequently is not as smooth as they expect. They face obstacles—legal, taxes, hiring, and management—from start to finish. While some eventually attain a steady state, others struggle, and a few even wind up shutting their operations.

The failures of these captive subsidiaries have led to the evolution of a new business model in the offshore services industry called a build-operate-transfer (BOT). In this model, a firm contracts with an offshore partner to build a shared services or offshore development center and operate it for a fixed interim period. The logic behind the BOT model: the offshore partner can initiate operations and reach operating stability much faster than it can with an in-house effort.

A typical BOT is built and managed in three phases:

1. *Build*: The offshore partner provides clients with a complete solution for building a presence in a particular country. The clients receive their own office space and establish their own brand identity at a lower price than comparable offshoring arrangements. Vendors take care of all administrative and legal issues, from real estate, utilities, and permits, to computers, communications, and office supplies. The vendor also provides the professional support staff and operating licenses to run functions such as call centers.
2. *Operate*: The offshore partner provides a comprehensive set of operational management services, from HR and staffing, to accent training, accounting, payroll, legal, facilities, and security. The clients are able to focus their management time on their core business rather than on operational issues.
3. *Option to transfer*: The offshore partner cannot lock in clients. The clients have the option to bring the operation in-house at any time. Typically, the outsourcing contract includes a clause that states the client has the option to buy the entire operation after a fixed period.

Building a subsidiary in a foreign country requires much knowledge and information about the country and culture, as well as the right personnel. Traditionally, the BOT model is usually found in the civil and construction engineering business, especially in the maintenance of highways and airports. Now the BOT model is becoming popular in the offshore outsourcing world. A BOT model provides customers with bottom-line enhancements and fully offloaded costs, risks, and ownership of the new venture. The risk of execution is minimized, and companies can spend their money on core functions.

The BOT model can also appear in different variations: one of which is called BOOT (i.e. Build-Operate-Option to Transfer). In this variant, the client prefers to set-up after 3–4 years a 100% operation for R&D, while continuing to have the BOOT unit operate independently under the Indian services company. In this variation, the 100% subsidiary focuses on strategic and sensitive R&D work while the BOOT unit does less strategic work. The BOT model is less risky than a joint venture and more rewarding, particularly over the first 5 years. The BOT model has not been tested in the Life Science space. In addition there are no examples of MNCs who have used BOT to enter into the life science sector in India. Therefore BOT will be the model, which we will focus on in greater detail in this report.

Benefits of BOT Model

BOT offers attractive business benefits over the traditional subsidiary/Joint venture/3rd party vendor path:

- *Rapid scaling of operations:* Ability to hire and retain 100 molecular biotechnologists in as little as 3 months!
- *Lower infrastructure set-up costs:* Lease lab space for as little as $2 per sq. ft/month, with no outlay on deposits and capital investments.
- *Shared infrastructure:* Client can access expensive capital equipment which is less frequently used on time share basis from the Indian operator.
- *Share risk and upside:* Allows the client to gradually evolve from a low to a high volume business with financial risk taken by Indian operator.
- *Better IPR protection than a 3rd party vendor:* Each team member works exclusively for the client while entering into a 1:1 direct NDA with them.
- Reduced time to operations through utilization of knowledgeable Indian operator management resources responsible for:
  - Real Estate
  - Government rules and regulatory compliance
  - Legal
  - Cultural transition
  - IT infrastructure procurement
  - Security
  - BOT model is more conducive medium in assisting a company to set-up a wholly owned subsidiary in the long run.

Risks Involved in BOT Model

- Close proximity of client facility to competitor's facility run by the Indian operator could pose risk to confidentiality and IPR
- Business continuity risk—change of ownership of the Indian operator could cause uncertainty in the continuity of the project.

Example: Struggling to reduce the development costs of new software products and to bring those products to market faster, JD Edwards signed a 6-year contract with Covansys, a global consulting and technology services company, in February, 2003, before it was acquired by PeopleSoft later that year. The maker of application enterprise software bet that 60 full-time Covansys developers devoted to quality assurance, testing, and maintenance of JD Edwards products would decrease the time it took for the company to deliver new products.

In hiring Covansys, JD Edwards freed up its internal testing and maintenance teams for strategic, new software development. By taking advantage of Covansys' development operations in Chennai, India, JD Edwards reduced the initial expense of establishing a new offshore operation.

According to the six-year agreement, JD Edwards can increase the number of Covansys developers annually. It can also assume ownership of the infrastructure that Covansys created and even take over the physical lease for the Chennai facility held by Covansys. If it does not work out quite the way JD Edwards intended, the company can walk away, an option that PeopleSoft may choose to exercise. Either way, the BOT arrangement minimizes the risk for JD Edwards.

Full Service Outsourcing Model

Clinical outsourcing strategies gaining footholds in the market today are innovative and offer companies options to drive their time to market and decrease costs. These strategies have come in various forms throughout the years and have been uniquely structured based on the needs of the sponsor company and service provider. There have been several strategies (or also referenced as structures/models) called: strategic alliances, strategic partnerships, preferred providers, staff augmentation, etc. The consensus seems to be that no one strategy works the best for everyone and that even at the same company, a different model is appropriate at different times.

In the nonclinical realm, the trend is toward a full-service model, often referred to as the one-stop shop. In simple terms, a full-service model (one-stop shop) may be the best approach when there are not enough internal resources to manage various providers or where global geographic reach is critical. The one-stop-shop model in recent years reflects two major trends in the pharmaceutical industry. The first is the renewed support for early-stage companies developing new drug candidates and their focus on getting to proof-of-concept (positive results at Phase IIA) as quickly as possible. Venture-backed early-stage companies account for over 50% of the new drug candidates in early development (preclinical through Phase IIA), and their development programs are geared toward achieving proof-of-concept as quickly and cheaply as possible. Most of these companies lack the facilities and breadth of scientific and development know-how to manage a program to proof-of-concept, let alone to commercialization. The full-service nonclinical CROs are promising these early-stage companies a quick and cost-effective route to proof-of-concept by providing a turnkey offering with complete nonclinical capabilities and project-management skills to tie it all together.

The second trend is the interest of private equity investors in the pharmaceutical services market. The nonclinical contract services business is highly fragmented and presents many acquisition opportunities for private equity investors looking to build a large CRO operation by buying up a number of smaller operations. The full-service CRO presents a logical model around which to build an acquisition strategy.

Clinical research organization (CRO) also called as contract research organization is defined by USFDA and code of federal regulation as "a person (i.e. a legal person which may be a corporation) that assumes, as an independent contractor with the sponsor, one or more of the obligations of a sponsor examples design of a protocol, selection or monitoring of investigations, evaluation of reports and preparation of material to be submitted to the FDA."[21 CFR 312.3(b)].

Functions

It is one of the organizations involved in clinical trials along with sponsors and volunteer patients, it gets the trial conducted on behalf of the sponsor, data management set-ups, independent auditors, and ethics committees. Its major functions are:

- Provide the right number of resources with the right competencies.
- Handling protocol development.
- Site selection and management.
- Study monitoring.
- Data management.
- Medical writing.
- Quality assurance.
- Look after some regulatory affair tasks.

Factors Affecting the Selection of CRO

- Core technical competence.
- The ability of the vendor to understand the objective of the trial.
- The capability of the CRO to match the sponsors budget.
- Local presence of the vendor's project management.
- Rapport shared with the vendor.
- The breadth of service offered.
- Global presence and brand image.
- Credibility of the vendor.
- Cultural gaps.

- IT issues.
- The ability to ensure compliance with both local and global regulations.
- Immediate cost gains.
- Transparency, to build confidence in this relationship.

Advantages of Outsourcing Trials to CROs

- Higher compliance with planned timeliness.
- Flexible capacity so as to manage peaks and valleys in a better way.
- Better ability to build the product development pipeline.
- Better compliance with regulatory requirement.
- Obvious cost savings.
- Projects utilizing CROs at higher levels tend to reduce cycle time by two to four weeks.

Challenges

- Biggest challenge for CROs is that there is more and more thinning of availability of resources in developing countries and as functional outsourcing picks up steam in the coming 1–2 years, there will be near-term lack of qualified resource available.
- CROs over promise and under deliver. They need to focus more on quality and less on cost.
- Are unresponsive once deal is signed.
- Are inexperienced and overpriced.
- Lack of defined expectations by sponsors is a significant problem for CROs.
- Poor communication between CRO and sponsor personnel is a significant problem for any project.
- Mismatched expectations between sponsor and CRO are often the cause of difficulties in relationships between outsourcing partner.

Conclusion

The presence of CROs with niche skills and the ability to rapidly provide the right number of resources with the right competencies has made the big pharma re-evaluate their strategies.

Chapter 26

Paramedical and its Scope in Healthcare

"What gets measured gets managed and what gets managed gets accomplished"

Paramedicals are the backbone of hospital and healthcare industry. A doctor cannot survive without paramedicals. The Indian healthcare fraternity has excelled than many of those in the most developed nations. However, the current healthcare education system has not able to keep pace with the growing healthcare professionals demand across the country. Moreover, the brain drain has led to acute shortage of qualified healthcare workforce.

PARAMEDICAL SCIENCES: COURSES WITH GREAT SCOPE

In modern world, paramedical sciences have emerged as important branches of medical science.

Without paramedics, the entire health industry is out of gear and is almost nonfunctionary.

A paramedic is a professional who helps the doctors in specialized areas and facilitates for better diagnosis, treatment and therapy. Be a Paramedic to discover the great realms of human health and earn good money. It is a hidden treasure, which is not known to many.

The increase in number of patients, variety of diseases and the demand for immense treatment has paved the way for paramedical professionals who are expert technicians or therapists providing better quality to human healthcare.

The planning commission report states that India is short of 6 lakh paramedicals. There is an increasing realization on the importance of paramedical personnel in the health sector. Paramedics are a boon to nursing homes and a dream for students, who have not been able to become full-fledged medical professionals. Healthcare delivery systems are undergoing rapid changes and the demand for skilled paramedical personnel is on the rise.

Almost all the diagnostic procedures are carried out by the paramedical staff and they have emerged a vital cog in the wheel of the healthcare delivery system. The population explosion coupled with the mushrooming of private and corporate hospitals has provided numerous opportunities for skilled paramedics.

Now, what is important is to know more about such 'Professionals' who do a Blood Test or a massage or a therapy and aid the doctor for better treatment of the patient and hence make healthcare easy and effective. These professionals are called as 'Paramedics.'

Paramedics are the key players in the health and medical sector. Without paramedics, the entire health industry is out of gear and is almost non-functionary. If there are no paramedics, then there is neither money nor any profit for doctors, hospitals, private clinics, etc.

So, be a paramedic and discover the great realms of 'Human health' and earn huge money. It is a hidden treasure which is not known to many. A few who found the hidden treasure are now the masters in the field of healthcare and medical sciences. Currently, they have better opportunities and bright prospects than a MBBS/BDS graduate.

Institution will need to attract more and more students and increase its pool of potential entrants and also ensure greater diversity from within the population. With corporate expanding business by reaching out to markets beyond metros and cities, there is a greater need for manpower in these areas. It would be extremely essential to have locally trained and skilled manpower to fuel this growth. Hence, educational institutes will need to increase the bouquet of offerings and reach to larger populations.

PARAMEDICAL: THE BACKBONE OF MEDICAL SCIENCE

In modern world, paramedical science has emerged as an important branch of medical science. It is proved as a milestone in the treatment of communicable, noncommunicable diseases. In other words, we can say that paramedical science is a backbone for medical science because right diagnosis of any disease is necessary to prevent fatal diseases.

With the advancement in the modes of medical treatment and the risen demand for diagnosis, automation and new life support systems, paramedics professionals are high in demand.

Plato (428 BC–348 BC) said, "The direction in which education starts a man will determine his future life." A good degree course module recognizes the wisdom in what was stated by the great philosopher hundreds of years ago!

Education is today identified among basic needs, as essential for an individual's survival as 'food, clothing and shelter.' The need for education has been recognized in all parts of the country and among all sections of society. Education brings success and success translates into social recognition. Though we have developed well in higher education system, a limited infrastructure facilities is there in most of the educational institutions.

From the first Five-Year Plan onwards India's emphasis was to develop a pool of scientifically inclined manpower. India's National Policy on Education (NPE) provisioned for an apex body for regulation and development of higher technical education, which came into being as the All India Council for Technical Education (AICTE) in 1987 through an Act of the Indian Parliament. The statutory All India Council for Technical Education (AICTE) was established for proper planning and co-coordinated development of technical education system through out the country. The Indian Institutes of Management are also among the Nation's premier education facilities. Several Regional Engineering Colleges (REC) have been converted into National Institutes of Technology. The UGC has inter-university centers at a number of locations throughout India to promote common research, e.g. the Nuclear Science Center at the Jawaharlal Nehru University, New Delhi, India.

The quality of education of these institutes have managed to change the outlook of India so much that this ancient country which was earlier known for yoga and mediation is now known for computer engineers. However, it does not mean that the challenge of making technical education accessible to the rural populace and other under developed sections of the society has been overcome. The literacy level in India is the highest compared to anywhere else in the world. The reason for the growth of literacy is because of the umpteen numbers of various types of Colleges and Universities offering different kinds of education in various fields beginning from Medicine to Engineering to Astronomy and Forestry India is, therefore, fast moving up the value chain in all aspects of scientific and financial research from software to medical to biomedics. The demand for professional courses is growing rapidly.

In India, both public and private institutions operate simultaneously. It is also likely that most of the growth in the rapidly expanding higher education sector took place in private unaided college or in self-financing institutions. It is felt that as of now more than 50% of the higher education in India is imparted through private institutions, mostly unaided.

Who is a Paramedic?

Paramedical science is that field of science which helps in providing assistance to Doctors in treating their patients. The stream of paramedical science ranges from diagnostics to procedures to therapies.

If a person completes a two- or three-year course and becomes an authorized person to work as a technician in a specific area of medical industry, s/he is called a paramedic. The professional is an integral part of the hospital and becoming one is highly rewarding both in India and abroad. Paramedical courses for those who have passed Class 10+2.

Name of paramedical courses: Laboratory technology, imaging technology, optometry technology, dental technology, dialysis technology, cardiac care technology, physiotherapy, occupational therapy, speech therapy, biotechnology, biomedical waste, radiation therapy, critical care technology, operation theater technology, etc.

New and latest paramedical courses: Mortuary technician, medical record technician, hospital linen and laundry technician, dental technician, infection control technician, etc.

CURRENT ROLE OF PARAMEDICAL

Paramedics are the key players in the health and medical sector. Without paramedics, the entire health industry is out of gear and is almost nonfunctionary.

A paramedic is a professional who helps the doctors in specialized areas and facilities for better diagnosis, treatment and therapy. The increase in number of patients, variety of diseases and the demand for immense treatment have paved the way for paramedical professionals who are expert technicians or therapists providing better quality towards human healthcare. Thus, the field of paramedical sciences is gaining ever increasing importance and demand, offering lucrative careers in the health sector.

The paramedical staff plays vital role in any hospital other than doctors. Any doctor before he starts treatment to the patient, he has to take the guidance and reports of various tests conducted on patients to know about his/her condition. These tests are carried out by the experienced paramedical staff. The continuous expansion of the healthcare industry brings a more demand for trained paramedical professionals.

FACTS AND FIGURES : PARAMEDICALS

Red Flag Warning: Currently, india requires 12 lakh doctors and 96 lakh paramedical and supportive staff *(Source : Survey 2013—Six Sigma Healthcare)*

Global scenario/shortage of paramedical staff

Country	Shortage	Number of Indian paramedical working there (Approx)
India	6.45 Lakh	
China	4.12 Lakh	574
Canada	66,000	1298
US	2.14 Lakh	1445
Russia	2.67 Lakh	677
Sri Lanka	1.24 Lakh	234
Australia	43,000	350

Note: For Indian paramedical, there is a huge scope in all above countries

OPPORTUNITIES FOR PARAMEDICALS

Paramedical science is emerging as a multidimensional branch of service which is filled with great opportunities. As paramedical is only capable of removing and diagnosing different diseases, it has given way to career opportunities and played an important role in improving the health conditions of people.

After completing the basic course in any of the paramedical streams, the candidate can take up a job in a hospital, nursing home, clinic, health departments, etc. With the opening of corporate hospitals, the scope for these professionals has increased tremendously. The candidates can also choose for teaching as a profession. Besides, they can open their own laboratories/clinics.

Employment opportunity for paramedical professionals is increasing day by day not only in India rather in the western countries such as the USA, Canada, UK, UAE, etc. Their role is to help doctors to provide the correct diagnosis of a disease to enable its best possible treatment. Paramedical sciences have their own value and significance.

Paramedical science is emerging as a multidimensional branch of service which is filled with great opportunities. As paramedical is only capable of removing and diagnosing different diseases, it has given way to career opportunities and played an important role in improving the health conditions of people.

Almost in every Primary Health Centre (PHC), there are many vacancies of pathology technicians, X-ray technicians, pharmacists, and dental technicians.

Recruitment in PHC and Description Hospital.

Recruitment in International Health Agencies such a WHO, UNICEF, Red Cross.

Recruitment in Radiological and Atomic Research Centre.

Remuneration

The average starting salary for paramedical professional varies from ₹ 20,000 to 30,000 per month. It may go to ₹ 40,000 and more depending on personal skills and experience and the hospital.

Paramedical Institutes

- All India Institute of Medical Sciences (AIIMS), Delhi
- Global Institute of Healthcare Management, New Delhi
- Postgraduate Institute of Medical Education and Research (PGIMER), Chandigarh

How paramedical staff hired in India in the absence of any paramedical council or regulatory body?

Medical sciences cannot take even a single step without paramedical science. At present every hospital depends on paramedical staff and there is a huge shortage of paramedicals in India or across the globe. The movement or shortage of paramedical staff is very high and it is tough to take any legal action on paramedical staff in the absence of any registering body or paramedical council. Since there is no paramedical council till date, its very difficult to control the negligence of paramedicals in India. This field is highly unregulated.

Current Process of Hiring Paramedical Staff

- Hospitals inviting direct application for the job in the leading news papers and selecting the candidate as per need.
- Hospital takes paramedical staff by doing campus placements in the respective institutes.
- Placement through placement agencies or consultants.

Recommendations

- Government should formulate uniform syllabus, regulations for paramedical courses.

- Establish a centralize monitoring body for paramedical staff and their welfare.
- Establish paramedical council of India.
- To start registration of paramedical staff.
- Establishment of paramedical university in every state.
- Development of current paramedical Institutes.

List of Paramedical Courses

S. No.	Courses offered	Eligibility	Duration
1.	Certificate in Healthcare Waste Management	10+2	6 Months
2.	Diploma in Medical Lab Technology	10+2 with PCB/PCM 10th with Science	2 Years 3 Years
3.	Diploma in Ophthalmic Technology	10+2 with PCB/PCM 10th with Science	2 Years 3 Years
4.	Diploma in Operation Theatre Technology	10+2 with PCB/PCM 10th with PCB/PCM	2 Years 3 Years
5.	Diploma in ECG Technology	10+2 with PCB/PCM 10th with PCB/PCM	2 Years 3 Years
6.	Diploma in Radiography Technology	10+2 with PCB/PCM 10th with PCB/PCM	2 Years 3 Years
7.	Bachelor of Physiotherapy	10+2 with PCB/PCM	4 Years
8.	Bachelor of Occupational Therapy	10+2 with PCB/PCM	3 Years
9.	Bachelor of Medical Lab Technology	10+2 with PCB/PCM	3 Years
10.	Bachelor of Radiation Technology	10+2 with PCB/PCM	3 Years
11.	Bachelor of Optometry and Ophthalmic Technology	10+2 with PCB/PCM with english and with 45% aggregate marks	4 Years
12.	PG diploma in Geriatric Medicine	MBBS	1 Year
13.	PG diploma in Maternal and Child Health	MBBS	1 Year
14.	PG Diploma in Drug Regulatory Affairs	Graduate with science	1 Year
15.	Master of Physiotherapy (MPT)	BPT/BOT	2 Years
16.	Master of Occupational Therapy	BPT/BOT	2 Years
17.	Master of Medical Lab Technology	BPT/BOT/BMLT	2 Years
18.	Master of Radiation Technology	BRT/BPT/BOT/Graduate in concerned branch	2 Years

Contd...

Contd...

S. No.	Courses offered	Eligibility	Duration
19.	Master of Optometry and Ophthalmic Technology	BOOT/BPT/BOT/ Graduate in concerned branch	2 years
20.	B.Sc. (Biotechnology/microbiology/ biochemistry/mathematics/ general sciences/ physics/chemistry)	10+2 with PCM/PCB	3 years
21.	M.Sc. (Biotechnology/microbiology/ biochemistry/mathematics /general sciences/ physics/chemistry)	Graduate in related fields	2 years
	POSTGRADUATE DIPLOMA/ ADVANCE CERTIFICATE		
22.	Healthcare and Hospital Management (PGDHHM)	Graduate	1 year
23.	Medicolegal Management (PGDMLM)	Graduate	1 year
24.	Healthcare Materials Management (PGDHMM)	Graduate	1 year
25.	Nursing Administration (PGDNA)	Graduate/Diploma in Nursing	1 year
26.	Healthcare Leadership Management (HLM)	Graduate	1 year
27.	Medical Records Management (MRM)	Graduate	1 year
28.	Healthcare Finance Analyst (HFA)	Graduate	1 year
29.	Pharmacy Management (PM)	Graduate	1 year
30.	Certificate in Management Consulting	Postgraduate	6 months
31.	Certificate in Healthcare Management Consulting	Postgraduate	6 months
32.	Six Sigma Green Belt Programme in Healthcare	10+2, Science	7 days
33.	Six Sigma Black Belt Programme in Healthcare	10+2, Science	5 days
34.	Diploma in Mortuary Technician	10+2, Science	1 year
35.	Diploma in Infection Control	10+2, Science	1 year
36.	Diploma in Hospital Linen and Laundry	10+2, Science	1 year
37.	Diploma in Gas Manifold Technician	10+2, Science	1 year
38.	Diploma in Pharmacy Assistant	10+2, Science	1 year
39.	Diploma in Dialysis Technician	10+2, Science	1 year
40.	Diploma in Hospital and Health Architecture	Graduation	1 year

Source: www.gihmdelhi.com

Chapter 27 Plan for a Start-up Business

The business plan consists of a narrative and several financial worksheets. The narrative template is the body of the business plan. It contains more than 150 questions divided into several sections. Work through the sections in any order that you like, except for the *Executive Summary,* which should be done last. Skip any questions that do not apply to your type of business. When you are finished writing your first draft, you will have a collection of small essays on the various topics of the business plan. Then you will want to edit them into a smooth-flowing narrative.

The real value of creating a business plan is not in having the finished product in hand; rather, the value lies in the process of researching and thinking about your business in a systematic way. The act of planning helps you to think things through thoroughly, study and research if you are not sure of the facts, and look at your ideas critically. It takes time now, but avoids costly, perhaps disastrous, mistakes later.

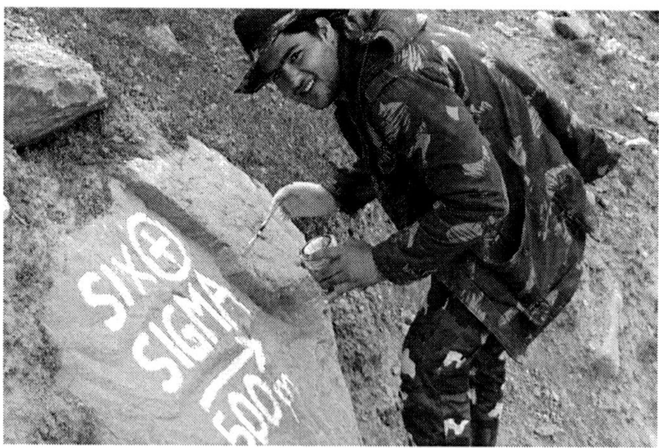

Leadership is Action, not Position

This business plan is a generic model suitable for all types of businesses. However, you should modify it to suit your particular circumstances. Before you begin, review the section titled *Refining the Plan*, found at the end. It suggests emphasizing certain areas depending upon your type of business (manufacturing, retail, service, etc.). It also has tips for fine-tuning your plan to make an effective presentation to investors or bankers. If this is why you're creating your plan, pay particular attention to your writing style. You will be judged by the quality and appearance of your work as well as by your ideas.

It typically takes several weeks to complete a good plan. Most of that time is spent in research and rethinking your ideas and assumptions. But then, that's the value of the process. So make time to do the job properly. Those who do never regret the effort. And finally, be sure to keep detailed notes on your sources of information and on the assumptions underlying your financial data.

If you need assistance with your business plan, contact the SCORE office in your area to set-up a business counseling appointment with a SCORE volunteer or send your plan for review to a SCORE counselor at www.score.org. Call 1-800-634-0245 to get the contact information for the SCORE office closest to you.

SAMPLE BUSINESS PLAN

EXECUTIVE SUMMARY

- Write this section last.
- We suggest that you make it two pages or fewer.
- Include everything that you would cover in a five-minute interview.
- Explain the fundamentals of the proposed business: What will your product be? Who will your customers be? Who are the owners? What do you think the future holds for your business and your industry?
- Make it enthusiastic, professional, complete, and concise.
- If applying for a loan, state clearly how much you want, precisely how you are going to use it, and how the money will make your business more profitable, thereby ensuring repayment.

GENERAL COMPANY DESCRIPTION

What business will you be in? What will you do?

Mission statement: Many companies have a brief mission statement, usually in 30 words or fewer, explaining their reason for being and their guiding principles. If you want to draft a mission statement, this is a good place to put it in the plan, followed by:

Company goals and objectives: Goals are destinations—where you want your business to be. Objectives are progress markers along the way to goal achievement. For example, a goal might be to have a healthy, successful company that is a leader in customer service and that has a loyal customer following. Objectives might be annual sales targets and some specific measures of customer satisfaction.

Business philosophy: What is important to you in business?

To whom will you market your products? (State it briefly here—you will do a more thorough explanation in the *Marketing Plan* section).

Describe your industry. Is it a growth industry? What changes do you foresee in the industry, short-term and long-term? How will your company be poised to take advantage of them?

Describe your most important company strengths and core competencies. What factors will make the company succeed? What do you think your major competitive strengths will be? What background experience, skills, and strengths do you personally bring to this new venture?

Legal form of ownership: Sole proprietor, Partnership, Corporation, Limited liability corporation (LLC)? Why have you selected this form?

PRODUCTS AND SERVICES

Describe in depth your products or services (technical specifications, drawings, photos, sales brochures, and other bulky items belong in Appendices).

What factors will give you competitive advantages or disadvantages? Examples include level of quality or unique or proprietary features.

What are the pricing, fee, or leasing structures of your products or services?

MARKETING PLAN

Market Research–Why?

No matter how good your product and your service, the venture cannot succeed without effective marketing. And this begins with careful, systematic research. It is very dangerous to assume that you already know about your intended market. You need to do market research to make sure you are on track. Use the business planning process as your opportunity to uncover data and to question your marketing efforts. Your time will be well spent.

Market Research–How?

There are two kinds of market research: primary and secondary.

Secondary research means using published information such as industry profiles, trade journals, newspapers, magazines, census data, and demographic profiles. This type of information is available in public libraries, industry associations, chambers of commerce, from vendors who sell to your industry, and from government agencies.

Start with your local library. Most librarians are pleased to guide you through their business data collection. You will be amazed at what is there. There are more online sources than you could possibly use. Your chamber of commerce has good information on the local area. Trade associations and trade publications often have excellent industry-specific data.

Primary research means gathering your own data. For example, you could do your own traffic count at a proposed location, use the yellow pages to identify competitors, and do surveys or focus-group interviews to learn about consumer preferences. Professional market research can be very costly, but there are many books that show small business owners how to do effective research themselves.

In your marketing plan, be as specific as possible; give statistics, numbers, and sources. The marketing plan will be the basis, later on, of the all-important sales projection.

Economics

Facts about your industry:

- What is the total size of your market?
- What percent share of the market will you have? (This is important only if you think you will be a major factor in the market.)
- Current demand in target market.
- Trends in target market—growth trends, trends in consumer preferences, and trends in product development.
- Growth potential and opportunity for a business of your size.
- What barriers to entry do you face in entering this market with your new company? Some typical barriers are:
  - High capital costs
  - High production costs
  - High marketing costs
  - Consumer acceptance and brand recognition
  - Training and skills
  - Unique technology and patents

- Unions
- Shipping costs
- Tariff barriers and quotas
- And of course, how will you overcome the barriers?
- How could the following affect your company?
  - Change in technology
  - Change in government regulations
  - Change in the economy
  - Change in your industry.

Product

In the *Products and Services* section, you described your products and services as you see them. Now describe them from your customers' point of view.

Features and Benefits

List all of your major products or services.

For each product or service:

- Describe the most important features. What is special about it?
- Describe the benefits. That is, what will the product do for the customer?

Note the difference between features and benefits, and think about them. For example, a house that gives shelter and lasts a long time is made with certain materials and to a certain design; those are its features. Its benefits include pride of ownership, financial security, providing for the family, and inclusion in a neighborhood. You build features into your product so that you can sell the benefits.

What after-sale services will you give? Some examples are delivery, warranty, service contracts, support, follow-up, and refund policy.

Customers

Identify your targeted customers, their characteristics, and their geographic locations, otherwise known as their demographics.

The description will be completely different depending on whether you plan to sell to other businesses or directly to consumers. If you sell a consumer product, but sell it through a channel of distributors, wholesalers, and retailers, you must carefully analyze both the end consumer and the middleman businesses to which you sell.

You may have more than one customer group. Identify the most important groups. Then, for each customer group, construct what is called a demographic profile:

- Age
- Gender
- Location
- Income level
- Social class and occupation
- Education
- Other (specific to your industry).

For business customers, the demographic factors might be:

- Industry (or portion of an industry)
- Location
- Size of firm
- Quality, technology, and price preferences
- Other (specific to your industry).

Competition

- What products and companies will compete with you?
  List your major competitors: Names and addresses
- Will they compete with you across the board, or just for certain products, certain customers, or in certain locations?
- Will you have important indirect competitors?
  For example, video rental stores compete with theaters, although they are different types of businesses.
- How will your products or services compare with the competition?
  Use the competitive analysis (Table 27.1) to compare your company with your two most important competitors. In the first column are key competitive factors. Since these vary from one industry to another, you may want to customize the list of factors.

In the column labeled Me, state how you honestly think you will stack up in customers' minds. Then check whether you think this factor will be a strength or a weakness for you. Sometimes it is hard to analyze our own weaknesses. Try to be very honest here. Better yet, get some disinterested strangers to assess you. This can be a real eye-opener. And remember that you cannot be all things to all people. In fact, trying to be causes many business failures because efforts become scattered and diluted. You want an honest assessment of your firm's strong and weak points.

Table 27.1 Competitive analysis

Factor	Me	Strength	Weakness	Competitor A	Competitor B	Importance to customer
Products						
Price						
Quality						
Selection						
Service						
Reliability						
Stability						
Expertise						
Company reputation						
Location						
Appearance						
Sales method						
Credit policies						
Advertising						
Image						

Now analyze each major competitor. In a few words, state how you think they compare.

In the final column, estimate the importance of each competitive factor to the customer. 1 = critical; 5 = not very important.

Now, write a short paragraph stating your competitive advantages and disadvantages.

Niche

Now that you have systematically analyzed your industry, your product, your customers, and the competition, you should have a clear picture of where your company fits into the world.

In one short paragraph, define your niche, your unique corner of the market.

Strategy

Now outline a marketing strategy that is consistent with your niche.

Promotion

How will you get the word out to customers?

Advertising: What media, why, and how often? Why this mix and not some other?

Have you identified low-cost methods to get the most out of your promotional budget?

Will you use methods other than paid advertising, such as trade shows, catalogs, dealer incentives, word of mouth (how will you stimulate it?), and network of friends or professionals?

What image do you want to project? How do you want customers to see you?

In addition to advertising, what plans do you have for graphic image support? This includes things like logo design, cards and letterhead, brochures, signage, and interior design (if customers come to your place of business).

Should you have a system to identify repeat customers and then systematically contact them?

Promotional Budget

How much will you spend on the items listed above?
Before start-up? These numbers will go into your start-up budget.
Ongoing? These numbers will go into your operating plan budget.

Pricing

Explain your method or methods of setting prices. For most small businesses, having the lowest price is not a good policy. It robs you of needed profit margin; customers may not care as much about price as you think; and large competitors can under price you anyway. Usually you will do better to have average prices and compete on quality and service.

- Does your pricing strategy fit with what was revealed in your competitive analysis?
- Compare your prices with those of the competition. Are they higher, lower, the same? Why?
- How important is price as a competitive factor? Do your intended customers really make their purchase decisions mostly on price?
- What will be your customer service and credit policies?

Proposed Location

Probably you do not have a precise location picked out yet. This is the time to think about what you want and need in a location. Many start-ups run successfully from home for a while.

You will describe your physical needs later, in the *Operational Plan* section. Here, analyze your location criteria as they will affect your customers.

- Is your location important to your customers? If yes, how?
- If customers come to your place of business:
- Is it convenient? Parking? Interior spaces? Not out of the way?
- Is it consistent with your image?
- Is it what customers want and expect?
- Where is the competition located? Is it better for you to be near them (like car dealers or fast food restaurants) or distant (like convenience food stores)?

Distribution Channels

How do you sell your products or services?

- Retail
- Direct (mail order, web, catalog)
- Wholesale
- Your own sales force
- Agents
- Independent representatives
- Bid on contracts.

Sales Forecast

Now that you have described your products, services, customers, markets, and marketing plans in detail, it is time to attach some numbers to your plan. Use a *sales forecast spreadsheet* to prepare a month-by-month projection. The forecast should be based on your historical sales, the marketing strategies that you have just described, your market research, and industry data, if available.

You may want to do two forecasts: 1) a 'best guess', which is what you really expect, and 2) a 'worst case; low estimate that you are confident you can reach no matter what happens.

Remember to keep notes on your research and your assumptions as you build this sales forecast and all subsequent spreadsheets in the plan. This is critical if you are going to present it to funding sources.

OPERATIONAL PLAN

Explain the daily operation of the business, its location, equipment, people, processes, and surrounding environment.

Production

How and where are your products or services produced?

Explain your methods of:

- Production techniques and costs
- Quality control
- Customer service
- Inventory control
- Product development.

Location

What qualities do you need in a location? Describe the type of location you will have.

Physical requirements:

- Amount of space
- Type of building
- Zoning
- Power and other utilities.

Access

- Is it important that your location be convenient to transportation or to suppliers?
- Do you need easy walk-in access?
- What are your requirements for parking and proximity to freeway, airports, railroads, and shipping centers?

Include a drawing or layout of your proposed facility if it is important, as it might be for a manufacturer.

Construction: Most new companies should not sink capital into construction, but if you are planning to build, costs and specifications will be a big part of your plan.

Cost: Estimate your occupation expenses, including rent, but also including maintenance, utilities, insurance, and initial remodeling costs to make the space suit your needs. These numbers will become part of your financial plan.

What will be your business hours?

Legal Environment

Describe the following:

- Licensing and bonding requirements
- Permits

- Health, workplace, or environmental regulations
- Special regulations covering your industry or profession
- Zoning or building code requirements
- Insurance coverage
- Trademarks, copyrights, or patents (pending, existing, or purchased).

Personnel

- Number of employees
- Type of labor (skilled, unskilled, and professional)
- Where and how will you find the right employees?
- Quality of existing staff
- Pay structure
- Training methods and requirements
- Who does which tasks?
- Do you have schedules and written procedures prepared?
- Have you drafted job descriptions for employees? If not, take time to write some. They really help internal communications with employees.

For certain functions, will you use contract workers in addition to employees.

Inventory

- What kind of inventory will you keep: raw materials, supplies, finished goods?
- Average value in stock (i.e., what is your inventory investment)?
- Rate of turnover and how this compares to the industry averages?
- Seasonal build-ups?
- Lead-time for ordering?

Suppliers

Identify key suppliers:

- Names and addresses
- Type and amount of inventory furnished
- Credit and delivery policies
- History and reliability
  - Should you have more than one supplier for critical items (as a backup)?
  - Do you expect shortages or short-term delivery problems?
  - Are supply costs steady or fluctuating? If fluctuating, how would you deal with changing costs?

Credit Policies

- Do you plan to sell on credit?
- Do you really need to sell on credit? Is it customary in your industry and expected by your clientele?
- If yes, what policies will you have about who gets credit and how much?
- How will you check the creditworthiness of new applicants?
- What terms will you offer your customers; that is, how much credit and when is payment due?
- Will you offer prompt payment discounts? (*Hint*: Do this only if it is usual and customary in your industry)
- Do you know what it will cost you to extend credit? Have you built the costs into your prices?

Managing Your Accounts Receivable

If you do extend credit, you should do an aging at least monthly to track how much of your money is tied up in credit given to customers and to alert you to slow payment problems. A receivables aging looks like the following table:

	Total	Current	30 days	60 days	90 days	Over 90 days
Accounts receivable aging						

You will need a policy for dealing with slow-paying customers:

- When do you make a phone call?
- When do you send a letter?
- When do you get your attorney to threaten?

Managing Your Accounts Payable

You should also age your accounts payable, what you owe to your suppliers. This helps you plan whom to pay and when. Paying too early depletes your cash, but paying late can cost you valuable discounts and can damage your credit (*Hint*: If you know you will be late making a payment, call the creditor before the due date).

Do your proposed vendors offer prompt payment discounts?

A payables aging looks like the following table:

	Total	Current	30 days	60 days	90 days	Over 90 days
Accounts payable aging						

MANAGEMENT AND ORGANIZATION

- Who will manage the business on a day-to-day basis?
- What experience does that person bring to the business?
- What special or distinctive competencies?
- Is there a plan for continuation of the business if this person is lost or incapacitated?

If you'll have more than 10 employees, create an organizational chart showing the management hierarchy and who is responsible for key functions.

Include position descriptions for key employees. If you are seeking loans or investors, include resumes of owners and key employees.

Professional and Advisory Support

List the following:

- Board of directors
- Management advisory board
- Attorney
- Accountant
- Insurance agent
- Banker
- Consultant or consultants
- Mentors and key advisors.

PERSONAL FINANCIAL STATEMENT

Include *personal financial statements* for each owner and major stockholder, showing assets and liabilities held outside the business and personal net worth. Owners will often have to draw on personal assets to finance the business, and these statements will show what is available. Bankers and investors usually want this information as well.

START-UP EXPENSES AND CAPITALIZATION

You will have many *start-up expenses* before you even begin operating your business. It is important to estimate these expenses accurately and then to plan where you will get sufficient capital. This is a research project, and the more thorough your research efforts, the less chance that you will leave out important expenses or underestimate them.

Even with the best of research, however, opening a new business has a way of costing more than you anticipate. There are two ways to make allowances for surprise expenses. The first is to add a little "padding" to each item in the budget. The problem with that approach, however, is that it destroys the accuracy of your carefully wrought plan. The second approach is to add a separate line item, called contingencies, to account for the unforeseeable. This is the approach we recommend.

Talk to others who have started similar businesses to get a good idea of how much to allow for contingencies. If you cannot get good information, we recommend a rule of thumb that contingencies should equal at least 20% of the total of all other start-up expenses.

Explain your research and how you arrived at your forecasts of expenses. Give sources, amounts, and terms of proposed loans. Also explain in detail how much will be contributed by each investor and what percent ownership each will have.

FINANCIAL PLAN

The financial plan consists of a 12-month profit and loss projection, a 4-year profit and loss projection (optional), a cash-flow projection, a projected balance sheet, and a break-even calculation. Together they constitute a reasonable estimate of your company's financial future. More important, the process of thinking through the financial plan will improve your insight into the inner financial workings of your company.

12-month Profit and Loss Projection

Many business owners think of the *12-month profit and loss projection* as the centerpiece of their plan. This is where you put it all together in numbers and get an idea of what it will take to make a profit and be successful.

Your sales projections will come from a sales forecast in which you forecast sales, cost of goods sold, expenses, and profit month-by-month for one year.

Profit projections should be accompanied by a narrative explaining the major assumptions used to estimate company income and expenses.

Research notes: Keep careful notes on your research and assumptions, so that you can explain them later if necessary, and also so that you can go back to your sources when it is time to revise your plan.

4-year Profit Projection (Optional)

The 12-month projection is the heart of your financial plan. *The 4-year profit projection* is for those who want to carry their forecasts beyond the first year.

Of course, keep notes of your key assumptions, especially about things that you expect will change dramatically after the first year.

Projected Cash Flow

If the profit projection is the heart of your business plan, cash flow is the blood. Businesses fail because they cannot pay their bills. Every part of your business plan is important, but none of it means a thing if you run out of cash.

The point of this worksheet is to plan how much you need before start-up, for preliminary expenses, operating expenses, and reserves. You should keep updating it and using it afterward. It will enable you to foresee shortages in time to do something about them—perhaps cut expenses, or perhaps negotiate a loan. But foremost, you should not be taken by surprise.

There is no great trick to preparing it: The cash-flow projection is just a forward look at your checking account.

For each item, determine when you actually expect to receive cash (for sales) or when you will actually have to write a check (for expense items).

You should track essential operating data, which is not necessarily part of cash flow but allows you to track items that have a heavy impact on cash flow, such as sales and inventory purchases.

You should also track cash outlays prior to opening in a pre-start-up column. You should have already researched those for your start-up expenses plan.

Your cash flow will show you whether your working capital is adequate. Clearly, if your projected cash balance ever goes negative, you will need more start-up capital. This plan will also predict just when and how much you will need to borrow.

Explain your major assumptions, especially those that make the cash flow differ from the *Profit and Loss Projection.* For example, if you make a sale in month one, when do you actually collect the cash? When you buy inventory or materials, do you pay in advance, upon delivery, or much later? How will this affect cash flow?

Are some expenses payable in advance? When?

Are there irregular expenses, such as quarterly tax payments, maintenance and repairs, or seasonal inventory build-up, that should be budgeted?

Loan payments, equipment purchases, and owner's draws usually do not show on profit and loss statements but definitely do take cash out. Be sure to include them.

And of course, depreciation does not appear in the cash flow at all because you never write a check for it.

Opening Day Balance Sheet

A balance sheet is one of the fundamental financial reports that any business needs for reporting and financial management. A balance sheet shows what items of value are held by the company (assets), and what its debts are (liabilities). When liabilities are subtracted from assets, the remainder is owners' equity.

Use a start-up expenses and capitalization spreadsheet as a guide to preparing a balance sheet as of opening day. Then detail how you calculated the account balances on your *opening day balance sheet.*

Optional: Some people want to add a *projected balance sheet* showing the estimated financial position of the company at the end of the first year. This is especially useful when selling your proposal to investors.

Break-even Analysis

A *break-even analysis* predicts the sales volume, at a given price, required to recover total costs. In other words, it is the sales level that is the dividing line between operating at a loss and operating at a profit.

Expressed as a formula, break-even is:

$$\text{Break-even sale} = \frac{\text{Fixed costs}}{\text{1-variable costs}}$$

(Where fixed costs are expressed in dollars, but variable costs are expressed as a percent of total sales).

Include all assumptions upon which your break-even calculation is based.

APPENDICES

Include details and studies used in your business plan; for example:

- Brochures and advertising materials
- Industry studies
- Blueprints and plans
- Maps and photos of location
- Magazine or other articles
- Detailed lists of equipment owned or to be purchased
- Copies of leases and contracts
- Letters of support from future customers
- Any other materials needed to support the assumptions in this plan
- Market research studies
- List of assets available as collateral for a loan.

REFINING THE PLAN

The generic business plan presented above should be modified to suit your specific type of business and the audience for which the plan is written.

For Raising Capital

For Bankers

- Bankers want assurance of orderly repayment. If you intend using this plan to present to lenders, include:
  - Amount of loan
  - How the funds will be used
  - What this will accomplish—how will it make the business stronger?
  - Requested repayment terms (number of years to repay). You will probably not have much negotiating room on interest rate but may be able to negotiate a longer repayment term, which will help cash flow.
  - Collateral offered, and a list of all existing liens against collateral.

For Investors

- Investors have a different perspective. They are looking for dramatic growth, and they expect to share in the rewards:
  - Funds needed short-term
  - Funds needed in two to five years
  - How the company will use the funds, and what this will accomplish for growth
  - Estimated return on investment
  - Exit strategy for investors (buyback, sale, or IPO)
  - Percent of ownership that you will give up to investors
  - Milestones or conditions that you will accept
  - Financial reporting to be provided
  - Involvement of investors on the board or in management.

For Type of Business

Manufacturing

- Planned production levels
- Anticipated levels of direct production costs and indirect (overhead) costs—how do these compare to industry averages (if available)?
- Prices per product line
- Gross profit margin, overall and for each product line
- Production/capacity limits of planned physical plant

- Production/capacity limits of equipment
- Purchasing and inventory management procedures
- New products under development or anticipated to come online after start-up.

Service Businesses

- Service businesses sell intangible products. They are usually more flexible than other types of businesses, but they also have higher labor costs and generally very little in fixed assets
- What are the key competitive factors in this industry?
- Your prices
- Methods used to set prices
- System of production management
- Quality control procedures. Standard or accepted industry quality standards
- How will you measure labor productivity?
- Percent of work subcontracted to other firms. Will you make a profit on subcontracting?
- Credit, payment, and collections policies and procedures
- Strategy for keeping client base.

High Technology Companies

- Economic outlook for the industry
- Will the company have information systems in place to manage rapidly changing prices, costs, and markets?
- Will you be on the cutting edge with your products and services?
- What is the status of research and development? And what is required to:
  - Bring product/service to market?
  - Keep the company competitive?
- How does the company:
  - Protect intellectual property?
  - Avoid technological obsolescence?
  - Supply necessary capital?
  - Retain key personnel?

High-tech companies sometimes have to operate for a long time without profits and sometimes even without sales. If this fits your situation, a banker probably will not want to lend to you. Venture capitalists may invest, but your story must be very good. You must do longer-term financial forecasts to show when profit take-off is expected to occur. And your assumptions must be well documented and well argued.

Retail Business

- Company image
- Pricing
  - Explain markup policies
  - Prices should be profitable, competitive, and in accordance with company image.
- Inventory
  - Selection and price should be consistent with company image
  - *Inventory level*: Find industry average numbers for annual inventory turnover rate (available in RMA book). Multiply your initial inventory investment by the average turnover rate. The result should be at least equal to your projected first year's cost of goods sold. If it is not, you may not have enough budgeted for start-up inventory.
- *Customer service policies*: These should be competitive and in accord with company image.
- *Location*: Does it give the exposure that you need? Is it convenient for customers? Is it consistent with company image?
- *Promotion*: Methods used, cost. Does it project a consistent company image?
- *Credit*: Do you extend credit to customers? If yes, do you really need to, and do you factor the cost into prices?

Case Study: Introduction

"FOR LOVE NOT MONEY" is an inspiring story of 'entrepreneurship'. This can be said to be fairy tale in the world of entrepreneurs. This is about a person who entered entrepreneurship by accident and defied his failures to raise his company to new heights. This company is "Marketics" and the leader of this tale is "Shankar Maruwada". Marketics is a specialist marketing analytics firm, which tackles business questions for top marketers across the world, using a wide variety of quantitative techniques. Shankar Maruwada cofounded Marketics, which was purchased by WNS in 2007 for an estimated $65 million. He joined UIDAI in July 2009 where he heads the marketing and communication efforts for the project, which is aimed at providing every Indian resident a unique identification number called as AADHAAR, The division he heads at the UIDAI is called as Demand generation, communication and awareness.

SUMMARY

The Beginning

Marketics has been on a roller coaster ride ever since its inception. The whole idea of Marketics came into being when Shankar Maruwada's batch mate who was working with a VC came up with a business plan. He needed someone to help with the marketing side of things and without thinking too much Shankar quit his job at P&G where he worked for four years, to enter into this unknown domain at that time. There were three partners—Malini, Shankar and Shailendra Malani, the prime mover behind the venture. The team launched a website revolving around consumer reviews. This was *apnaguide.com*. It was a community based site with utility value.

To keep their focus on this new venture, the partners quit their jobs, put in a bit of their own money and then got angel funding.

The Letdown

However their plan could not survive for long and they saw failure in this venture within the span of less than 6 months. And that was the first learning, "Things do not always go as per plan." This was the time when the team decided to do something else. With the help of Malani who had a technical background, they got the idea of making a Customer Relationship module out of the Apnaguide software. The product took six months to build, though it was a good product but only one company actually bought it—a leading Indian bank. Apnaguide.com came across another company Intercept started by a couple of ex-P&G colleagues—Ramki and Kimi. Since both the companies had same domain, Apnaguide merged and became part of Intercept in October 2001. However the biggest challenge followed this merger was to sell this module in Indian market along with the company's exhausting funds. This let down was soon followed by apnaguide mentors walking out of the company. However the tough times were not yet over with the original team getting disbanded as Malini and Shailendra quit this venture forever.

Something New

Just after an year the three partners on board—Shankar, Ramki and Vinay Mishra, an IIML graduate and colleague at Intercept came together to start something new from the ashes of the past failures, and this 'something new' was Marketics. After a long struggle to make a mark in entrepreneurship world, Marketics came as a blessing. The first decision made by them was—"not to sell their products in India". P&G USA was Marketics' first client.

The Strategy Followed

- The USP of Marketics was that it had people who had used analytics to make better decisions. And they knew that kind of service was not being provided by MR companies.
- Provided top quality work to the clients, who in turn gave top quality money to the company.
- Worked with only top notch clients-fortune 100 companies and developed client referral network to get new clients.
- Marketics believed that intellectual capital was more important than monetary capital and thus it made another wise decision to hire only young people and groom them.

New Merger

As commonly said "raise the money when you do not need it", the same way was what Marketics felt when they were having happy clients and enough cash pouring in. Somewhere down the line Marketics realized that they need to diversify their services. It was also advised to the company to align with somebody larger so that they can leverage the platform built by Marketics and make the company much bigger, much faster. As fate would have it, WNS came into the picture. Marketics was bought out at $65 million in 2007.

KEY LEARNINGS

- Follow the passion in your work, the money will just flow
- Have courage to transform your idea into reality
- Stick to your choices, even if they go wrong
- Have an attitude to make right things happen to you
- Changing roles is a part of an entrepreneur's life—at times playing contrasting roles might just prove good for the company
- To feed your idea, you need funds. Look for angel funding as an option better than VCs.

Chapter 28

Healthcare Management Consultancy Services

INTRODUCTION

A consultant is one who gives professional advice or services. You work in a particular field and offer your expertise to help others with their problems in the field that you know best. It is almost like training a new employee to take over your job. You simply share the tips, tricks, and techniques you have acquired over the years.

Anyone can be a consultant—as long as you have the experience, skill, and knowledge in your chosen field. You do not need to be recognized as the ultimate best in your field to become a consultant. It is also not necessary that you have been a CEO in a top company or even held a titled position. You also do not need to have owned or operated a business to become a successful business consultant. You will, however, need the ability to sell yourself, and an up-to-date understanding of the area in which you intend to be involved with. Look over your educational strengths and combine them

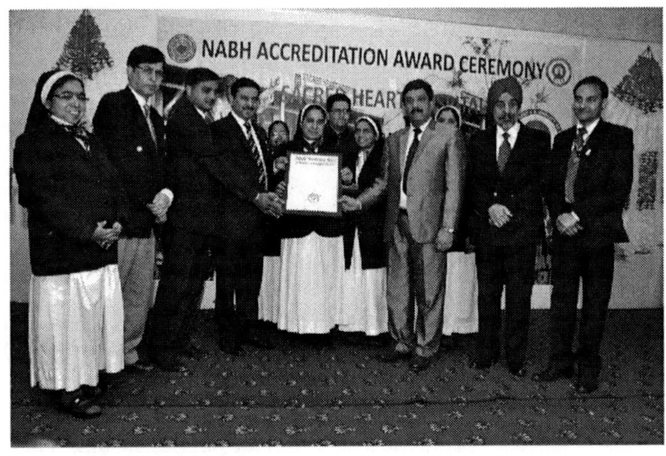

Quality Accreditation Consultancy Services in a Hospital

with any training and on-the-job experience gained in the marketplace. Insight, thorough study, and common sense can be joined together as a substitute for years of experience in a field.

If you want to become a consultant, the first step is to take an honest look at your own training and experience. You may have worked all your life in a particular field and received special training and education along the same lines. If you have worked as a special event coordinator for an exclusive island resort, you can offer your services as a consultant who helps plan, develop and execute theme parties for corporations and other hotels.

You may also qualify as a consultant if you taken any advanced academic degrees, certifications or special studies in your area of expertise. There are a number of fields that require certifications and special licensing before you can begin operating as a consultant. If you are computer networking specialist, you must pass the Microsoft Certified Systems Engineer (MCSE) certification at the very least. If you want to work as a fund raising consultant, it will help if you could be certified through the National Society of Fund Raising Executives, even through certification is not required to practice the profession.

GOOD MANAGEMENT

Good management is the key to success and good management starts with setting goals. Set goals for yourself for the accomplishment of the many tasks necessary in starting and managing your business successfully. Be specific and Write down the goals in measurable terms of performance. Break major goals down into sub-goals, showing what you expect to achieve in the next two-to-three months, the next six months, the next year, and the next five years. Beside each goal and sub-goal place a specific date showing when it is to be achieved.

Plan the action you must take to attain the goals. While the effort required to reach each sub-goal should be great enough to challenge you, it should not be so great or unreasonable as to discourage you. Do not plan to reach too many goals all at one time. Establish priorities.

Plan in advance how to measure results so you can know exactly how well you are doing. This is what is meant by "measurable" goals. If you cannot keep score as you go along you are likely to lose motivation. Re-work your plan of action to allow for obstacles which may stand in your way. Try to foresee obstacles and plan ways to avert or minimize them.

- *Getting started*: Before starting out, list your reasons for wanting to go into business. Some of the most common reasons for starting a business are:

  - You want to be your own boss.
  - You want financial independence.
  - You want creative freedom.
  - You want to fully use your skills and knowledge.
- *Next you need to determine what business is "right for you." Ask yourself these questions*:
  - What do I like to do with my time?
  - What technical skills have I learned or developed?
  - What do others say I am good at?
  - Will I have the support of my family?
  - How much time do I have to run a successful business?
  - Do I have any hobbies or interests that are marketable?
- *Then you should identify the niche your business will fill. Conduct the necessary research to answer these questions*:
  - What business am I interested in starting?
  - What services or products will I sell?
  - Is my idea practical, and will it fill a need?
  - What is my competition?
  - What is my business's advantage over existing firms?
  - Can I deliver a better quality service?
  - Can I create a demand for my business?
- *The final step before developing your plan is the prebusiness checklist. You should answer these questions*:
  - What skills and experience do I bring to the business?
  - What will be my legal structure?
  - How will my company's business records be maintained?
  - What insurance coverage will be needed?
  - What equipment or supplies will I need?
  - How will I compensate myself?
  - What are my resources?
  - What financing will I need?
  - Where will my business be located?
  - What will I name my business?

Your answers will help you create a focused, well-researched business plan that should serve as a blueprint. It should detail how the business will be operated, managed and capitalized.

One of the most important cornerstones of starting a business is the business plan. Once you have completed your business plan, review it with a friend or business associate. When you feel comfortable with the content and structure, make an appointment to review and discuss it with your banker. The business plan is a flexible document that should change as your business grows.

"I'm sailing away, set an open course for the virgin sea
I've got to be free, free to face the life that's ahead of me
On board, I'm the captain, so climb aboard
We'll search for tomorrow on every shore
And I'll try, oh Lord, I'll try to carry on"

("Come Sail Away", Dr Pradeep Bhardwaj)

A consultant is a knowledge worker. Therefore, the first thing you need to ensure is that you have a sound *educational background* in your area of practice. In many areas of consultancy practice you also need to acquire a professional *certification* in your field. Each profession would have its own requirement for certification. The national nodal professional body for your profession will provide the necessary information in this regard.

A consultant is a person who works by selling their specialist knowledge. So you need to make sure you have this knowledge and have the propensity and appetite to develop it as the industry it serves changes. You may also need to acquire a professional qualification or certification. So make sure you have the requisite bits of paper. As soon as you do quit your job you will need to figure out your own balance between the time you spend marketing and the time you spend delivering. If you are delivering a lot then you will have little time for marketing. Do not neglect this or else when you run out of work to deliver there will be nothing in the future.

How Important is Hands on Experience for a Start-up?

Can you Learn to Drive a Car by Reading the Instruction Manual?

While it is possible to think the big things through by going to a research stint, it gives little experience with the tactical skills and in dealing with ground realities. It is possible from a research perspective to come up with sound strategies and business ideas; but you may get severely hampered when it comes to actually implementing them. There is no denying that fact that you need a few years of hands on experience where you hone not only your technical skills, but also the people issues within the organization and outside.

Mentoring

Any business, including consultancy practice, is fraught with uncertainties. You may need to take decisions regarding issues beyond your immediate area of expertise. You will be buffeted by changing business realities due to myriad reasons, such as, competition, obsolescence, business cycles, regional and global geopolitics, and many more. To guide you through this jungle it is prudent to adopt a seasoned *mentor*. Ideally, he is a person whose professional background and expertise is from your area of consultancy practice, he has hands on experience in running a company and has a wide network of professional contacts. Adopt him, use him as a sounding board, treat him as your friend, philosopher and guide.

Entrepreneurial Thought Processes

Entrepreneurs think differently. The life of an entrepreneur is one of seeking and seizing opportunity. They have historically been known as risk takers. Learning to think in an entrepreneurial way could allow you to stay one step ahead of the competition, whether it be in your business or with other aspects of your life.

You should go out and reach for the stars. While you may not be successful in plucking one, you would not come up with a handful of mud either. It is a painful thing to start on your own. A 9–5 job gives a sense of security alright. But that security is given to you by those who take risks. And when you give that kind of security to others, the feeling is hard to describe. Makes you a humble and a fuller being.

Business Development

Once you are through with the initial phase of the start-up, you need to focus on the business development aspect of your consultancy practice.

A very important part of starting or growing a business is making contacts and creating a web of resources for your company. Creating both personal and professional bonds with other people is critical and could open doors for a budding consultant. To do this one could try to find common ground with new acquaintances and make some sort of connection with them. Always having business cards on hand and using them as a way to casually exchange phone numbers. One should try to go to as many social and business functions as possible. Making contacts is crucial to the future success of your business.

Some suggestions for doing this are: Make a list of individuals that you would like to meet. Then determine your common interests. Think of every possible connection you could have with these people. Are your children at the same middle school? Do you belong to the same religious/social organization? Are you both members of a certain club? Will they be attending an upcoming industry conference? Try to find the common link that will create a casual and relaxed first meeting. Once you do have the opportunity to meet, make a note of the place you met and the discussion you had. Pay attention to their interests and things that are important to them, whether they are business-oriented or personal. It is appropriate to touch base with them or extend an invitation to some sort of gathering once every six months, just to keep the lines of communication open. To help you in your effort it could be useful to use a contact management program such as MS Outlook or Act! that allows you to keep updated information on contacts. These programs will also allow you to create notes on each individual and record your discussions. Creating a personal relationship with these individuals is the way to gain their trust and business. Keeping in touch with people is the way to maintain professional and personal relationships and the best way to promote your practice.

You never know how helpful the web of relationships could be to you in the future.

Conclusion

While you are contemplating at starting a consultancy practice, you may use these ideas to help you develop your thoughts. However, you must remember that each business is unique and there is no predefined roadmap for success. Ultimately, your convictions based on your unique experience, training, background and opportunities are the best guide. Best of luck!

It is a great idea for a business start-up in these economically challenging times to sell your own knowledge and expertise as a consultant. Independent consulting is one of the fastest growing and most profitable business models around. More and more people are enjoying the independence and extra money it brings as well as the change in the quality of life through being in control of what you do and with whom you work.

WHAT IS A CONSULTANT?

A consultant is someone who offers help to someone or a business trying to solve a problem. Consultants work in a specific field of knowledge and provide expert knowledge to help solve problems. This will be a field that you are most familiar with.

In theory almost anyone can be a consultant—as long as you have what a client wants. This usually means skill and knowledge to solve a problem. It is not necessary to be the world's leading expert in a particular field. Nor do you need to have been in the same line of business yourself, nor any other kind.

Among other things you will need to be able to 'sell yourself', and have a very good appreciation and understanding of how to solve the problem that needs to be solved. This is normally good knowledge combined with experience and good communication skills.

Select something which you know about and something which you like. Can you communicate the benefits of your skills to a lay person? Can you write about what you know in a way that is easy for a person to understand? Can you explain how your knowledge and skill could solve a problem? These are all essential talents you will need to have in addition to the basic knowledge of the area in which you are offering expertise.

Save up as much money as possible before starting any organization

All too often, people go into business without any savings, exclusively using loan money from friends, banks, or the SBA. They except to be able to start paying the loans back right away with their profits. What these business owners do not realize is that it can take months or years to make a profit. And once a lender discovers a business isn't as profitable as expected, the lender is likely to call in the loan or refuse to renew it for another year. Often new business owners then have to take out home equity loans or use credit cards to pay off their loans (which puts their home and credit rating at risk).

A better plan is to save up as much of the needed investment money as possible, including your living expenses for the first year, or even two. Odds are that your business would not be profitable for one to two years. Even if you get plenty of business coming your way—and your customers pay you on time, which is not always a sure thing—you will want to be able to invest most of that money back in the business for space, equipment, advertising, and insurance needs.

Steps

Here are some steps that you will need to take to set-up your consultancy define your market before you do anything else. Who is it you are selling your consultancy and knowledge to and what do they want? Everything else rests on this. There is no point in doing anything until you can answer these questions. Where are the people you will be selling to and how do you know what it is they want. My point is this: however clever or knowledgeable you are about something is no guarantee that someone will pay you for it. So find out what they want first (related to your area of expertise of course) then go from there. This goes whether you are setting up as a sole trader or with others to create accompany. A mistake that many make is that they feel they are good at something and that the world owes them a living. Lots of businesses of all kinds go down the tubes for this reason. They invent or create a product and then look for someone to buy it. No! Look for something that people want then go away and create it!

Plan once you have answered the above question, prepare your business plan. A business plan will help you work through your vision and strategy for keeping the business working. What is the rationale that your business can succeed? Provide evidence! What exactly are your products and services (you may have a main one but develop other 'back end products too'. What is it that you want to achieve by when. How much do you want to make be when? Be realistic and bold. What is your evidence that this figure can be reached. How are you going to market? What is your financial plan? Do you need to borrow? How will you convince lenders? There are lots more things that should be in a plan and each of these needs to be unpacked and detailed. Brainstorm these, then start putting them to a time-line.

Make a space to work where are you going to work from? Many sole traders start from home. This is a good idea as it keeps overheads down. But if you do this make sure you inform the insurers of your house as turning your home into a workplace without telling them will render your insurance null and void. Choose a space in your home that is comfortable and warm. Obviously you will need phone access, internet access, a place for your computer, files and books (consultants always have lots of books).

What about Marketing?

If you do not have clients or customers then you do not have a business. Usually, it pays to ensure that you have some before you leave your paid employment. The next thing to do is to inform them that you are ready and available for work.

Your marketing should narrow in on you being the expert that people need to solve their problems. A good way to do this is publish a few articles on the internet with links to your site (you must have a site!) which answers a question related to your field (you could go to Answers. Yahoo.com and look for a question to answer. Show your practical value to your potential customers. People need to get the idea that you are an expert, the expert. There are tons of ways you can market yourself and get your name out there. Here are 7 things you need to be thinking about:

1. *Networking*: Going to events where your target market congregates is one of the most effective. You will need business cards if you go to these. Also be prepared to speak to a wide range of people with a wide range of potential issues they may be looking for answers to. Start with the people you already know—your former colleagues and bosses, your friends and existing industry contacts. If there are name badges make sure you have the right information on yours. Talk to as many people as you can and collect business cards. Online networks are also important. These are

known as forums. Join the ones that form you target market. But do not abuse these through blatant marketing or you will just get banned. Use these to build relationships.

2. *Ask for referrals*: If you get work and it is successful ask your client for a referral or two. Normally people will be happy to recommend you. Ask for a quote you can put on your website. Even if the person to whom you are referred does not have any work for you at the present time ask if they too could refer you to other potential clients.
3. *Public presentations*: Consultants are usually good at communicating. You need to be able to talk about your area of expertise to all sorts of people. Speaking at events offers a great opportunity to get your message out there. This can terrify some. But fear not. Practice with a friend what you want to say. Use visual aids to detract attention from yourself. Keep what you want to say short and to the point and ask the audience questions frequently to maintain attention and interest and interaction. Volunteer to offer them free information. Contact you chamber of commerce, organizations and forums in your locality. See what possibilities there are at local colleges, universities and libraries.
4. *Ads and articles*: Try to get a short article in a publication or trade journal that your target market reads. This is good for your reputation and gets your message out there among potential purchasers. Make it interesting and engaging—not just an in-your-face advert. Approach a journalist or editor to write something for you. They are usually happy to have new information to provide. Put together a short e-book and put it on your website to sell.
5. *Direct mail*: You can distribute direct mail as sales letters, ad mailings, or brochures. The thing is to create a document that attracts the attention or your recipient, engages their interest, provokes their curiosity ultimately compels them to take action. It is absolutely imperative that you emphasize the benefits that your client will receive as a result of buying your services. Concentrate less on everything else.
6. *Cold calling*: Yes, I know—it sounds a pain and few people like it but do not neglect it. Practice cold techniques. Learn the first names of the people you want to speak to so that it sounds to the gatekeepers—of which there will be plenty—that you know them. Understand that the person you assume is the decision maker may not be. It could be the person above or below them or even along from them! Make your aim of a call to get an appointment. Keep it short, keep it clear and do it early in the morning—sometimes the person you want to speak to will be in before the secretary and may well answer the phone instead.

7. *Your website*: It is true that much of your business will be generated from face to face relationships. Some think that this means you do not really need a website. Think again! Your website is your presence on the web. A place for all those who do not know a person who can solve their problem personally—so they look online. It is a place where all those internet articles you are going to write can be stored so that people can see at a glance your expertise. It is a place where you offer back-end products and services, related business products and so on in addition to your consultancy service. Your site has the potential to send your income through the roof. Apart from having your contact details on there you absolutely must have lots of great copy (Yes, 'sales copy'), and for goodness sake have an opt-in section so that you can collect all the e-mail addresses of people who are interested in what you do.

Starting a consulting business or selling your knowledge takes not only your specialist expertise but also business knowledge and wisdom, tactics and patience. It relies on good communication and marketing, the ability to build rapport and to understand the needs of your potential clients.

BEING A CONSULTANT IS BEING IN BUSINESS

The days of spending large sums of money on advertising have gone. That was last century's way of building business. These days, the focus is on building contacts, creating a reputation by helping people and solving their problems. All of this can be done at very low cost.

One of the biggest mistakes that new consultants make is to focus too much on being the expert and not enough on marketing themselves. You can be the most knowledgeable person in your field, but without marketing yourself, you are unlikely to win a consistent pipeline of clients that are ready to pay you for your consulting services.

Below is a list of key points that you should keep in mind each and every day. All of these simple statements can be put into practice with little or no money, yet together they can help you build a successful consulting business.

- Select a niche and remain focused
- Commit to yourself to being the undisputed expert in your niche
- Agree with yourself that you are in this business for the long-haul
- Be sure you have guts, determination and the ability to succeed
- Move away from negative people
- Listen and learn from those successful consultants who have trod before you

- Preserve your time and money
- Help people and give away an abundance of free advice
- Accept help from smart people when they offer it
- Never forget that you will need to consistently market yourself
- Do not make the mistake of selling. Instead, help people solve their problems.

Out of all the above, you might still be asking the question; "are you sure I do not need a large budget to market my consulting business?" I can fully appreciate that concern, especially when there is so much advertising in newspapers, magazines and TV these days.

I can assure you that plenty of very successful consultants all over the world have attained their success without a large advertising budget. In fact some of the principles of advertising are so simple, they are overlooked by most.

Knowing these simple marketing principles can make the difference between a successful consultant and a failed consultant who has to go back to working for someone else, all because they neglected the importance of marketing. Knowing your subject might be sufficient to 'get a job,' but it is very insufficient if you want to be a successful independent consultant.

There are some very good resources on the internet and books on the subject of consulting. Some spend more time discussing business cards, premises and tax than on the more critical success factors such as marketing. However there are some excellent resources available that will show you how to market yourself as an independent consultant using a small budget.

If you are committed to succeeding and are prepared to listen to the right people, there is no reason why you cannot become a successful consultant.

TIPS FOR INTERNAL CONSULTANCY

From our considerable experience of internal consultancy work, we have listed below a few of what we feel are the key tips for anyone working in this field. We hope that you find them helpful.

– Fred Sherwin

1. *Success in consultancy is as much about managing relationships as content*: Of course, for some "expert" assignments the content is crucial. However, for most it is the building and maintaining of relationships—particularly between consultant and client—that leads to successful assignments.
2. *What all clients want?:* Each client is different—in the way they see your role, in the level of involvement they wish, and in the sort of results

they seek. With experience, one learns to read the situation, adapt, and establish an agreed working relationship. However, the following are common to virtually all clients:

- *No unexpected surprises*: More anything else, this needs to be the touchstone that governs any consultancy assignment. If anything is going amiss, clients want to know in case it impacts on something else they or others are doing.
- *A success*: It is easy to forget this at times, but almost all clients want a success—it reflects on them just as much as it reflects on you. But how does your client define success?
- *Clarity and flexibility*: They want to be clear what your role is and what you are planning to do, but also expect you to be flexible and able to adapt to changed circumstances. Thus, work to define your role and then stay in it, but be prepared to flex and adapt when needed.
- *Your interest*: They expect you to be interested in their work, their ideas, their people, and the issues they face.

3. *Have a consultancy process*: You need to have in mind a consultancy process that you expect to progress through, as a game-plan for both yourself and the client. Not just because it is tidy but because it helps you to manage the client relationship. The one that we use envisages an assignment as progressing through five broad stages:
   - *Entry*: Where one builds the initial relationship with the client and carries out an initial survey or scoping to establish what the assignment is about, what it should aim to achieve, the likely time and effort required, and possible risks and difficulties.
   - *Contracting*: Where one agrees with the client what the task is, what the consultant's role is, and how it should be tackled.
   - *Diagnosis*: Gathering information and ideas to arrive at options and a plan of action.
   - *Intervention*: Taking actions to deliver the results, be it a report or organizing the changes.
   - *Withdrawal:* Ensuring that the client organization can carry on without you and leaving the ground clear for your future involvement. This is a general model and you may find it best to amend it to something that suits your own particular work and style. You may need to customize a process for a particular assignment.
4. *On the practice of consulting*
   - *The "golden rule"—start with an initial survey or scoping:* The initial meeting between client and consultant is crucial. If the client is in a rush or under pressure, there is a danger that you might be agreeing

to a brief, resources and timescales without knowing very much at all about the issues and difficulties. An initial survey followed by a brief proposal and a further meeting, gives both you and the client a much better basis for moving forward.

- *If you are unsure or wish to change the brief—go back to the client:* During the assignment, if you become at all unsure about the brief or feel that it needs to be changed, go back to the client and discuss it. If you feel that way then the likelihood is that the client feels the same. If things are deviating from what the client expects— tell them. What they want most of all is no unexpected surprises.
- *Be organized:* If you are acting as a consultant, the client expects that you will be professional. To maintain that image, you do need to be well organized. If you start to make errors or miss meetings, then that image will be eroded. Plan and project manage your assignment well.
- *Managing expectations is key:* When assignments do start to flounder, in most cases it is because a mismatch develops between the client's expectations and the consultant's plans and activities. This is why in many assignments, regular stock-takes, perhaps by note or phone, are needed.
- *Get connected and stay connected:* If you want to get and retain the client's confidence and respect, you need to convince them that you are connected—that you understand their world. Some key pointers are:
  - Get to know the client's business so that you understand their pressures, concerns and priorities
  - Be aware of other projects going on so that you have a similar context to them
  - Try to keep connected with the daily happenings in the team, e.g. concerns and priorities.
- *Consciously build your own reputation with the client:* The more respect that the client has for you and your work, the more impact you will have and the more they will ask you to input. It also means that at the end you can withdraw to return.

5. *Learning to read situations*: If managing relationships is the key to success in consulting, then it is the behavior and interpersonal skills of the consultant that make that happen. All really skilled consultants have excellent interpersonal skills. They need them in order to:
   - Read situations
   - Build empathy with clients and others
   - Gain the trust and respect of those they are working with

- Facilitate meetings
- Influence others
- Tailor communications to suit the audience
- Predict peoples' reactions
- Avoid or get out of difficult situations

These skills-listening, observing, questioning, challenging, influencing, negotiating—are fundamental to good consulting and can all be developed through training and experience. They form a key element of our consultancy skills training.

6. *About you as a consultant*
   - *Where is your consulting "comfort zone"?* Your comfort zone is the style that you are personally most comfortable with. For some it is "process consulting", for others "facilitation", for yet others it is "expert advice". We can all flex and operate outside of this comfort zone—but only within limits. What is your comfort zone and what are the limits?
   - *What are your strengths and weaknesses?:* Planning, organizing, interpersonal skills, creativity? Identify them and then major on your strengths and start to develop to remedy your weaknesses.
   - *What is your organizational role?:* Internal consultants often have a dual role. They consult but they are part of a group with functional responsibilities which carry a monitoring accountability, e.g. internal audit. Such dual roles can make uneasy bedfellows and confuse both you and the client.
7. *Consultancy ethics*: And finally—consultancy can be a seductive role. One can be in a situation of having influence and knowledge far beyond what people in the client's team have. Some consultants can be tempted to misuse this. But as a consultant you do need a set of ethics to work to. If a client invites you into their operation to help them, they have the right to expect that you:
   - Respect the client's knowledge
   - Be careful not to be over-prescriptive or judgmental
   - Respect confidentiality
   - Avoid becoming involved in the internal politics
   - Remain in the role that the client expects you to fulfill.

Internal Consultancy Skills Case Study

For four years we supported a central government department with the introduction of their "professionalism through quality" initiative to their thirty local operating sites located all over the UK.

After an initial survey, we developed a proposal to run training workshops for members of change teams based at their thirty local operating sites.

- The teams were to start and lead local initiatives.
- The workshop covered both process and service improvement techniques and consultancy skills for change agents.
- The teams would be guided by a national steering group which also sponsored UK-wide improvements.

The whole program was highly successful. We ran workshops across the UK covering one hundred and fifty members of PTQ teams who then "kickstarted" and led local initiatives.

Thereafter we advised senior managers and the steering group, developed a self-assessment "health-check" to help to steer progress at each operating site, and introduced further training as required . The momentum and interest grew and by the end of that period every site in the UK had an active team working on identifying local customer improvements.

Outcome

All the PTQ teams were able to return to their sites and develop a local initiative. These led to numerous improvements in working practices and procedures to improve customer service.

Consulting Skills

A workshop to train participants in the consultancy skills needed to successfully work with clients. It covers:

- Operating as a consultant
  - The consultancy phases
  - What clients want and building a relationship
- Entry and contracting
  - Managing initial contacts
  - Key skills and behaviors
  - Client and consultant roles
- Diagnosis
  - Research and analysis
  - Stakeholder and clients needs
  - Establishing the issues
- Intervention
  - Different intervention styles
  - Scoping the project
  - Developing proposals

- *Withdrawal and the future role:* Includes key interpersonal skills of listening, questioning, and influencing.

Facilitation Skills

A workshop to train participants in the key interpersonal skills of facilitation. It covers:

- The facilitation process and role
- Establishing and building the relationship
- Facilitating meetings
  - How groups develop and behave?
- Intervention strategies
  - What to use; when and how?
- Key interpersonal skills
  - Observing
  - Listening, questioning
  - Challenging, and influencing.

A self-assessment helps participants to identify their own strengths and weaknesses.

Research, Analysis and Problem-solving

Aimed at all who wish to become better acquainted with the approaches, tools, and techniques of structured problem solving. It covers:

- Scoping the problem
- Collecting the information required—hard and soft information
- Establishing the "real" problem—the root causes
- Tools and techniques
  - Brainstorming, mind maps
  - Fishbone analysis, process mapping and beyond
- Finding solutions
  - Tools for creativity
- Implementing
  - Roadblocks and how to remove them.
  - Plans, pilots and implementation.

We have taken that framework as the structure of this consultancy skills toolkit.

TOOLKIT

Overview	The key aspects of the consultancy role and approach
Working with clients	The skills to work with and manage clients and their expectations
Delivering projects	The skills to manage consultancy projects to the client's requirements
Dealing with people	The interpersonal skills to work with and deal with people

Consultancy Process

You need to have in mind a consultancy process that you intend to progress through. You need it as a game-plan both for yourself and the client. Not just because it is tidy, but because it helps you to manage the client relationship. The one that we use envisages an assignment as progressing through five broad stages (Fig. 28.1):

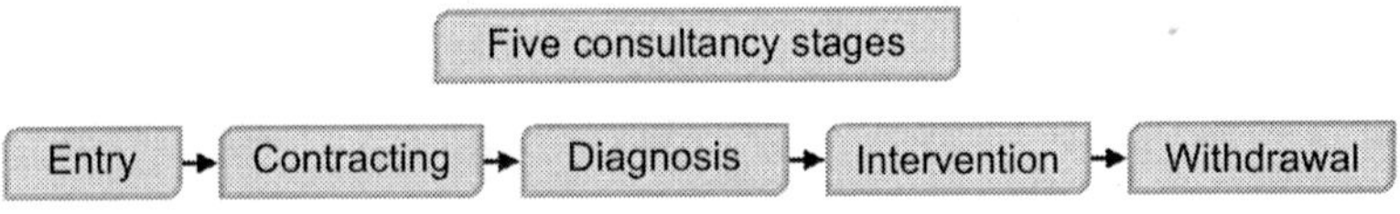

Fig. 28.1 Stages of consultancy

1. *Entry:* Where one builds the initial relationship with the client and carries out a survey or scoping to establish what the assignment is about, what it should aim to achieve, the likely time and effort required, and possible risks and difficulties.
2. *Contracting:* Where one agrees with the client what the task is, what the consultant's role is, what the client's role is, and how the work should be tackled?
3. *Diagnosis:* Gathering information and ideas to arrive at options and a plan of action.
4. *Intervention:* Taking actions to deliver the results, be it a report or organizing the changes.
5. *Withdrawal:* Ensuring that the client organization can carry on without you and leaving the ground clear for your future involvement.

This is a general model and you may find it best to amend it to something that suits your own particular work and style or for a particular assignment.

What all Clients Want?

Each client is different—in the way they see your role, in the level of involvement they wish, and in the sort of results they seek. With experience, one learns to read the situation, adapt, and establish an agreed working relationship. However, the following are common to virtually all clients:

- *No unexpected surprises:* More anything else, this need to be the touchstone that governs any consultancy assignment. If anything is going amiss, clients need to know. In particular in case it impacts on something else they or others are doing.
- *Success:* You want success but so do your clients—it reflects on them just as much as it reflects on you. But how does your client define success? Spend some time in the early days establishing just that.
- *Clarity and flexibility:* They want to be clear what your role is and what you are planning to do, but also expect you to be flexible and able to adapt to changed circumstances. Thus, work to define your role and then stay in it, but be prepared to flex and adapt when needed.
- *Your interest in them:* They expect you to be interested in their work, their ideas, their people, and the issues they face. Try to exhibit that.

About you as a Consultant

Consultancy Styles

There are a variety of consultancy styles—each suited to different people and different situations (Fig. 28.2). For example:

- Some consultants adopt the *Expert* style—they see themselves as bringing a knowledgeable, independent approach to the client—a depth of knowledge and expertise that the client lacks. A style often employed by medical practitioners, technical/IT consultants, and business strategy analysts. Extremely useful in some situations but absolutely inappropriate in others.
- Others see their prime contribution as working on and helping with the *Process*. Sometimes working with the client to help them to decide what is to be done and how it is to be achieved, sometimes working

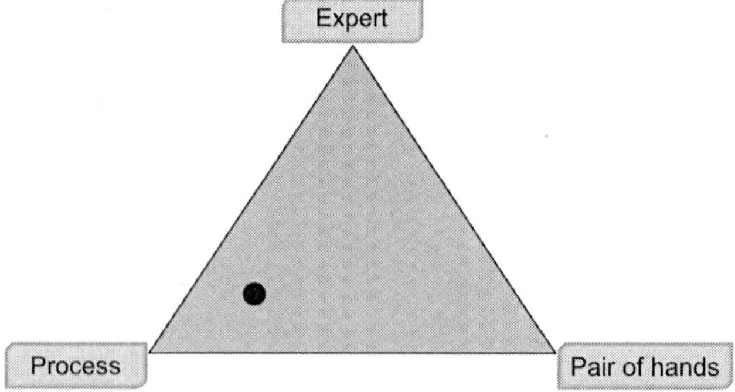

Fig. 28.2 Consultancy style pyramid

with a manager to help them review their management style, or at other times working with a team to help them work together more effectively. Coaching, counseling, and organizational development all fall under this heading.

- Yet others see themselves as essentially a *Pair of Hands*. Their task is to help the client to implement the client's strategies, plans, and decisions. A style often employed by some of the larger consultancy bureaus.

So, which style is the best one? Clearly it depends on what the situation and the client requires. In some situations, the expert style may be most effective, whereas in others the process style would be best employed.

In practice consultants rarely work within one single style—their position is somewhere within the triangle above. The dot in the triangle depicts someone who has a strong preference for process working but who can flex into other styles as the situation requires.

For practicing consultants the message from this is quite simple:

- Try to establish your own preferred style of consultancy—essentially where you lie within the triangle—and then develop your ability to flex and operate in your less preferred styles. *(Note: Process consulting is covered best in books by Edgar Schein who pioneered the field.)*
- When starting an assignment, consciously assess what style of consultancy the situation and the client require and what you can provide. Attempt to avoid a style mismatch, e.g. working in a process mode with a situation and client that requires an expert mode.
- In your contracting, ensure that you agree this with the client—so that they are clear about the style you will be adopting.

Consultancy Development: Key Points

- *Where is your consulting "comfort zone"?*: Your comfort zone is the style that you are personally most comfortable with. For some it is "process consulting", for others "facilitation", for yet others it is "expert advice". We can all flex and operate outside of this comfort zone—but only within limits. What is your comfort zone and what are the limits?
- *What are your strengths and weaknesses?*: Planning, organizing, interpersonal skills, creativity? Identify them and then major on your strengths and start to develop to remedy your weaknesses.
- *What is your organizational role?*: Internal consultants often have a dual role. They consult but they are part of a group with functional responsibilities which carry a monitoring accountability, e.g. internal audit. Such dual roles can make uneasy bedfellows and confuse both you and the client.

Working with Clients

If there is anything that distinguishes the excellent consultant from the average it is the way that they relate to and work with (and in fact manage) their clients.

This does not simply happen automatically and without effort. To really work effectively with a client the consultant has to invest time and effort in:

- Understanding the clients world—their business and organization, and the pressures they face
- Understanding how it feels to be the client dependant on the consultants efforts
- Keeping in touch with the dynamics of the clients situation
- Keeping the client in touch with how the consultant is progressing
- Sorting out those things that need to be brought to the clients attention from those which would only confuse and distract.

This section contains some models and analyzes from the field of customer service that our own clients have found valuable. Use them to think through what you feel your clients' requirements are.

Professional Versus Mass Services

Clearly good customer service is vital in any consultancy assignment. However, when thinking about customer service in consultancy, it is vital to distinguish between:

- A *mass service* as provided by a fast food restaurant or a shop.
- A *professional service* as provided by a solicitor, architect, or doctor.

Most customer service ideas are based on providing a mass service. Although there are elements in common, there are also significant differences, summarized in the Table 28.1.

Table 28.1 Significant differences of customer services between the mass and professional services

Mass services	Professional services
• Has customers	• Has clients
• Usually a one-off contact	• Regular or repeating contact
• Brief contact—a transaction	• Extended client contact—a project
• Customers with similar needs	• Clients with varying needs
• Pre-prepared service	• Service created/customized for particular client
• Customer often knows exactly what they want	• Clients often does not have the technical expertise to know what they want—they just want a solution to their problem

KEY CONCLUSION

Serving clients is different to serving customers.

Each client is unique with particular needs and all consultants need to invest time and effort in building and maintaining the relationship. In particular:

- In understanding their clients situation
- In building trust and a relationship with them
- In ensuring that their client is up-to-date with progress
- In ensuring their client keeps them up-to-date on relevant developments
- In ensuring that their client understands sufficiently the professional or technical options available—even at times coaching or training their client in this.

KEY POINT

Clients and professionals, by nature, tend to have different views as to what the service is. Professionals tend to emphasize the core specialist elements, clients value the softer "helpful" peripheral elements.

Successful professionals recognize this and adapt their style to suit. In particular they invest time and effort in ensuring that they have a good grasp of the clients world and perspective, and attempt to accommodate to that.

Its all about perceptions and expectations. A survey was carried out of accountancy practices in three countries—UK, Sweden, and Canada. The researchers identified eight elements of service provided by such practices:

- Technical expertise
- Taxation advice
- Statutory
- Peace of mind/confidence
- Problem solving
- Ideas testing
- Financial advice
- Prestige

Each practice and their clients were asked to score these for importance.
The key points were as follows:

- *In all cases the professionals providing the service rated the core technical elements as being the features that the client valued most (financial advice, technical expertise)*
- *Whereas the actual clients placed much more emphasis on the softer peripheral elements (peace of mind, confidence, statuary, tax advice).*

Surveys of solicitors gave similar results, with clients rating approachability highest.

What it feels Like to be a Buyer?

The following was taken from a slide presentation about buyers reviewing competitive tender proposals. It summarizes some of the thoughts that go through a buyers head when making such decisions and choices.

It is particularly relevant to consultants when an assignment is being established, but also some of the feelings described continue during the progress of the assignment.

Dealing with People—Interpersonal Skills

If managing relationships is the key to success in consulting, then it is the behavior and interpersonal skills of the consultant that make that happen. All really skilled consultants have excellent interpersonal skills. They need them in order to:

- Read situations
- Build empathy with clients and others
- Gain the trust and respect of those they are working with
- Facilitate meetings
- Influence others
- Tailor communications to suit the audience
- Predict peoples' reactions
- Avoid or get out of difficult situations.

These skills such as listening, observing, questioning, challenging, influencing, negotiating are fundamental to good consulting and can all be developed through training and experience. They form a key element of our consultancy skills training.

Active Listening

But do not we all listen? Yes certainly but there are different types of listening, in particular:

- *Normal listening:* Here the listener is just listening to enjoy the story or argument being told—almost coasting. This is the listening we might use in a restaurant, bar, or meeting. The listener is joining in the conversation whilst sometimes half-listening, sometimes thinking about other topics, sometimes thinking about their own next comment.
- *Competitive listening:* Where the listener is more interested in promoting his or her point of view instead of considering the speaker's thoughts. The listener listens, but also looks for breaks in the conversation to deliver their own point of view, perhaps even attacking any points they may not agree with.

- *Active listening:* Here the listener moves onto another level. Not just enjoying the story but actively working with the speaker to understand the speakers story, how the speaker feels, what they think, and actively showing their interest and understanding through their body language, questions, responses, etc.

Active listening style is a very effective way to gain a deep understanding of the speakers knowledge, beliefs, thoughts and feelings. It is used widely by counsellors, psychologists and psychiatrists in their daily work, and in consultancy work it is an invaluable skill. It focuses on two elements:

1. *Creating an atmosphere that makes it easy for the speaker to talk about the topic and the issues concerned.*
   The best atmosphere in terms of physical location/environment and lack of distractions, but in particular in the behavior of you as the listener—a behavior of listening that:
   - Encourages them to talk
   - Shows that you are paying attention
   - Ensures that they realize that you are listening noting what they are saying
   - Helps them to say what they want to say.
2. *Using communication skills to steer and guide the conversation in the direction that you wish it to go, and providing the context and detail you need.*
   This is achieved mainly through the following communication skills:
   - Questions obtaining information by the use of questions.
     - *Open questions*: What should we do to ...?
     - *Specific questions*: How much are we talking about?
     - *Closed questions*: Was she late?
     - By asking closed questions to check assumptions—yours and theirs.
   - *Summarizing*: In order to check your understanding of what they have said.
   - *Supporting*: Encouraging communication by using supporting statements:—I see. And then?
   - *Listen and paraphrase*: Use their words to demonstrate that you were listening. (Perhaps using their words to form questions.)
   - *Main points*: Identifying the main points they make and how they differ from yours.
   - *Facts V opinion*: Distinguishing fact from opinion in the other person's statements.

Tips for Active Listening

It really is all about self-discipline and the use of some very simple tactics. The following summarize the key points.

- *First and foremost, stop talking!*: It is difficult to listen and speak at the same time.
- *Put the other person at ease*: Give them space and time and "permission" to speak their piece. How we look at them, how we stand or sit, makes a huge difference. Relax, and let them relax as well.
- *Show the other person that you want to hear them*: Look at them. Nod when you can agree, ask them to explain further if you do not understand. Listen to understand them and their words, rather than just for your turn.
- *Remove distractions*: Good listening means being willing to turn off the TV, close a door, stop returning emails or reading your mail. Give the speaker your full attention, and let them know they are getting your full attention.
- *Empathize with the other person*: Especially if they are telling you something personal or painful, or something you intensely disagree with, take a moment to stand in their shoes, to look at the situation from their point of view.
- *Be patient*: Some people take longer to find the right word, to make a point or clarify an issue. Give the speaker time to get it all out before you jump in with your reply.
- *Watch your own emotions*: If what they are saying creates an emotional response in you, be extra careful to listen carefully, with attention to the intent and full meaning of their words. When we are angry, frightened or upset, we often miss critical parts of what is being said to us.
- *Be very slow to disagree, criticize or argue*: Even if you disagree, let them have their point of view. If you respond in a way that makes the other person defensive, even if you "win" the argument, you may lose something far more valuable.
- *Ask lots of questions*: Ask the speaker to clarify, to say more, give an example, or explain further. It will help them speak more precisely and it will help you hear and understand them more accurately.
- *Stop talking*: This is both the first and the last point, because all other tools depend on it. Nature gave us two ears and only one tongue, which is a gentle hint that we should listen twice as much as we talk.

Specialized Consultancy as Medicolegal Consultants

Medicolegal is the term, which incorporates the basics of two sister professions, i.e. Medicine and Law. Everybody talks about "the law" but few, aside from lawyers, judges and law teachers, have more than the vaguest notion of what constitutes "law". The average layman often has about as much accurate information about "the law" as he has about medicine-or life on Venus. And, unfortunately, two professional groups suffer from more ignorance of law and medicine than is good for them: lawyers, at least those who do not constantly deal with medical issues in their legal practice, know very little about the medical profession and its problems; physicians frequently comprehend very little about the law and how it affects them in the practice of their profession. Medicolegal experts can provide a link between these two professions for their smooth and effective functioning in a scientific manner.

MEDICAL PRACTICE IN TODAY'S SCENARIO

As you know the practice of medicine has a long history of changes and has now been declared as business. Doctor-patient relationship has been drastically changed in the last one decade and medical fraternity is facing very tough time because of growing number of cases. This trend is disturbing the doctor who wants to practice honestly and ethically. Doctors in general, are very sensible people and the nature of their work makes them very vulnerable to litigation. Few common factors of growing litigation against the doctors are as under:

- Awareness of consumer right has increased today at very large.
- Consumer Protection Act is implemented upon the doctors where the complainants get many advantages.
- Competition in profession has also laid to this problem.
- The patient/relative is misguided by the materialistic society.
- The media hype about lawsuits and violence against the doctors which encourage other to follow the example.
- The cost of treatment which has increased with the development of medical services.
- Failure on the part of doctors to establish report and communication with the patient/relative.
- Unethical and greedy attitude of some doctors, which tarnishes the reputation of entire doctor's community, etc.

MEDICAL NEGLIGENCE

Medical negligence is the breach of the duty owned by a doctor towards the patient, to exercise reasonable degree of care and skill which results in some physical, mental and financial disability or losses. Hence, it is a civil or criminal mistake (error) arising out of the contract between doctors and patients relationship.

CONSUMER FORUMS

Consumer forum is quasi judicial authority framed under the law in order to safeguards the interest of the consumers. CPA was enacted in 1986 and is now well known to everyone. After the landmark judgment of the Supreme Court in IMA versus VP Santa in 1995 the doctor's fraternity has been taken finally under purview of CPA.

SERVICE OFFERED

Medicolegal Aspects

Medicolegal advice during routine working in Hospital, Healthcare, Institution, Maternity Home, Nursing Home, Individual Doctor including General Practitioner.

Examples

- Advice on giving Medicolegal information to police after hearing facts of individual case.
- Decisions regarding issuing of cause of Death Certificate.
- Decisions regarding sending body for the post-mortem, examination in certain cases.

Legal Aspects

- Civil cases by Hospital or Nursing Home or Individual Doctor.
- Defending in civil cases on Hospital or Nursing Home or Individual Doctor.
- Criminal cases by Hospital or Nursing Home or Individual Doctor or defending in criminal cases on Hospital or Nursing Home or Individual Doctor.

Legal Proceeding in Respect of the Consumer Protection Act, 1981

- Cases on Hospital or Nursing Home or Individual Doctor.
- Cases by Hospital or Nursing Home or Individual Doctor.
- In District consumer forum, State Consumer Commission or National Consumer Commission.

Labor or Human Resource Problems

- Enquiry of employee of misconduct.
- Filling or defending cases in labor courts for or on behalf of Hospital, Nursing Home or Individual Doctor.
- Providing assistance to prepare and formulate agreement in between Employer and Employees of Hospitals, Nursing Homes or other institution.
- Issues relating to Provident Fund, Bonus payable, Gratuity or any other compensation Act or Benefits under Maternity Benefit Act.
- Drafting of Employments Bonds.
- Issues relating to payment of wages Act and minimum wages Act, etc.

Issues Relating to Property

- Drafting of various convincing Legal drafts for transfer of Rights in immovable Property such as Agreement, Deed, Purchase Deed, Lease Deed, Leave and License Deed, Rent Deed, Mortgage Deed, etc.
- Property issues such as Tresspass, Adverse Possession, and Encroachment of immovable property.
- Any other matters of immovable property with Revenue Department, Local Authority such as Municipal Corporation or Collector of District.

Recovery of Money Receivable to the Hospital, Nursing Home or Individual Doctor

- Cases of Dishonor of negotiable instruments such as Cheque, promissory note or bill of exchange.
- Filling cases in civil courts or defending the cases in money matter.

Legal issues arising under Nursing Home Registration Act, 1949, PNDT Act, MTP Act, Drugs and Cosmetics Act and getting institutions registered or renovation of Licensees under the said Acts.

Legal issuing arising under Environment Protection Act, 1986 and relating to Biomedical Waste Managements Rules.

Legal issues arising under various medical laws, acts like:

- The Indian Medical Council Act
- The Indian Medicine Central Council Act
- The State Act
- The Pharmacy Act
- The Dentists Act
- Drugs and Cosmetics Act, etc.

Legal issues relating to Charitable Trust Act, 1950 and The Societies Registration Act, 1860 including registration of Institutions, Associations or Organization as Public Trust or Societies.

Arranging various slides shows, demonstration, lectures relating to various legal aspects in medical profession for Hospitals/Nursing Homes, various Medicos Associations, and societies and for individual practitioner for creation of legal awareness amongst Medicos.

Issuing of legal notices and filing and defending the cases of Hospitals, Nursing Homes, Individual Medico in lowest court and up to the Apex Court of India, i.e. The Supreme Court of India.

1. *Medical negligence cases*: We prepare and draft opinions in medical negligence cases for review in medical council/police investigation teams/consumer courts/civil courts/criminal courts. We offer defence experts to assist you in fighting your case in every legal proceeding.
2. *Medicolegal reports and postmortem reports examination*: We offer highly qualified experts to interpret medicolegal reports and post-mortem reports for defence or prosecution side. Our reports are highly scientific and our expert would appear as defence expert witness before court to assist you in your legal proceedings.
3. *Forensic science reports/DNA fingerprinting*: We offer highly qualified experts to examine all forensic reports such as viscera report, documents reports, hand-writing analysis, ballistic reports, chemical analysis reports, etc. Our experts can examine DNA fingerprinting reports to assist you in cases of disputed paternity, divorce cases, maintenance cases, etc.
4. *Private medicolegal investigations*: We offer our services in private medicolegal investigations where we can assist government agencies or investigative agencies/on your behalf and desired results can be achieved through our scientific expertise.
5. *Hospital and nursing home care*: We offer medicolegal consultancy services to hospitals, nursing homes or polyclinic either on retainer-ship basis or on consultation basis. We offer to design forms to avoid negligence suits. We also offer our services for better medical record keeping.
6. *Consultancy to insurance companies*: We offer consultancy services to insurance companies to verify claims involving healthcare matters.

CRIMINAL NEGLIGENCE CASES AND ITS REASONS

When a Criminal Case Occurs Against Doctor?

- Sudden death after injection
- Death in intensive care unit/ICCU

- Death in operation theater
- Abortion cases, septic, death
- PNDT cases—female child
- MTP cases—places and doctor not registered
- Disabilities such as Gangrene and Amputation after IV/IM injection
- Death after delivery/LSCS.

WHAT IS THE MAIN DIFFERENCE BETWEEN CIVIL AND CRIMINAL LAW?

- Under criminal law usually a police complaint is registered u/s 154 and Police may arrest a Doctor or leave him on bail (recent Supreme Court view is not to arrest Doctor).
- Police applies wrong sections due to their ignorance about Medical Law and Doctors are harassed.
- Doctors have to attend Criminal Court on each date.
- Final Judgment levies fine and imprisonment, if doctor is found guilty.

What You Need to Start?

Below are some of the steps that you need to take to set-up your consulting business:

1. *Choose your legal structure*: It is best to formalize your business structure right from the start, both for legal and tax considerations. The three most common forms of business are sole proprietorship, partnership and corporations. Many self-employed consultants prefer to set-up their business as sole proprietorship, which is the easiest business form to set-up. However, you may be susceptible to legal liabilities since any liabilities incurred by your business become personal liability.
2. *Prepare your business plan*: Like any other business, it is important that you prepare your own business plan. Even though you will not present the plan to potential investors, the business plan can help you think through your strategies for keeping the business afloat and profitable, marketing and getting your expertise known to your customers, organizing your business, and generating and managing your finances. There is a number of books and business plan software in the market that could help you prepare your business plan.
3. *Create your home office*: If you are starting this business on a shoe-string budget, you can start-out by working from your home. This is particularly important, if you are embarking on this business on a part-time basis. You can work from a spare room, a garage or loft converted into an office, or even a small corner tucked in the hallway. The design of your office

will largely depend on various factors: (a) the kind of consulting field you are in (e.g. an interior designer may need a bigger space than a an online marketing consultant); (b) the equipment and supplies that you need; and (c) whether you expect to entertain and meet with clients in your home. If you expect to meet clients regularly in your home office, better check the zoning regulations in your area as neighbors may complain on the increased number of traffic in your vicinity.

You may want to read the following articles for a more detailed discussion of steps that you need to take as you start your business:

Marketing Your Consulting Business

Once you have set-up your consulting business, the next step is to let people know that you are available for work. You must now find someone willing and able to pay you for your expert advice.

Your marketing should focus on packaging you as an expert in your field and highlighting the value-added that you could provide your clients. You must let people know that you are a professional with the expertise, they need—you can help the clients solve their problems, supplement their staff, act as a catalyst, teach their organization, create new business or influence other people.

Some of the most effective ways of increasing awareness about your consulting business and finding your customers include:

1. *Networking*: Interacting with players in your targeted industry is one of the most, if not the most, effective way of marketing your consulting business. Simply put, the more contacts you have, the greater your chances of getting clients for your consulting business. Start with the people you already know—your former colleagues and bosses, your friends and existing industry contacts.

   You should also actively participate in every networking opportunity that you can find: participation in industry organizations and events, breakfast gatherings, chamber of commerce activities, professional groups and social clubs. The more visible you are, the greater the chances that your name will be on top of the potential clients' heads when they look for a person with your expertise.
2. *Referrals*: A pleased and satisfied client can be a very effective marketing tool for your consulting business. Once you have completed your projects with clients, and they are extremely satisfied with your performance, make sure that you ask for referrals and recommendations! They will only be too pleased to help spread the word about how great you are and the quality of your work. Strong word of mouth from a fellow business

owner is so much more effective than any kind of advertising in the world.

3. *Cold calling*: It would be great, if clients knock on your door all the time. Alas, that is not always the case. There will be times when you have to go out there to look for them. You may dread the idea of cold calling; but selling is an integral part of operating a business.

   To succeed in cold calling, you must practice techniques for getting past the cordon sanitaires of secretaries and assistants to reach the decision-makers. Note that the top boss may not always be the decision-maker in the organization: it can be the human resource director who recommends and decides on consultants who will be hired; or the marketing personnel. The key is to research carefully the power structure of the organization, and get that appointment.

   Prepare yourself thoroughly by practicing and harnessing your sales pitch and improving your closing techniques. Read books, attend training and seminars, or get a coach to help you improve your cold-calling techniques.

4. *Public speaking*: As a consultant, you are presenting yourself as an expert. As an expert, you need to be visible talking about your expertise. Public speaking is an excellent opportunity to present your expertise to an interested audience. If you are nervous about the idea of speaking in public, you can start small. Public libraries often arrange for events that utilize speakers. Volunteer to share your knowledge in their forums. You may also want to contact organizations and clubs in your area to offer your expertise. If you have built an impressive enough resume, you can even get an agent to look for possible speaking engagements for you.

5. *Books, articles and newsletters*: Getting published can greatly help in establishing a reputation for excellence in your field. Contact editors of both print and online publications in your field, and pitch story ideas to them. Submit regular articles, or even start a column. You can take this a step further by starting your own newsletter, or even a book. Becoming an author of a book (and if you are lucky, a best selling one at that!) can make it very easy for you to get new clients for your business.

6. *Advertising*: You can pick-up some customers, regardless of the area of your specialization, by advertising in your area's most popular newspaper or trade and specialized business publications. Examine the editorial styles and types of advertising the publications carry, then select the single publication that most corresponds with your needs. Unless a publication reaches the people to whom you are trying to sell, do not advertise in it regardless of style, quality, or advertising rates.

Avoid radio and television advertising; they are not only costly but generates the least amount of return for your advertising dollars.

7. *Direct mail advertising*: Direct mail solicitation can be done through postcard, sales letter mailings or brochures. Whatever, the length of your sales piece, the key is to follow the AIDA formula of copywriting: attracting the Attention, Interest, Desire, and Action on the part of the reader. You must appeal to the needs and wants of your target audience: why should they hire you and how will your services benefit them?

   Starting a consulting business involves more than expertise in your field: it takes business savvy, loads of financial smarts, excellent people and communication skills, and marketing know-how to succeed. Most of all, you need to gather your courage and start the business now. You will find consulting to be a very rewarding and personally fulfilling career.

Top Healthcare Consultancy

Six Sigma Star Healthcare, Delhi (*www.sixsigmahealth.org*)

USEFUL BOOKS ON CONSULTANCY

- Management Consultancy—a handbook of best practice. Edited by Philip Sadler, Kogan Page.
- Consultancy Services in India—Perspectives and Export Prospects by Dr SP Agarwal, Professor and Head, Centre for International Trade in Technology, Indian Institute of Foreign Trade, Bookwell, New Delhi
- Management Consulting—A Guide to the Profession. Edited by Milan Kubr, International Labour Office, Geneva
- The Overnight Consultant by Marsha D Lewin by John Wiley and Sons, Inc.,
- Getting the most from consultants—A Manager's guide to choosing and using consultants by Martin Wilson, Pitman Publishing.
- Getting Started in Consulting by Alan Weiss, John Wiley and Sons, Inc.
- Great Consulting Challenges and how to Surmount Them—Powerful Techniques for the Successful Practitioner by Alan Weiss, Jossey-Bass/Pfeiffer, A Wiley Imprint
- How to Market Design Consultancy Services? by Shan Preddy, Gower.
- Process Consulting—How to Launch, Implement, and Conclude Consulting Project by Alan Weiss, Jossey-Bass/Pfeiffer, A Wiley Company
- Developing a Consulting Practice—By Robert O Metzger, Sage Publications

- Getting the Most Out of Your Consultant—A Guide to Selection through Implementation by Gordon W Fuller, CRC Press
- Handbook for Users of Consulting Services by Consulting Services Division, Central Projects Services Office, Asian Development Bank, Manila, Philippines (Fourth Edition, 1993)
- How to succeed as an Independent? Consultant by Timothy RV Foster, Kogan Page
- The Flawless Consulting—A Guide to understanding your expertise by Peter Block Assisted by Andreu M Markowitz. Pefiffer, A Wiley Imprint
- The Seven Cs of Consulting—Your complete blueprint for any consultancy assignment by Mick Cope, Prentice Hall of India.
- Financial and Consultancy Services—Issues in International Trade edited by VL Rao, Jan ter Wengel, Sage Publications
- Smart Things to know about—Consultancy by Patrick Forsyth
- Management Consulting in Practice—A casebook of International Best Practice by Fiona Czerniawka and Paul May.

Annexure

LIST OF MANAGEMENT JOURNALS/ MAGAZINE/NEWSPAPERS

1. Six Sigma Health Express
2. Academy of Management
3. Academy of Management Journal
4. Academy of Management Review
5. Accounting and Business Research
6. Accounting, Organizations and Society
7. The Accounting Review
8. ACM Transactions on Information Systems
9. Johnson at Cornell University—Administrative Science Quarterly (ASQ)
10. American Economic Review
11. American Journal of Sociology
12. American Sociological Review
13. ASCI Journal of Management
14. Asian Case Research Journal
15. Energy Asia
16. Asian Review of Accounting Information
17. Asian Venture Capital Journal
18. Bank Accounting and Finance
19. The Banker—Unrivalled Coverage of Global Finance and Banking
20. Banking Statistics—RBI
21. Banking Strategies
22. Banking Technology
23. The British Accounting Review
24. British Academy of Management
25. Brookings Papers on Economic Activity
26. Business Ethics Network
27. California Management Review

28. The China Business Review
29. Contemporary Accounting Research
30. Monetary and Credit Information Review—Reserve Bank of India
31. CRISIL—Rating Publications, hand-outs
32. Decision—The IIMC Journal—Indian Institute of Management Calcutta
33. Decision Support Systems
34. Econometrical
35. Economic Intelligence Service
36. The Economic Journal
37. Economica
38. Energy Policy
39. Entrepreneur
40. Entrepreneurship and Regional Development
41. Entrepreneurship Theory and Practice
42. European Journal of Operational Research
43. European Journal of Purchasing and Supply Chain Management
44. European Management Journal
45. European Venture Capital Journal
46. Executive Leadership
47. Finance India
48. Financial Management Association International
49. Foreign Affairs
50. Global Finance Journal
51. Group and Organization Management
52. Handbook of Business Strategy
53. Harvard Business Review
54. Harvard Management Update
55. Hedge Fund Strategies: A Global Outlook
56. Human Relations
57. Human Resource Management
58. IBM Research
59. The ICFAI Journal of Applied Finance
60. IEEE Spectrum
61. IEEE Transactions on Engineering Management
62. IIC Monthly News
63. IIE Solutions
64. IMF Staff Papers
65. The Economy of India
66. Indian Economic Review
67. Indian Export Bulletin

68. Indian Journal of Commerce
69. The Indian Journal of Economics
70. Indian Journal of Industrial Relations
71. Indian Institute of Public Administration
72. Indian Journal for Training and Development
73. Indian Journal of Transport Management
74. Industrial Marketing Management
75. Journal of Industrial Relations
76. INFOR: Information Systems and Operational Research
77. Information and Management
78. Information and Organization
79. The Information Society Journal
80. Information Systems Management
81. Information Systems Research
82. Information Technology and People
83. Insurance Chronicle
84. Interfaces
85. International Financial Statistics
86. International Journal of Business Performance Management
87. The International Journal of Accounting
88. The International Journal of Advanced Manufacturing Technology
89. International Journal of Computer Integrated Manufacturing
90. Computers and Operations Research
91. International Journal of Electronic Commerce
92. International Journal of Entrepreneurship and Innovation
93. International Journal of Human Resources Development
94. International Journal of Innovation Management
95. International Journal of Manufacturing Technology and Management
96. International Journal of Production Economics
97. International Journal of Production Research
98. International Journal of Research in Marketing
99. International Journal of Services Technology and Management
100. International Journal of Technology Management
101. International Journal of Transport Economics
102. International Social Security Review
103. Investment Dealers Digest
104. Journal of Accountancy
105. Journal of Accounting Research
106. Journal of Accounting and Economics
107. Journal of Advertising
108. Journal of Advertising Research

109. Journal of Applied Corporate Finance
110. Journal of Applied Probability
111. Journal of Applied Psychology
112. Journal of Applied Statistics
113. Journal of Banking and Finance
114. Journal of Business
115. Journal of Business and Economic Statistics
116. Journal of Business Ethics
117. Journal of Business Strategy
118. Journal of Business to Business Marketing
119. Journal of Business Venturing
120. Journal of Conflict Resolution
121. Journal of Consumer Research
122. Journal of Corporate Finance
123. Journal of Cost Management
124. Journal of Derivatives
125. Journal of Development Economics
126. Journal of Development Studies
127. Journal of Economic Behavior and Organization
128. Journal of Economic Literature
129. Journal of Economic Perspectives
130. Journal of Economics and Business
131. Journal of Economics and Management Strategy
132. Journal of Educational and Behavioral Statistics
133. Journal of Empirical Finance
134. Journal of Engineering and Technology Management
135. Journal of Entrepreneurship
136. Journal of Experimental Social Psychology
137. Journal of Finance
138. Journal of Financial and Quantitative Analysis
139. Journal of Financial Economics
140. Journal of Financial Management and Analysis
141. Journal of Financial Markets
142. Journal of Financial Research
143. Journal of Forecasting
144. Journal of General Management
145. Journal of Human Development
146. Journal of Indian School of Political Economy
147. Journal of Industrial Economics
148. Journal of Intellectual Capital
149. Journal of Interactive Marketing

150. Journal of International Business Studies
151. Journal of International Economics
152. Journal of International Marketing
153. Journal of Knowledge Management
154. Journal of Law, Economics and Organization
155. Journal of Leadership and Organizational Studies
156. Journal of Macroeconomic Dynamics
157. Journal of Macroeconomics
158. Journal of Macromarketing
159. Journal of Management Information Systems
160. Journal of Management Inquiry
161. Journal of Management Studies
162. Journal of Marketing
163. Journal of Marketing Education
164. Journal of Marketing Management
165. Journal of Marketing Research
166. Journal of Monetary Economics
167. Journal of Money, Credit and Banking
168. Journal of Operations Management
169. Journal of Organizational Behavior
170. Journal of Pension Economics and Finance
171. Journal of Personality
172. Journal of Personality and Social Psychology
173. Journal of Political Economy
174. Journal of Portfolio Management
175. Journal of Product Innovation Management
176. Journal of Public Policy and Marketing
177. Journal of Retailing
178. Journal of Service Research
179. Journal of Social Psychology
180. Journal of Strategic Information Systems
181. Journal of Structured and Project Finance
182. Journal of Supply Chain Management
183. Journal of the Academy of Marketing Science
184. Journal of the American Statistical Association
185. Journal of the Operational Research Society
186. Journal of the Royal Statistical Society Series A: Statistics in Society
187. Journal of the Royal Statistical Society Series B: Statistical Methodology
188. Journal of Transport Economics and Policy
189. Journal of World Trade: Law, Economics and Public Policy
190. Knowledge and Process Management

191. Leader to Leader
192. Leadership Quarterly
193. Leadership Strategies
194. Long Range Planning
195. Management and Change
196. Management Accountant
197. Management International Review
198. Management Review
199. Management Science
200. Managerial and Decision Economics
201. Manufacturing and Service Operations Management
202. Marketing Health Services
203. Medgate Today
204. Marketing Management Magazine
205. Marketing Research Magazine
206. Marketing Science
207. Mathematical Finance
208. McKinsey Quarterly
209. Mergers and Acquisitions Service
210. MIS Quarterly
211. MIT Sloan Management Review
212. Money and Finance
213. Networks
214. New Technology Work and Employment
215. NSE News
216. Operations Research
217. Operations Research Letters
218. OR/MS Today
219. Organization Science
220. Organization Studies
221. Organizational Behavior and Human Decision Processes
222. Oxford Economic Papers
223. Pacific-Basin Finance Journal
224. Pensions and Investments
225. Personality and Social Psychology Bulletin
226. Personnel Psychology
227. PM Journal
228. PM Network
229. Portfolio Organizer
230. Power in Asia
231. Private Equity Week

232. Production and Operations Management
233. Production and Inventory Management Journal
234. Production Planning and Control
235. Professional Banker
236. Project Finance International
237. Psychological Bulletin
238. Psychology and Marketing
239. Purchasing
240. Quality Progress
241. Quantitative Finance
242. Quarterly Journal of Economics
243. Research and Development Management
244. Research and Journal of Economics
245. RBI Bulletin
246. Readers' Subscription Service
247. Research Policy
248. Review of Economic Studies
249. Review of Economics and Statistics
250. Review of Financial Studies
251. Review of Urban and Regional Development Studies (RURDS)
252. SAM Advanced Management Journal
253. Six Sigma Health Express
254. Social Psychology Quarterly
255. Strategic Management Journal
256. Strategic Organization
257. Strategy and Leadership
258. Supply Chain Management
259. Supply Chain Management Review
260. Systems Research and Behavioral Science
261. Technological Forecasting and Social Change
262. Technology Analysis and Strategic Management
263. Theory and Decision
264. Training and Development Journal
265. Transportation Journal
266. Transportation Science
267. Treasury Management
268. Venture Capital Journal
269. Venture Capital: The Journal of Entrepreneurial Finance
270. Vikalpa
271. World Bank Economic Review
272. World Development

Glossary

SIX SIGMA
Ref: Chapter 14

A

- **Adjusted R-squared:** Modification of R-squared used in regression and multiple regression to compare models with different number of explanatory terms. Adjusted R-squared is more useful only if the R-squared is calculated based on a sample not the entire population.
- **Analysis of variance (ANOVA):** Statistical technique for analyzing experimental data.
- **Attribute data:** Pass/fail or go/no-go information. The control charts based on attribute data include percent chart, number of affected units chart, count chart, count-per-unit chart. Commonly used attribute control charts are also called C, U, P, NP charts.
- **Availability:** One of three components used to calculate the Overall Equipment Effectiveness (OEE). Availability can be expressed by the ratio of the uptime divided by the schedule time which is the same as the uptime plus downtime.

B

- **Benchmarking:** Comparing a process or product to the others to determine improvement plan. Trying to obtain all similar concepts from worse to best to make decisions on improvements.
- **Blocking:** Used in design of experiments (DOE) to neutralize background variables that cannot be eliminated by randomizing through spreading them across the experiment.
- **Box-plot:** Also known as a box and whisker diagram is a graphing tool that displays centering, spread, and distribution of a continuous data set.

- **Brainstorming:** A technique that teams use to generate ideas on a particular subject. Each person in the team is asked to think creatively and write down as many ideas as possible. The ideas are not discussed or reviewed until after the brainstorming session.

C

- **C-chart:** Count chart for attribute data.
- **Capability index (Cp, Cpk, Pp, Ppk, Cpm, Cpkm)** all assume normal data. Pp and Ppk are rarely used compared to Cp and Cpk. They should only be used as relative comparisons to their counterparts.
  - *Cp:* A short-term process capability index. The best process can perform. A function of the standard deviation that numerically describes variation relative to the tolerance or specifications. Used to establish baseline measurement in the measure phase of a DMAIC project and final score in the control phase. The Cp is the best process can perform if that process is centered on the midpoint and the Cp = Cpk.
  - *Cpk:* A short-term process capability index that is a function of the mean and standard deviation, very commonly used.
  - *Pp:* Numerically describes the long-term capability (Cp is short-term indicator) of a process assuming it was analyzed and stays in control. Similar to Cp, this capability index is only a function of the standard deviation, not a nominal (target) value that may be historical or provided by the customer.
  - *Ppk:* Numerically describes the long-term capability. Account for centering of the process among the midpoint of the specifications. However, this performance indice may not be optimal if the customer wants another point as the target other than the midpoint. The calculation of Cpm accounts for the addition of a target value.
  - *Cpm:* Cpm is a capability index, also known as the Taguchi capability index, that is a function of the specification limits, mean of the process, sample standard deviation, and a provided target, T.
- **Cause-and-effect diagram:** A tool for seeking out all the causes, regardless of magnitude, that are contributing to the effect, Y. It is also referred to as the Ishikawa diagram after developer Kaoru Ishikawa and the Fishbone Diagram due to its configuration as the skeleton of a fish. This diagram is one of the seven tools of quality and is one of frequently used subjective screening tools in a DMAIC Six Sigma project.
- **Central limit theorem:** States that given a distribution with a mean and variance, the sampling distribution of the mean approches a

normal distribution with a mean and variance/N as N, the sample size, increases. Also referred to as the Law of Large Numbers in the insurance and risk management field of study.

- **Check sheet:** "Sheet" used to collect data in real-time and at the location where the data is generated. Data can be of any type and is the first steps to any improvement project which can be either quantitative or qualitative (attribute, discrete, variable, continuous).
  - *Classification:* A trait such as a defect or failure mode must be classified into a category.
  - *Location:* The physical location of a trait is indicated on a picture of a part or item being evaluated.
  - *Frequency:* The presence or absence of a trait or combination of traits is indicated. Also number of occurrences of a trait on a part can be indicated.
  - *Measurement:* A measurement scale is divided into intervals, and measurements are indicated by checking an appropriate interval.
  - *Check list:* The items to be performed for a task are listed so that, as each is accomplished, it can be indicated as having been completed.
- **Coefficient of correlation:** It measures only a linear relationship between two variables and is denoted by an "r" value. The "r" value is used to measure the correlation and it will always range from -1.0 (anticorrelation) to +1.0. As the value approaches 0 their is less linear correlation, or dependence) of the variables.
- **Coefficient of determination:** The COD ranges from 0–1 (0–100%) represented by R-squared. The proportion of variability of the dependent variable (Y) accounted for or explained by the independent variable (X) equal to the coefficient of correlation value squared.
- **Common causes:** Causes of variation that are inherent in a process over time. They affect every outcome of the process and everyone working in the process. (See also "special causes.")
- **Conformance:** An affirmative indication or judgment that a product or service has met the requirements of a relevant specification, contract or regulation.
- **Continuous improvement:** The ongoing improvement of products, services, or processes through incremental and breakthrough improvements.
- **Control chart:** A chart with upper and lower control limits on which values of some statistical measure for a series of samples or subgroups are plotted. The chart frequently shows a central line to help detect a trend of plotted values toward either control limit, the LCL or UCL.

- **Control limit:** Control limit for points above the central line in a control chart. There is a lower control limit (LCL) and an upper control limit (UCL) and this is provided by the process where as the specification limits (used in process capability assessments) are provided by the customer.
- **Corollary:** An inference derived from axioms or propositions that follow from axioms or other proven propositions.
- **Corrective action:** The implementation of solutions resulting in the reduction or elimination of an identified problem.
- **Critical to quality (CTQ):** Key measurable characteristics of a product or process whose performance standards, or specification limits, must be met in order to satisfy the customer. Sought in the Define phase of Six Sigma projects as a part of gathering the Voice of the Customer (VOC). They align improvement or design efforts with critical issues that affect customer satisfaction.
- **Cumulative sum control chart:** A control chart on which the plotted value is the cumulative sum of deviations of successive samples from a target value. The ordinate of each plotted point represents the algebraic sum of the previous ordinate and the most recent deviations from the target.
- **Customer delighter:** Delighter features are used in Kano Model that are characteristics that pleasantly surprise and exceed customer expectations.
- **Customer satisfaction:** The result of delivering a product or service that meets customer requirements.

D

- **Defect:** A nonconforming characteristic for a product, process, or service. A defective unit may have one or more defects.
  - Class 1 = Very serious
  - Class 2 = Serious
  - Class 3 = Major
  - Class 4 = Minor

Causes that have higher lower class of defect are often given higher subjective scores relative to their impact on the effects. Such as 'severity' scoring withing the FMEA creation process.

F

- **Factor:** Also known as a predictor variable (x, PIV). This input variable may be controlled or uncontrolled variable whose influence is being studied.

- **F-distribution:** The F-value is a measurement of distance between individual distributions. As F goes up, P goes down saying that there is more confidence in there being a difference between two means and to accept the alternative hypothesis. To calculate, take the mean square of X divided by the mean square of error. Compare this value to the F-critical value found in a table is another way to test hypothesis used in ANOVA.

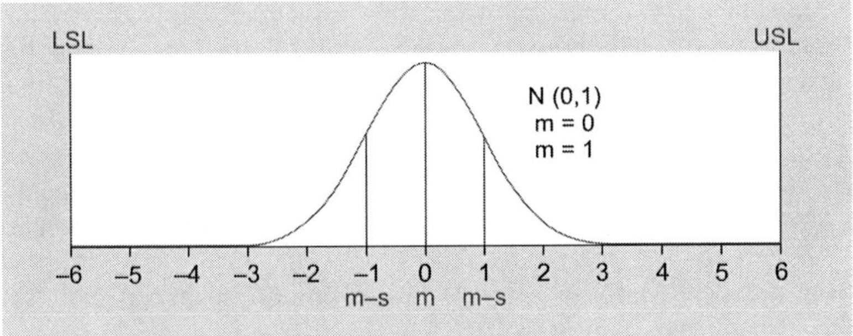

- **FIT:** Predicted value of the response variable provided a specific combination of factor settings.

G

- **Gantt chart:** Visual project planning device used for production scheduling. It is a horizontal bar chart that serves as a visual tool for project management. It illustrates dependent steps and where the project is at any given time. The chart was developed by Henry Laurence Gantt, born in 1861.

I

- **Inference space:** Operating range of factors that are being analyzed.

K

- **Kurtosis:** Measure of peakness or flatness of a distribution.

L

- **Linearity:** Variation between a known standard across the low and high end of the gage. It is the difference between an individual's measurements and that of a known standard or truth over the full range of expected values.

M

- **Multicollinearity:** When two or more predictor variables (x, input variables) are found to be correlated with each other.

R

- **R-squared:** The amount of variation explained by the regression equation. Used in inference space to predict future outcomes on the basis of other related information. It is the sum of the squares of the regression model divided by total sum of squares. The square root of it is the correlation coefficient, r.
- **Residual:** Difference between an actual and fitted (predicted) experimental value. Term commonly found when using regression or multiple regression.
- **Response variable (Y, KPOV):** Process output. This is linked to the customer critical to quality (CTQ) characteristics.
- **Rolled throughput yield (RTY):** The probability of the entire process producing zero defects. RTY is more important as a metric to use where the process has excessive rework. RTY is the product of each process's throughput yield, TPY.

S

- **Seven tools of quality:** Commonly used tools in just about every DMAIC Six Sigma project to help understand an existing process and drive most effective improvements.
  - Fishbone diagram (finding all the root causes)
  - Check sheet (collecting data)
  - Flow chart (Process map—what is really happening)
  - Control chart (determining the initial and final state of process)
  - Histogram (determining the data distribution)
  - Pareto chart (finding the vital few)
  - Scatter diagram (for correlation/regression).
- **Shewhart cycle:** Named after father of statistical control and creator of the cotnrol chart, Walter Shewhart. Also called 'plan-do-check-act cycle', or PDCA cycle, or PDSA cycle representing 'plan-do-study-act'.
- **Signal-to-noise (S/N) ratio:** A mathematical equation that indicates the magnitude of an experimental effect above the effect of experimental error due to chance fluctuations.

- **Six-Sigma quality:** A term used to generally indicate that a process is well within specifications or has received "perfection". Process can be better than six-sigma. Technically the specification range is ±6 standard deviations.
- **Specification:** A document or customer provided evidence that states the requirements to which a given product or service must conform. Commonly found as the lower specification limit (LSL) and/or the upper specification limits (USL). Customer may also provide a target that may or may not be in the middle of the LSL and USL.
- **Stability:** Represents variation due to elapsed time. It is the difference between an individual's measurements taken of the same parts after an extended period of time using the same techniques.

T

- **Throughput yield (TPY):** The number of acceptable pieces at the end of the end of a process divided by the number of starting pieces excluding scrap and rework (meaning they are a part of the calculation).

U

- **U-chart:** Count per unit chart used with attribute data.

ALTERNATIVE THERAPY

Ref: Chapter 22

A

- **Acupuncture** is the practice of inserting very thin needles in specific acupuncture points or combinations of points on the body.
- **Alternative medical systems** is the name of a National Center for Complementary and Alternative Medicine (NCCAM) classification for those forms of alternative medicine that are built upon a "complete system of ideas and practice". It can include:
  - Ayurveda
  - Chiropractic
  - Homeopathy
  - Naturopathic medicine
  - Osteopathy
  - Traditional Chinese medicine.
- **Anthroposophical medicine** was invented in the early twentieth century by Rudolf Steiner and Ita Wegman. Practitioners supplement anthroposophical ideas with conventional therapies and homeopathic remedies. Anthroposophical doctors must have a recognized medical degree (MD, DO, or equivalent).
- **Anthroposophic pharmacy** is the process of developing treatments according to anthroposophic theories. Anthroposophic medicinal products are primarily used within anthroposophic medicine.
- **Aromatherapy** is the use of essential oils and other aromatic compounds, primarily to affect mood.
- **Attachment therapy** is a form of therapy aimed at children with alleged 'attachment disorders', usually fostered or adopted children. It is substantially based on outdated notions of suppressed rage due to early adverse experiences. Traditionally, it uses a variety of confrontational and physically coercive techniques of which the most common form is holding therapy, accompanied by parenting methods which emphasize obedience. Following implication in a number of child death and maltreatment cases in the USA there has been a recent move away from coercion by some leading theorists and practitioners. It is largely unvalidated.

B

- **Bates method** is related to the visual acuity. It is based on the belief that errors in visual accommodation are due to mental strain, and that vision may be improved by appropriate relaxation techniques.
- **Biologically based therapy**, is the precise name of an NCCAM classification, for alternative treatments that use substances found in nature and/or some other natural therapy. It can include:
  - Chinese food therapy
  - Fasting
  - Herbal therapy
  - Macrobiotic lifestyle
  - Natural health
  - Natural therapy
    - Diet and food
    - Dietary supplements
    - Exercise
  - Naturopathy
  - Orthomolecular medicine
  - Urine therapy.
- The **Biomedical model of health** is a conceptual model of illness that excludes psychological and social factors and includes only biological factors in an attempt to understand a person's illness. According to this model, health constitutes the freedom from disease, pain, or defect, thus making the normal human condition health. The model's focus on the physical processes, such as the pathology, biochemistry and physiology of a disease, does not take into account the role of social factors or individual subjectivity. The model also overlooks the fact that the diagnosis (that will affect treatment of the patient) is a result of negotiation between doctor and patient.
- **Body work** is any therapeutic, healing, or personal development work that involves some form of touching, energetic work, or the physical manipulation of a practically oriented physical and somatic understanding of the body.

C

- **CAM** is an acronym for **complementary and alternative medicine**, a large range of treatments and theories on the nature of health and illness, many of them unrelated, which have in common that they are not commonly employed by the conventional medical establishment.

See also: List of branches of alternative medicine, List of famous people in alternative medicine, and History of alternative medicine.

- **Chelation therapy** is the use of chelating agents such as Ethylenediaminetetra acetic acid (EDTA) to remove heavy metals from the body. While in conventional medicine, chelation therapy is used only to treat heavy metal poisoning, some alternative practitioners advocate the use of chelation therapy to treat coronary artery disease.
- **Chinese medicine**—the group of philosophies embodied by Chinese medicine are, more accurately, referred to as Oriental Medicine with roots in many different Asian countries. This millennia-old Asian medical tradition works to bring balance to the body through acupuncture, massage, Eastern herbalism, diet; and lifestyle changes such as martial arts and meditation.
- The practice of **Chiropractic** is a manual therapy involving the manipulation of the vertebral subluxation to restore proper, motion, biomechanics, and nerve flow from the brain to the body.
- **Christian science** a religious movement founded by Mary Baker Eddy (1821–1910) which augments and modifies Christianity with her own ideas. Christian Scientists believe the material world is an illusion and so illness too is not real, but an 'error' which can be corrected with special kinds of prayer, and not by medicine.
- **Color puncture** is an alternative medicine practice asserting that light can be used to stimulate acupuncture points for the purpose of balancing energy in the body and promoting healing and better health. It is also called color light acupuncture in North America. It is a form of color therapy.
- **Complementary medicine** refers to treatments that are used *along side* ("complementary to") conventional medicine.

D

- **Diet-based therapy** uses a variety of diets in order to improve health and longevity, to control weight, as well as to treat specific health conditions like high cholesterol.
  - Breatharian
  - Fruitarianism
  - List of diets
  - Living foods diet
  - Macrobiotic lifestyle
  - Okinawa diet
  - Ovo-lacto vegetarian

- Raw foodist
- Vegan
- Vegetarianism
- Low-fat diet
- Low-carb diet (Zone diet, Atkins diet).

- The **Doctrine of signatures** was developed around 1500 and claims that a plant's physical appearance reveals its medical value. The Doctrine of Signatures is often associated with Western herbalism.

E

- **Eclectic medicine** was a nineteenth-century system of medicine used in North America that treated diseases by the application of single herbal remedies to effect specific cures of certain signs and symptoms.
- **Energy medicine** is the name of a NCCAM classification, for alternative treatments that involve the use of veritable (which can be measured) and putative (which have yet to be measured) energy fields. It can include:
  - Magnet therapy
  - Reiki
  - Shiatsu
  - Therapeutic touch
  - Eden Energy Medicine approach developed by Donna Eden.
- **Exercise-based therapy** uses a variety of traditional forms of physical movement, in order to improve health and longevity, to increase, lengthen and tone muscle mass, gain flexibility, as well as to treat specific health conditions and to relieve stress. It can include:
  - Aerobic exercise
  - Aerobics
  - Bodybuilding
  - Feldenkrais method
  - Martial arts
  - Physical culture
  - Pilates
  - PNF stretching
  - Stretching
  - Some forms of Qigong
  - T'ai chi
  - Walking
  - Weight training
  - Yoga.

F

- **Feldenkrais method** is an educational system centered on movement, aiming to expand and refine the use of the self through awareness.
- **Flower essence therapy** is regarded by some as a sub-category of homeopathy, which uses homeopathic dilutions of flowers. This practice was begun by Edward Bach with the Bach flower remedies but is now practiced much more widely.
- **Folk medicine** is the collection of procedures traditionally used for treatment of illness and injury, aid to childbirth, and maintenance of wellness.

G

- **Grahamism,** named for Sylvester Graham, recommended hard mattresses, open bedroom windows, chastity, cold showers, loose clothing, pure water and vigorous exercise.

H

- **Herbalism** is the practice of making or prescribing herbal remedies for medical conditions.
- **Heroic medicine** is any medicine or method of treatment that is aggressive or daring in a dangerously ill patient. It generally includes the pre-scientific treatments of 18th-century doctors, such as bloodletting.
- **Holism** is the study and advocacy of wholeness in health, science, politics, or any other area of life.
- **Hydrotherapy** is the external use of water in the medical treatment of disease, such as through the use of baths, the application of hot and cold compresses or sheet packs, and shower sprays. These applications typically use water as a medium for delivery of heat and cold to the body, capitalizing on the thermoregulatory properties of the body for therapeutic effect.

I

- **Integrative medicine** as defined by National Center for Complementary and Alternative Medicine combines conventional medical treatments and CAM treatments for which there is some claimed scientific evidence of their safety and effectiveness. Integrative medicine also adopts the term 'integrative health' which incorporates mental, spiritual and community wellness with personal health.

- **Iridology** (also known as iridodiagnosis) is an alternative medicine technique whose proponents believe that patterns, colors, and other characteristics of the iris can be examined to determine information about a patient's systemic health. Practitioners match their observations to *iris charts* which divide the iris into zones corresponding to specific parts of the human body.

L

- **Life extension** is a movement the goal of which is to live longer through intervention, and to increase maximum life span or average life span, especially in mammals. Researchers of life extension are a subclass of biogerontologists known as 'biomedical gerontologists'. *See also the* List of life extension related topics.
- **Lifestyle** is the particular attitudes, habits, or behaviors associated with an individual.
- **Lifestyle diseases** are diseases that appear to increase in frequency as countries become more industrialized and people live longer.

M

- **Manipulative and body-based methods**, is the precise name of a NCCAM[2] classification, for alternative treatments that are based on manipulation and/or movement of one or more parts of the body. It can include:
  - Acupressure
  - Alexander technique
  - Body work
  - Bowen technique
  - Chiropractic
  - Feldenkrais method
  - Manipulative therapy
  - Massage therapy
  - Medical acupuncture
  - Metamorphic technique
  - Myofascial release
  - Naprapathy
  - Osteopathy
  - Rolfing
  - Shiatsu
  - Somatics

- Taijiquan
- Trager approach
- Tui na
- Zero balancing.

- **Manual lymphatic drainage (MLD)** is a type of gentle massage which is believed by proponents to encourage the natural circulation of the lymph through the body.
- **Mind-body connection** idea says that the causes, development, and outcomes of an illness are determined as much from the interaction of psychological and social factors as they are due to the biological factors of health. Many mind-body therapists take the definition of 'mind-body connection' further and state that the *root cause* of illness is actually in the mind and spirit, and that for complete and permanent eradication of an illness, the cause must be addressed and cure focused there.
- **Mind-body intervention** is the name of a NCCAM classification, that covers a variety of techniques designed to enhance the mind's capacity to affect bodily function and symptoms. It can include:
  - Aromatherapy
  - Art therapy
  - Autosuggestion
  - Bach flower therapy
  - Buteyko method
  - Eutony
  - Feldenkrais method
  - Hatha yoga
  - Hypnotherapy
  - Metamorphic technique
  - Journaling
  - Meditation
  - Music therapy
  - Nia technique
  - Reiki
  - Self-hypnosis
  - Support groups
  - Taijiquan
  - Trager approach
  - Visualization
  - Vivation
  - Yoga.

N

- **Nature cure** is the progenitor of naturopathy in Europe. It postulates that all disease is due to violations of nature's laws, and that true healing consists in a return to natural habits.
- **Natural health** is an eclectic self-care system of natural therapies that purports to build and restore health by working with the natural recuperative powers of the human body.
- **Naturopathy** is the eclectic practice of Naturopathic Doctors (ND) using many different natural therapies as treatment. The original method of treatment of Naturopathy was the water cure.
- **Natural therapy** is the treatment method used by advocates of natural health.
- **NCCAM classifications**—The National Center for Complementary and Alternative Medicine, or NCCAM, has classified complementary and alternative therapies into five different categories, or domains:
  - Whole medical systems
  - Mind-body intervention
  - Biologically based therapy
  - Manipulative and body-based methods
  - Energy therapy.

Q

- **Qigong** is an exercise aspect of Chinese medicine. Qigong is mostly taught for health maintenance purposes, but there are also some who teach it, especially in China, for therapeutic interventions. There are hundreds of different schools, and it is also an adjunct training of many East Asian martial arts.

R

- **Reiki** is a form of treatment developed by Mikao Usui in Japan around 1922. Practitioners use their hands on or above the patient in order to control, increase or open up a postulated energy, "ki", in the body. Training is usually through short courses, after which one can become certified as a "Reiki master".
- **Reflexology**.

S

- **Siddha medicine**.
- **Systems medicine**, or systems health, looks at the dynamic systems of the human body as part of an integrated whole, incorporating biochemical,

physiological, and environment interactions that sustain life. Systems medicine draws on theories from holistic medicine, systems science and systems biology when developing a comprehensive approach that considers an individual's health in light of their genomics, behavior and the external environment.

T

- **Thalassotherapy**—the use of seawater as a form of therapy. Thalassotherapy was popular in England during the second half of the eighteenth century, with Doctor Richard Russell credited as playing a significant role in its popularity.
- **Therapeutic music**—music played live at the bedside of persons who are faced with physical, emotional, and spiritual challenges, generally in the person's home, a hospice or in a clinical setting.
- **Traditional Chinese Medicine (TCM)** is a system of healthcare which is based on the Chinese notion of harmony and balance inside the human body as well as harmony between the body and its outside environment. TCM can include or address the following components:
  - Acupressure
  - Acupuncture
  - Chinese martial arts
  - Chinese pulse diagnosis
  - Coin rubbing
  - Cupping
  - Five elements
  - Food therapy
  - Herbology
  - Jing
  - Meridian
  - Moxibustion
  - Neigong
  - Qigong
  - San Jiao
  - Shen
  - Tao Yin
  - TCM model of the body
  - Trigger point
  - Tui na
  - Yin and yang
  - Zang Fu theory
  - History of traditional Chinese medicine.

- **Traditional Japanese medicine**—Pre-Western Japanese medicine was strongly influenced by traditional Chinese medicine and is often seen as a sub-category of TCM. It includes the following practices:
  - Shiatsu
  - Japanese martial arts.

U

- **Unani.**
- **Uropathy** is a specialized branch of alternative medicine, including any sort of oral or external application of urine for medicinal or cosmetic purposes, see urine therapy.

W

- **Water cure (therapy)** in the therapeutic sense is a course of medical treatment by hydrotherapy. In the nineteenth century, the term "Water Cure" was used synonymously with "hydropathy", which itself is the 19th century term for hydrotherapy. Conceptually, water cures include a broad range of practices—essentially any therapeutic uses of water. *See Water cure (therapy) and Hydrotherapy for further discussion and links.*
- **Wellness** has been used in CAM contexts since Halbert L Dunn began using the phrase "high level wellness" in the 1950s, based on a series of lectures at a Unitarian Universalist Church in Arlington, VA. Wellness is generally used to mean a healthy balance of the mind-body and spirit that results in an overall feeling of well-being.

Y

- **Yoga** is a diverse and ancient East-Indian practice. There are many different styles and schools of yoga. It is generally a combination of breathing exercises, physical postures, and meditation, that calms the nervous system and balances body, mind, and spirit. It is thought to prevent specific diseases and maladies by relaxing the body, deepening respiration and calming the mind. Yoga has been used to lower blood pressure, reduce stress, and improve flexibility, concentration, sleep, and digestion. It has also been used as supplementary therapy for such diverse conditions as cancer, diabetes, asthma, and AIDS.

Index

Page numbers followed by *f* refer to figure and *t* refer to table.

D

E

F

G

H

I

Q

R

S